The Doctor's Handbook, Part 2

The Doctor's Handbook, Part 2

UNDERSTANDING THE NHS

Fourth Edition

TONY WHITE

PhD FRCS MB BS AKC

Consultant Otolaryngologist (retired)

Foreword by

JOHN BLACK

President, Royal College of Surgeons

Radcliffe Publishing

Oxford • New York

Radcliffe Publishing Ltd
18 Marcham Road
Abingdon
Oxon OX14 1AA
United Kingdom

www.radcliffe-oxford.com
Electronic catalogue and worldwide online ordering facility.

First Edition 1999
Second Edition 2001
Third Edition 2006

British Library Cataloguing in Publication Data
A catalogue record for this book is available from the British Library.

ISBN-13: 978 184619 459 7

The paper used for the text pages of this book
is FSC certified. FSC (The Forest Stewardship
Council) is an international network to promote
responsible management of the world's forests.

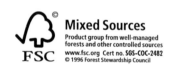

Mixed Sources
Product group from well-managed
forests and other controlled sources
www.fsc.org Cert no. SGS-COC-2482
© 1996 Forest Stewardship Council

FSC

Typeset by Pindar NZ, Auckland, New Zealand
Printed and bound by TJI Digital, Padstow, Cornwall, UK

Contents

Foreword

When you purchase a new computer there is never an instruction manual, other than brief instructions on the whereabouts of the on/off switch and how to clean the screen. This has led to bulging shelves in bookshops, packed with titles such as *Mac for Dummies: the manual you should have got with your computer but didn't*. At the onset of the two major steps in a medical career, namely into specialist training and consultant life, we could all do with an instruction manual, not about the clinical 'daytime job', difficult and challenging though it may be, but about the rest.

Part 1 is concerned with self-assessment and in the broadest terms improving professional communication at all levels. Much of this is taught in medical schools, but not brought together in an accessible way. Part 2 is a guide to the directorates, executive agencies, authorities, councils, departments, institutes and trusts that make up the modern NHS, together with insights into funding and a look into the future.

Every single thing in this book will turn up at some time in a specialist doctor's career, thankfully not all at once! Treat it as a *vade mecum* and guide to the complexities and frustrations of life as a medical specialist, which despite all remains an honourable and rewarding calling.

John Black
President
Royal College of Surgeons of England
May 2010

Preface

I often meet doctors who express the wish that they had received training earlier in their careers in a broader range of non-clinical aspects of their work. Others, who are committed to continuing professional development, seek learning material that will enable them to handle the wider issues they confront on a day-to-day basis, and for which initial medical education failed to prepare them. Many trainers can also find it difficult to access a single source that provides material for the non-clinical training of their juniors. This book, now in two parts, was written to address these and other needs revealed by research carried out by John Gatrell and me. Since publication I continue to be delighted with the positive feedback received from specialist registrars and other grades of doctors, including many consultants and surprisingly even NHS managers.

Before the first edition was published it was piloted extensively, working with doctors from many specialties. Many comments were received which helped to develop the first edition. John and I continued to receive positive feedback on the second and third editions and this has encouraged the publishers to go ahead with a fourth. With each new edition we have endeavoured to incorporate suggestions from readers. In this edition the chapters have been rearranged to allow new and existing material to be amalgamated where appropriate and make it easier to access information. It has been a difficult and rather subjective exercise which may not appeal to every reader.

Since the third edition, further changes in the structure, funding and governance of the NHS have continued, in addition to the changes that have occurred with the selection, training and appraisal of doctors. I have incorporated all these into this fourth edition, although inevitably there will be ongoing changes, for example, revalidation and Modernising Medical Careers (MMC), as they are carried through. At the time of writing many changes are imminent but not yet active; for example, the introduction of licensing and revalidation. This has obviously been a challenge in trying to be as up to date as possible between writing and publication.

To some extent I have tried to overcome this by referring the reader to the original source for current information. Indeed one of the striking changes in this edition compared to the original edition is the amount of information of value that is now available on various professional websites. Perhaps the most striking example is the information and guidance available from the General Medical Council website (www. gmc-uk.org) in almost all aspects of professional non-clinical work.

One criticism of the book is a lack of some references but the number of direct references in the text is deliberate, as I want the text to be readable and informative. The book is not designed to be academic but a useful handbook. Where no direct

reference is quoted you will find the sources of information in the related reading sections with each chapter.

I hope you will continue to find these books valuable in your current medical role
and a means of support in your future professional development.

Tony White
May 2010

About the author

Tony White is a retired consultant otolaryngologist appointed in Bath, where he was clinical director for seven years. He has a PhD from Bath University with a thesis on 'The Role of Doctors in Management'.

Together with John Gatrell he undertook a three-year research project into the non-clinical development needs of doctors that resulted in publication of the NHS Training Directorate report, *Medical Student to Medical Director*, which also formed a basis for this book.

He has written several books on medical management and contributed to and edited several other textbooks as well as writing numerous papers. He has lectured widely and organised many workshops on doctors' management development issues. He was a member of a number of national advisory committees to develop doctors' non-clinical skills and acted as regular tutor on training courses in various regions.

Abbreviations

Latin abbreviations continue to be found in textbooks and learned journals. It is useful to know their meaning and indeed they may be used, albeit cautiously, in writing. I would suggest for clarity it is often better to write 'see above' and 'see below' rather than 'v. sup.' and 'v. inf'.

ad fin.	(*ad finem*) – near the end (of the page).
c./ca./cca.	(*circa*) – around, about, approximately, used of uncertain dates.
cap	(*capitulum*) – capital, capital letter or chapter.
cf.	(*confer*) – compare; used to suggest that another work might usefully be consulted in relation to the subject under discussion.
ead./eadem	see *id.*
e.g.	(*exempli gratia*) – for example, but sometimes used similarly to 'including' when not listing everything.
et al./*et al.*	(*et alii*) – and others. Used in multi-author references, although it is customary to include all the authors in the first citation and/or in the bibliography. It can also stand for *et alia* – and other things, or *et alibi* – and other places.
etc.	(et cetera) (include &c. and &/c.) – and the others, and other things, and the rest.
ff.	(*foliis*) – from pages used in citations to mean 'and on succeeding pages'.
i.a.	(*inter alia*) – among other things.
ibid./ib.	(ibidem) – in the same place; used in citations as 'in the same place' and relates to the immediately prior source.
id.	(*idem*) – the same (man). Used to avoid repeating the name of a male author (in citations, footnotes, bibliographies, etc.). If quoting a female author, use the corresponding feminine form *ead.* (*eadem*), the same (woman).
i.e.	(*id est*) – that is, or 'in other words'.
l.c./loc.cit.	(*loco citato*) – in the place already mentioned. Relates to sources before the immediately prior citation.
NB/n.b.	(*nota bene*) – note well.
op. cit.	(*opere citato*) – in the work already mentioned. Relates to sources before the immediately prior citation (loc. cit and op. cit. are more or less identical). In citations used in a similar way to 'ibid.', though 'ibid.' is usually followed by a page number.
p.m.a.	(*post mortem auctoris*) – after the author's death.

p.p./pp/*per pro.*	(*per procurationem*) – through the agency of.
PS/p.s.	(*post scriptum*) – written after.
q.v.	(*quod vide*) – which see; used to cross-refer to material that can be found elsewhere within a piece of writing. Note cf. refers to external material.
	For more than one term or phrase, the plural is *quae videre* (qq.v.).
seq./seqq.	(*sequentia*) – the following.
sc./scil.	(scilicet = *scire licet*) – that is to say or namely.
sic	– indicates that text is literally transcribed from the original. Often written in parentheses following a misspelled word to indicate that the error is the original writer's mistake.
s.v.	(*sub voce*) – under the word (specified). Used with alphabetically arranged reference works.
v.	(*vide*) – see, look up.
v. inf.	(*vide infra*) – see below.
viz	(videlicet) – that is to say, namely. As distinct from i.e. and e.g., viz. is used to indicate a detailed description of something stated before, and when it precedes a list of group members, it implies near completeness.
v.s. v.sup.	(*vide supra*) – see above.
vs.	(versus) – against.

Acknowledgements

I remain especially grateful to Dr Hugh Platt, whose vision initiated and inspired the original work.

My thanks are also due to those readers who took the trouble to contact us with suggestions for this fourth edition.

I wish to thank those who provided wisdom and guidance over all the editions including medical royal colleges, postgraduate deaneries, medical defence organisations, health authorities and hospital and primary care trusts. I freely acknowledge that some ideas may have come from seeds sown during discussions with these people. I apologise if any reference is not attributed or is incorrectly acknowledged; any such errors are mine alone.

Particular thanks in this edition are due to Liz Jones for her help in finding, writing and checking material and for stepping in at a very late stage, working into the small hours, to write new material for clinical governance and quality. Jenny Barker, Managing Director, Wiltshire PCT, for advice and checking of facts. Tim Albert, writer and trainer, for general advice on writing skills. Gillian Nineham of Radcliffe Publishing, the midwife who coped with a rather difficult birth of this fourth edition.

Due to other commitments John Gatrell has not been able to act as co-author for this edition; in his place I have received help and guidance from colleagues working in the various subjects. But it is appropriate to express thanks for the efforts he has given to earlier editions and for his provision of useful new material such as that on Meyers-Briggs personality types, emotional intelligence and the writings of Frederick Herzberg.

Not least, I am grateful to my wife Anne not only for her efforts in checking and researching new material, but whose continued support, tolerance and encouragement has made the whole fourth edition possible.

Tony White

Introduction

These handbooks have three main aims:

- ○ to support the development of a range of mainly non-clinical skills related to professional development
- ○ to provide a basis for making the most of a number of learning opportunities that occur during training
- ○ to serve as a source of useful information to doctors in the NHS.

Sometimes it is difficult to ask for advice about non-clinical aspects of our work – it is often assumed that we should acquire this awareness through a kind of osmosis, picking it up along the way. The books try to provide answers to questions that you feel you ought to know, but perhaps do not like to ask. The books also provide assistance with the development of new skills and capabilities that we know are relevant to professional careers. It is intended to be a useful resource to help you with a particular problem and an opportunity to work through larger sections in order to learn more about specific aspects of your work.

Some kinds of learning can be achieved through reading textbooks, some through one-to-one instruction and others are better undertaken in group training sessions. All require opportunity, an element of underpinning knowledge with a commitment to learn. These handbooks are designed to cover the knowledge element that is the basis for developing professional skill and judgement. It should fit in with your work and be relevant to everyday needs. It supplements other training such as short courses which become available from time to time.

The books emerged from an extensive study of the non-clinical learning needs of doctors at all stages in their careers and has been further informed by a series of development programmes for doctors. The General Medical Council's 'Good Medical Practice Guidelines' remind us that a high level of clinical competence is only one aspect of professional medical practice. Personal insight, effective team working, good leadership, teaching others and skill in dealing with patients need to be supported by clear understanding of the complex structures and systems in the modern NHS.

Following the introduction of MMC, standardised multi-source feedback techniques have been introduced to improve the assessment of interpersonal skills exhibited by doctors in training. This is just one example of the increased breadth of assessment that modern medical trainees must be able to accommodate. Their world has increased in complexity through technological advances on the one hand and political intervention on the other. As future consultants they may be expected to play a much greater role in the organisations in which they work, yet have less power and influence than most of their predecessors. I have tried to cover a wide range of needs in these books. We hope you find it useful and enjoy the experience of using them as a learning resource.

Needs and experience change over time and it would be helpful if you let me know things that need to be included, things that could be omitted and things that need changing or moving from one section to another. This process of continuous development and review will ensure that it stays relevant for future readers.

Learning objectives

Key learning objectives of these handbooks are listed below. You might find it helpful to start by familiarising yourself with their contents as a whole. If you believe you are already competent in an area, study the action points in that section. This should help you to decide if you need to do more. You may feel that some sections are irrelevant at this stage in your career. Put them to one side, but make a note to return to them later. These books will also act as a reference document into which you can dip as the need arises.

On completion of the books you should be better able to do the following.

- Identify your preferred learning style and make better use of learning opportunities.
- Organise your time so that you can cope with work and enjoy available leisure time.
- Delegate tasks to others in a way that helps to develop them and permits you to make better use of your own abilities.
- Make effective presentations to small and large groups.
- Work efficiently in a team.
- Lead others in the achievement of team goals.
- Understand and deal with conflict.
- Deal with stress in yourself and others.
- Contribute usefully and effectively to meetings.
- Instruct and train others in skills and knowledge aspects of clinical tasks.
- Appraise and assess in the context of training and revalidation.
- Present clear and concise formal reports and other written communications.
- Undertake research and prepare articles for publication.
- Present yourself successfully in the selection process.
- Deal with patients and close family members when breaking bad news.
- Request a post-mortem.
- Appear at a coroner's inquest and as a witness in court.
- Support, advise and help to develop colleagues.
- Identify the key aspects of quality service delivery.
- Recognise trust and related national systems for risk management.
- Differentiate between audit and research and apply audit principles to a range of settings.
- Reflect on your personal values in the context of your career and work as a doctor.
- Understand something of the current structure and funding of the NHS.
- Have a clearer idea of the way healthcare is changing and developing.

Understanding the NHS

The aim of this chapter is to provide an outline of recent reforms and a brief summary of the structure of the NHS, both nationally and locally. It also reviews healthcare reforms in a worldwide context. Most of the following information can be downloaded from www.dh.gov.uk/PublicationsAndStatistics/fs/en; click on 'Statistics' but prepare to be overwhelmed by data. There are also other data sources for some information: for example NHS, British Medical Association (BMA) and medical college websites, although they do not always agree on statistics.

A statistical picture of the NHS

o Nationwide, the NHS employs more than 1.5 million people.
o Just short of half the workforce are clinically qualified, including some 90 000 hospital doctors, 35 000 general practitioners (working in about 10 000 practices), 315 410 qualified nurses and 16 000 ambulance staff.
o Only the Chinese People's Liberation Army, the Wal-Mart department store chain and Indian Railways directly employ more people.
o The NHS costs more than £1500 annually for every person in the country.
o .5 million people attended A&E departments including minor injury units (MIUs) and walk-in centres (WiCs) in the first quarter of 2009 (DoH 1) and 12.3 million from April 2007 to March 2008 (HES 1).
o Nearly 13 million people attend outpatients every year and a million patients have ward attendances which makes a total of almost 28 million people attending hospitals every day for outpatient treatments.
o There are 3 million day case operations per year or 3.6 million if day case treatments are included.
o There are nearly 9 million inpatient admissions every year.

○ On average the NHS deals with 1 million patients every 36 hours – that's 463 people a minute or almost 8 a second.

○ Every day, approximately 700 000 people visit their general practitioner and about 100 000 visit their dentist.

○ Every GP sees an average of 140 patients a week.

○ Every day, over 1700 babies are delivered.

○ A one-week stay in hospital costs £1100 and a night in intensive care costs £500.

○ Over 559 million prescriptions are dispensed each year, costing over £5 billion and representing 12% of all NHS expenditure.

○ There were 44 660 managers in the NHS in 2009, an increase of 11.9% on 2008 and 84% on 1999.

○ The total numbers of consultants in England are very difficult to ascertain but at September 2005 it was 31 993 (FTE = 29 613).

○ In 2008–09 the NHS employed 1600 management consultancies.

○ Doctors in 2006 made up 9% of the NHS workforce. Of the 106 432 doctors, 72 347 were hospital-based, and 34 085 general practice-based.

○ The NHS spent £584 million on agency staff in 2007–08.

○ The total number of GPs in the NHS is around 30 000 (in England, although 25% are part-time) working from about 10 000 practices (see below).

○ The vacancy rate for doctors and dentists posts in March 2009 was 5.2%.

○ NHS Direct received 240 000 calls and 9000 visits to its website during the Christmas holiday of 2004.

○ 77% of funding comes from general taxation, 12% from the NHS share of national insurance contributions and 2% from patient charges.

○ Just under half of NHS spending goes on acute services. This amounts to about £800 per person per annum.

○ The NHS spends £14 billion in Scotland and £7 billion in Wales.

○ Over 40% of total hospital and community health services expenditure is for people over 64 years of age, though they represent just 16% of the population.

○ OECD countries are spending record amounts on healthcare, largely due to the rising cost of pharmaceuticals and the diffusion of modern medical technologies.

○ Staff costs account for two-thirds of all NHS expenditure.

○ The NAO claims that 5000 people die each year from hospital-acquired infections, and that at any one time 9% of patients have a hospital-acquired infection.

○ The hospital-acquired infection problem is said to cost the NHS £1 billion a year.

○ The estimated cost of adverse events in the NHS is believed to be in excess of £2 billion a year.

○ The NHS spends an estimated £30 million a year on recruitment advertising.

○ The NHS spent over £584 million in 2007–08 on agency staff.

○ The Royal College of Nursing (RCN) reported that according to a Freedom of Information Act survey the government spent £350 million on external management consultants in the financial year 2008/09 (*Nursing Times* 10 May 2009). As a result the NHS is the fourth largest user of external consultancy and reducing the money spent on external management consultancy could deliver 11% of the expected reduction in government health spending announced in the 2009 budget. Indeed over three years (to August 2009) the DoH spent £470 million on some 100 contracts with management consultants.

o NHS WiCs, of which there are currently 93, treat around 3 million patients a year.

o 46 NHS-run Treatment Centres have been opened as of May 2009. More than 304 000 patients have been treated from April 2003 to March 2006.

o 21 Independent Sector Treatment Centres (ISTCs) and a mobile ophthalmology unit have been opened as of May 2009 in which 80 000 elective procedures and 38 000 diagnostic assessments have been carried out.

Problems with the statistics

Conflicts in quoted figures from different authorities appear to be common and I looked at the reason for this with regard to waiting lists. It is difficult to interpret but it gives a clue to the reason for the variations in published figures. There have always been differences between the official figures acknowledged for patient waiting times, those published by the Department of Health (DoH) and the waiting times taken from hospital episodes statistics (HES). These appear to be mainly because of the different ways in which the times were calculated.

HES waiting times are worked out as the maximum waiting time and timed from the date at which the decision is taken to put the patient on a waiting list, until the point at which they are admitted and the treatment takes place. But the HES waiting times include days when the patient isn't available for treatment; for example, due to illness or holidays. Such days are called suspensions or deferrals from the waiting list.

Before December 2003, all DoH official waiting times were worked out as the date a patient was put on a trust's waiting list to the date they were admitted. Unlike the HES waiting times, they did not include suspensions or deferrals. There were problems with the method for working out official waiting times due to the definitions for calculating the time when patients were suspended or deferred that were unclear. This led to inconsistencies and local interpretations. There were even suggestions that some trusts were using 'phantom' suspensions to keep patients off waiting lists so that government targets could be met. Another anomaly that arises is that the waiting list time does not include any investigations. So, for example, a patient referred for a replacement hip operation would not start their waiting list time clock until all investigations were completed. The system also gave no way of reflecting the overall waiting time if a patient moved from a waiting list at one trust to a list at another.

In December 2003 a Data Set Change Notice (DSCN 37/2003) was issued. The changes set out in this document attempted to ensure that the DoH official waiting times more closely reflect the patients' perceptions of how long they have waited. The DSCN and background documents give the official guidance on this. The new DoH official waiting times are worked out from the date at which the patient is placed on a waiting list at any provider until the date at which the patient is admitted for the treatment. This is regardless of which provider gives the treatment. For example, with their consent, the patient may be moved from the waiting list at one provider to that of another provider, who may be able to treat them more quickly. This might be as a result of the Patient Choice initiative decision.

The change to the official waiting times doesn't mean that they are calculated as the difference between the date when the patient is added to the waiting list and the operation date. However, if the treatment does not take place (e.g. if the patient is sent home with a cold), the waiting time continues to be counted until the date of the admission that does result in the treatment taking place. Patients can be suspended from a waiting list for short periods of time while they are unavailable for admission for social or medical reasons. Patients may also refuse at least two admission dates that they are offered. In this case they are considered to have self-deferred and the waiting time is then counted from the earliest date offered. The total number of days for periods in which the patient was suspended or was self-deferred can be subtracted from the total waiting time.

Patients may also cancel appointments or not turn up on an accepted admission date they had previously accepted. In this case the waiting time is reset to zero and the clock restarts from the date on which the patient failed to attend. Planned admissions are used where a patient is waiting for treatment for clinical reasons, rather than until resources become available. Such patients are usually excluded from waiting times calculations, although there is no reason why the time waited should not be recorded because the time between clinical events could have significance.

Comparing HES- and NHS-derived waiting times is difficult. It is possible for the HES waiting time to be greater than, equal to, or less than the NHS derived waiting time. Well, I said it was a complex business, but if you want to try to make sense of it go to HES online at www.hesonline.nhs.uk. This is a Hospital Episode Statistics data warehouse containing details of all admissions to NHS hospitals in England. It includes private patients treated in NHS hospitals, patients who were resident outside of England and care delivered by treatment centres (including those in the independent sector) funded by the NHS. HES also contains details of all NHS outpatient appointments in England.

HES is the data source for a wide range of healthcare analysis for the NHS, government and many other organisations and individuals. It contains admitted patient care data from 1989 onwards, with more than 12 million new records added each year, and outpatient attendance data from 2003 onwards, with more than 40 million new records added each year.

(The HES Service and the HES website are run by Northgate Information Solutions on behalf of The NHS Information Centre for Health and Social Care.)

A similar problem arose in trying to identify the number of GPs. The statistics do not often give a figure in context; for example, whether for UK or England alone, whether including GP retainers and GP registrars, or whether total number of whole-time equivalent (WTE) numbers. For example, www.dh.gov.uk/en/Publicationsandstatistics/Pressreleases/DH_4112146 gives a figure for the total number of GPs (excluding GP retainers and GP registrars) in England as at 31 December 2004 as 31 798. The NHS Information Centre at www.ic.nhs.uk/webfiles/publications/nhsstaff2008/gp/Bulletin Sept 2008.pdf gives a figure of 27 347 in 2008. And at www.

parliament.uk in a parliamentary answer in House of Commons in 2008 the latest available figure was given as 33 364 in 2007; see www.publications.parliament.uk/pa/cm200708/cmhansrd/cm080707/text/80707w0033.htm.

Overview of NHS

Since its launch the NHS has grown to become the world's largest publicly funded health service. It is also one of the most efficient, most egalitarian and most comprehensive. The system was born out of an ideal that healthcare should be available to all – and that principle remains at its core. With the exception of charges for some prescriptions and optical and dental services, the NHS still remains largely free at the point of use for anyone who is resident in the UK – more than 60 million people. It covers everything from antenatal screening and routine treatments for minor illness to major surgery, accident and emergency treatment and end-of-life care.

The NHS structure

I am aware that most doctors in training may not be greatly interested in the structure of the NHS. However, as you approach your consultant post, you will need to have a basic outline of the system if only to be primed for any questions in a consultant interview. I have tried to keep things as basic as possible just to give you an outline. I have moved the historical review (in case you need to identify old structures) towards the end of the chapter so I will first outline the current structure in England and then later deal briefly in this chapter with other parts of the UK, i.e.:

o NHS in Northern Ireland
o NHS in Scotland
o NHS in Wales
o Isle of Man
o Channel Islands (Jersey and Guernsey).

All have different or their own independent health service structures.

There are two major aspects of managing the NHS, dealing with:
o strategy, policy and managerial issues
o all clinical aspects of care.

The latter clinical part can be further divided as follows.
o Primary care at the frontline, involving GPs, pharmacists, opticians, dentists etc. Primary care trusts (PCTs) are in charge of primary care and have a major role around commissioning secondary care, providing community care services. They are now at the centre of the NHS and control 80% of the NHS budget. As they are local organisations, they are thought to be best positioned to understand the needs of their community, so they can make sure that the organisations providing health and social care services are working effectively.
o Secondary care, hospital-based, usually accessed via GP referral or ISTCs and

now also included are the ambulance services. Secondary care, sometimes known as acute healthcare, can be either elective or emergency. Elective usually follows referral from a primary or community health professional such as a GP. Other examples of secondary care services include specialist services for mental health, learning disabilities and older people.

○ Tertiary care through specialist hospitals treating particular types of illness such as cancer, or involving highly specialised doctors dealing with particularly difficult or rare conditions.

○ Community care through partnership with local social services departments.

Sometimes there is a separation of two further groupings.

○ Elective care, meaning planned specialist medical care or surgery, usually following referral from primary care. Elective care patients may be admitted either as an inpatient or a day case, or may be an outpatient consultation or clinic.

○ Emergency care, also known as Accident and Emergency, when patients attend hospital as a result of an accident or trauma and require emergency treatment. Some patients will come to A&E themselves and others will arrive in an ambulance.

The divisions between these sectors are becoming less distinct, with structural changes taking place. In particular, the NHS is moving towards local decision making, breaking down barriers between primary and secondary care and a change aimed at enabling greater patient choice (information on these reforms can be found in the document *Shifting the Balance of Power*, available online at www.publications.DH.gov.uk/shifting thebalance/index.htm).

The primary care trusts oversee 29 000 GPs and 18 000 NHS dentists.

There are at the time of writing 175 acute NHS trusts and 60 mental health NHS trusts, which oversee 1600 NHS hospitals and specialist care centres. There are currently 115 foundation trusts across England.

Emergency vehicles are provided by the NHS ambulance services trusts. There are 11 ambulance trusts in England. The Scottish, Welsh and Northern Ireland ambulance services provide cover for those countries.

NHS care trusts provide care in both health and social fields. There are few care trusts and they are based mainly in England. There are none in Scotland and the Scottish NHS has no plans to introduce them.

NHS mental health services trusts provide mental healthcare in England and are overseen by the PCT.

There are also a number of agencies under the umbrella of the NHS such as the National Institute for Health and Clinical Excellence (NICE) that are set out in detail later in this chapter.

The current structure is based on *Our Health, Our Care, Our Say: a new direction for community services*, the White Paper of 2006. This set a new direction for the whole health and social care system first outlined in the DoH Green Paper, *Independence, Well-being and Choice*. There was a radical shift in the way in which services were delivered, attempting a more personalised service to better accommodate people's lives. It attempted to give people a stronger voice so that they were the major drivers of service improvement.

This 2006 White Paper outlines the proposed changes for the provision of NHS community services, with four broad aims to:

o   improve health and well-being
o   provide convenient access to high-quality services
o   provide support for those with greatest need
o   place care provision in the most appropriate setting, closer to home.

Two significant themes evident throughout the document are the:

o   shift in emphasis to the community setting rather than the hospital for care delivery
o   increased emphasis on prevention.

Contributing to this trend are the:

o   increasing number of people living with chronic diseases
o   ageing of the population.

These demographic changes associated with escalating healthcare costs are unsustainable in the long term. In 2005 the World Health Organization felt that health services across the globe were inadequately prepared to meet these emerging challenges.

So this chapter describes some of the major players in the NHS hierarchy and how they relate to each other. You need to be aware, however, that details continue to change, it is changing even as I write, and where possible I will point you to an appropriate source to update your information. The one continuing feature has been not only change but also in the balance between central and local control.

Management of the NHS at national level

These are the organisations within the NHS that essentially have a strategic role.

Parliament

The NHS is financed mainly through taxation so it relies on Parliament for its funds, and has to account to Parliament for their use through the Secretary of State for Health, the cabinet member responsible for the service. In addition, Parliament scrutinises the service through debates, MPs' questions to ministers and Select Committees, procedures that mean the government has to publicly explain and defend its policies for the NHS.

Secretary of State and Health Ministers

The DoH has six ministers: the Secretary of State, two ministers of state and three parliamentary under-secretaries of state, one of whom is responsible for public health matters and one for social and community services, while the third sits in the House of Lords. The Secretary of State, often referred to as the 'Minister of Health' has overall strategic responsibility for NHS improvement, delivery, reform, finance and resources, while the other ministers each have specific areas of NHS activity assigned to them. The Department for Education and Skills has the lead for children's issues and works closely with the DoH.

Select Committees

Three Select Committees (the Health Committee, the Public Accounts Committee and the Public Administration Committee) each comprising backbench MPs representing the major parties, are particularly relevant to the NHS. They are all able to summon ministers, civil servants and NHS employees to give oral or written evidence to their inquiries, usually in public. Their reports are published throughout the parliamentary session.

Health Committee

The Health Committee, with a maximum of 11 members and the quorum for any formal proceedings being three, examines the expenditure, administration and policy making of the DoH and its associated bodies. It complements the work of the Public Accounts Committee and shadows the work of the DoH, carrying out inquiries into major health policy issues. This Committee follows up reports of the health service commissioner or ombudsman who is responsible for investigating areas of maladministration in the NHS, failure to provide a service and other complaints from the public. (*See* Chapter 6 in Part 1 for more detailed information.) The Health Committee's constitution and powers are set out in House of Commons Standing Order No.152. The members of the Committee are appointed by the House and unless discharged remain on the Committee until the next dissolution of Parliament. For more information see www.parliament.uk/parliamentary-committees/health-committee.cfm.

Public Accounts Committee

The Public Accounts Committee of 16 members, and traditionally chaired by a member of the Opposition, is more concerned with ensuring the NHS is operating economically, efficiently and effectively. Its inquiries are based on reports about the service's 'value for money', produced by the Comptroller and Auditor-General, who heads the National Audit Office. It tries to draw lessons from past successes and failures that can be applied to the future. The chief executive of the NHS may be called before the Committee to answer questions. For more information see either www.parliament.uk/parliamentary_committees/committee_of_public_accounts.cfm or www.nao.gov.uk.

Public Administration Committee

The Public Administration Committee has 11 members and examines reports from the Health Service Commissioner (better known as the Ombudsman, *see* p. 232 in Part 1).

See www.parliament.uk/parliamentary_committees/public_administration_select committee.cfm or www.ombudsman.org.uk.

The Audit Commission

Although not a strategic health service body, it is worth mentioning here as it is the independent body set up by Parliament with a role in auditing the NHS with particular reference to value for money. For further information, *see* Chapter 4, 'Funding and the NHS' or go to www.audit-commission.gov.uk.

Department of Health and its boards and committees

The DoH is responsible for running and improving the NHS, public health and social care in England. This organisation provides strategic direction, secures resources, sets national standards and invests in the service. There has been a large change programme that has seen radical alterations to the way the DoH operates. Some of the main changes include: a structural reorganisation; the introduction of flexible teams to improve the response to changing priorities; and a 38% reduction in core DoH staff, with half of these posts being transferred to arm's length bodies (ALBs; see below p. 15 onwards). For more details go to links at www.dh.gov.uk.

Secretary of State and Health Ministers

The Secretary of State for Health leads the NHS, along with five other Health Ministers. The Permanent Secretary and NHS Chief Executive (a role that was combined from 2000 until 2006) acts as the link between the DoH and the Secretary of State.

Department Health Board

The Department Health Board is responsible for managing DoH business and has as its priorities:

o providing advice to Ministers on developing the strategy and objectives for the health and social care system
o setting DoH standards
o establishing the framework of governance, assurance and management of risk
o approving:
  ‣ Departmental Business Plan
  ‣ DoH Resource Account for each financial year
  ‣ Departmental Report
  ‣ major expenditure commitments.

The Department Health Board members comprise:
o Permanent Secretary/NHS Chief Executive (Chair)
o Chief Medical Officer (CMO)
o Chief Nursing Officer (CNO)
o Director-General Social Care, Local Government and Care Partnerships
o Director-General DoH Finance and Operations
o three non-executive members.

They meet about six times a year. You can discover more about them at the DoH website: www.dh.gov.uk/en/Aboutus/HowDHworks/BoardsandCommittees/DH_088623.

Below the Department Health Board are three Management Boards, as follows.

1 Corporate Management Board (CMB)

This supports the DoH Permanent Secretary in his or her personal responsibility as Accounting Officer for Departmental Expenditure and provides leadership for the department.

Corporate Management Board members comprise:
○ Permanent Secretary (Chair)
○ NHS Chief Executive
○ Chief Medical Office
○ Chief Nursing Officer
○ Chief Information Officer
○ NHS Medical Director
○ Director-General, Health Improvement and Protection
○ Director-General, Research and Development
○ Director-General, Communications
○ Director-General, Finance and Chief Operating Officer
○ Director-General, Social Care, Local Government and Care Partnerships
○ Director-General, Policy and Strategy
○ Director-General, NHS Finance, Performance and Operations
○ Director-General, Commissioning and System Management
○ Director-General, Workforce.

Other regular attendees include:
○ Director of Operations
○ Director of Human Resources
○ Director of DoH Development and Delivery
○ Head of Internal Communications.

CMB meetings are scheduled around the annual business planning and quarterly performance management cycle, with additional ad hoc meetings as required (six or seven meetings a year). You can read about them in more detail online at www.dh.gov.uk/en/Aboutus/HowDHworks/BoardsandCommittees/DH_088624.

2 NHS Management Board and executive groups

The NHS Management Board supports the NHS Chief Executive in his or her responsibility as Accounting Officer for NHS expenditure and provides leadership for the NHS, ensuring effective two-way communication. It manages NHS performance and shapes policy and strategy for the NHS.

This Board currently brings together all strategic health authority (SHA) Chief Executives and the NHS Chief Executive's leadership team of Directors-General within the DoH on a monthly basis. Its members together provide leadership for the NHS and are responsible for ensuring that performance and financial delivery in the NHS is on track and recommending remedial action as necessary.

In summary it is a meeting chaired by the NHS Chief Executive with virtually all the CMB members plus Chief Executive of all SHAs, the Director, Office of the SHAs, the Chief of Staff, Chief Adviser to the NHS Chief Executive, and Director of NHS Communications.

They meet monthly. For further information go to the DoH website at www.dh.gov. uk/en/Aboutus/HowDHworks/BoardsandCommittees/DH_088625.

3 The National Leadership Council (NCL)

The National Leadership Council is a subcommittee of the NHS Management Board. The stated purpose of the NLC is to ensure that world-class leadership, talent and leadership development exists at every level of the healthcare system.

The NLC has 25 core members, 5 patrons and 14 fellows. For further information see www.dh.gov.uk/en/Aboutus/HowDHworks/BoardsandCommittees/DH_097657.

Various DoH committees

In addition there are a number of committees, all of which have pages on the DoH website. Go to www.dh.gov.uk/en/Aboutus/HowDHworks/index.htm.

Audit Committee

This advises the Accounting Officers and the Department's Board on risk management, corporate governance and assurance arrangements in the DoH and its subsidiary bodies.

Committee of the Regions

This supports the DoH presence in the regions in respect of the delivery of local health and social care.

Corporate Management and Improvement Committee

A subcommittee of the CMB, to which it reports, this committee is responsible for ensuring that, operationally, the DoH is managed in a consistent, efficient and effective manner, focusing on capability, planning, performance and risk management, corporate policy making, internal communication, environmental, reputational and social issues.

Performance Committee

The Performance Committee monitors performance against the DoH's Strategic Objectives, Public Service Agreements, critical programmes and projects and financial targets on behalf of the Departmental Board and provides a source of challenge on these to supporting boards.

Policy Committee

Another subcommittee of CMB (see above) and responsible for developing and implementing best practice in policy-making across the DoH, in particular an evidence-based approach to the development of policy. It also advises CMB on the relative priority of policies and their fit with departmental strategy.

Some key personnel in the Department of Health

The Permanent Secretary

The Permanent Secretary is answerable to the Secretary of State and Parliament for the way the DoH is run.

NHS Chief Executive

The Chief Executive ensures that the department provides strategic leadership for the NHS and social care. The Chief Executive's report to the NHS is published in December each year and outlines the service's progress towards meeting key objectives. The Chief Executive produces a weekly bulletin, emailed every Thursday to NHS and council chief executives and directors of social services, containing details of publications, circulars and announcements. For details see either www.publications.DH.gov.uk/nhsreport/index.htm or www.publications.DH.gov.uk/cebuiletin/index.htm.

The posts of Permanent Secretary and Chief Executive were combined between 2000 and 2006.

The Chief Medical Officer and Heads of Profession

Within the DoH, there are seven Heads of Profession providing the government with expert knowledge in their field. These individuals include:
○ Chief Medical Officer (the principal medical advisor to the government and the head of all medical staff in England)
○ Chief Nursing Officer
○ Chief Dental Officer
○ Chief Social Services Inspector
○ Chief Health Professions Officer
○ Chief Pharmaceutical Officer
○ Chief Scientist.

The CMO is the government's principal medical adviser and the professional head of all medical staff in England. The CMO produces an annual independent report on the state of the nation's health. For further information online go to www.dh.gov.uk/PublicationsAndStatistics/Publications/AnnualReports/CMOAnnualReportsArticle.

National clinical directors

National clinical directors are experts in their field and take the lead in implementing key national clinical priorities. Their roles vary but include chairing taskforces, promoting the work of their specialty, developing clinical networks and advising on clinical quality and governance. There are national directors for:

o Emergency Access and Service Configuration
o Mental Health
o Health and Work
o Transplantation
o Heart Disease and Stroke
o Primary Care
o Pandemic Influenza Preparedness
o Widening Participation in Learning
o Diabetes
o Kidney Services
o Cancer
o Equality and Human Rights
o Children, Young People and Maternity Services.

Some of the strategic agencies

There were a number of executive agencies within the DoH responsible for particular business areas, but in 2004 the department produced a paper with the object of reconfiguring the arm's length bodies (ALB) in an attempt to save £500 million. The review was prompted because many frontline staff reported that ALB activities generated considerable levels of bureaucracy, because of the amount of overlap and duplication in their functions. This saw the number of such bodies reduced from 38 to 20, with a 25% reduction in staff. The review covered 42 separate arm's length bodies, employing more than 22 000 staff. Thirty-eight of these bodies existed in 2003/04 and the review also looked at four future ALBs. The review and reconfiguration was to be completed by 2008, although further changes took place in 2009.

These ALB's are set up for ministers who want independent advice without direct influence from Whitehall departments. They work independently of ministers to whom they are nevertheless accountable. Civil servants do not staff them. There are four types of executive non-departmental public bodies (NDPB) but the DoH has only two types:

o NDPBs typically established in statute and carrying out executive, administrative, regulatory and/or commercial functions
o advisory NDPBs providing independent, expert advice to Ministers on a wide range of issues.

Below are further examples in more detail, although they all have their own websites where more information is available.

First let us consider some that are specific executive agencies of the DoH.

NHS Purchasing and Supply Agency (PASA)

The agency has been reshaped and is now taking on procurement and contracting functions from other ALBs. It advises on procurement policy and strategy, and contracts nationally for products and services critical to the NHS, using its purchasing power to achieve savings. PASA is attempting to ensure the best possible value for money when purchasing goods and services. For more information go to www.pasa.nhs.uk/PASAweb.

Medicines and Healthcare Products Regulatory Agency (MHRA)

MHRA continues to ensure that all medicines, medical devices and equipment on the UK market meet appropriate standards of safety, quality and performance. It also deals with adverse reports and incidents. It is the government agency responsible for guaranteeing that medicines and medical devices work, and are acceptably safe, based on the premise that no product is risk-free. They state that their judgements are underpinned by work that is robust and fact-based to make certain that the benefits to patients and the public justify the risks. Therefore they keep watch over medicines and devices, and take any necessary action to protect the public promptly if there is a problem. They also aim to make as much information as possible publicly available.

They attempt to enable greater access to products, and the timely introduction of innovative treatments and beneficial technologies. They therefore encourage everyone, public and healthcare professionals as well as industry, to report any problems with a medicine or medical device, so that they can investigate and take any necessary action.

A full explanation of how and what they do can be found in their publication *Medicines and Medical Devices Regulation: what you need to know*, available online at www.mhra.gov.uk/home/groups/comms-ic/documents/websiteresources/con2031677.pdf. Their website is at www.mhra.gov.uk/index.htm.

NHS Connecting for Health (NHS CFH)

This was formerly the NHS National Programme for IT (NPfIT) that in turn replaced the NHS Information Authority (NHSIA). The programme has its origins in the 1998 DoH strategy Information for Health that committed the NHS to lifelong electronic health records for patients, round-the-clock, online access to patient records for clinicians and information about best clinical practice.

Following the development of the NHS Plan a supporting document called *Building the Information Core: implementing the NHS Plan* was published in January 2001. This outlined the information and IT systems needed to deliver the NHS Plan and support patient-centred care and services.

In 2001, Derek Wanless, a commissioner with the Statistics Commission, was asked to examine future trends affecting the health service in the UK over the next two decades. The Wanless Report, published in April 2002, had several key recommendations for IT in the NHS. These included:

○ doubling and protecting of IT spend
○ stringent, centrally managed national standards for data and IT
○ better management of IT implementation in the NHS, including a national programme.

The Wanless Report coincided with the publication of *Delivering the NHS Plan* (2002), which developed the vision of 'a service designed around the patient', offering patients more choice of where and when to access treatment.

In June 2002 the DoH published its new strategy for developing IT in the NHS: *Delivering 21st Century IT Support for the NHS: a national strategic programme.*

This strategy laid the foundations for the National Programme for IT, including the creation of a ministerial taskforce and the recruitment of a Director-General. The programme was established formally in October 2002. Its task was to procure, develop and implement modern, integrated IT infrastructure and systems for all NHS organisations in England.

Two years later, following the review of its arm's length bodies, the DoH announced the creation of a new organisation, combining responsibility for the delivery of the National Programme with the management of the IT-related functions of the NHS Information Authority, which would close. This organisation was NHS Connecting for Health, a directorate that was established in April 2005 with the purpose of bringing in new computer systems and services.

The plan is attempting to move the NHS towards a single, central electronic care record for patients and to connect 30 000 general practitioners to 300 hospitals, providing secure and audited access to these records by authorised health professionals. NHS CFH is responsible for delivering this programme. In due course it is planned that patients will also have access to their records online through a service called HealthSpace. NHS CFH agency will create 'the world's biggest civil information technology programme'.

The DoH plans to provide an electronic patient records systems protected by the highest levels of access controls and other security measures, making a secure NHS network for exchanging information that is centrally monitored and strongly protected as well as a secure NHS email facility that encrypts all data in its system. Indeed the NHS has been put on notice after suffering a series of security breaches, putting private patient information at risk. Some 140 breaches were reported in the first four months of 2009, causing alarm at the office of the data regulator, the Information Commissioner. In some cases, computers were dumped in skips, in others passwords were written on encrypted discs or memory sticks that were then lost. At the time the Commissioner, Richard Thomas, said he had written to the DoH demanding immediate improvements and planned to send inspectors into hospitals to check compliance. At the time of writing some 14 NHS organisations have already faced action from the commissioner.

Other problems have related to the cost of the programme, together with its ongoing problems of management and the withdrawal or sacking of two of the four IT providers, placing it at the centre of ongoing controversy. The Commons Public Accounts Committee has repeatedly expressed serious concerns over its scope, planning, budgeting and practical value to patients. As of January 2009, while some systems were being deployed across the NHS, other key components of the system were estimated to be four years behind schedule and others had yet to be deployed outside individual trusts. The programme is in its seventh year and not due for completion until 2014/15 at the earliest. To date, expenditure on the programme was given in a parliamentary answer in 2008 as:

- ○ 2004/05 – £620 m
- ○ 2005/06 – £968 m
- ○ 2006/07 – £1.17 bn
- ○ 2007/08 – £1.19 bn
- ○ 2008/09 – £1.20 bn (forecast).

According to the National Audit Office (NAO), at the time of writing it will not be completed until 2014, four years late, and is expected to cost £12.4 billion. The cost could be further increased as the NHS has confirmed it is signing new deals with CSC and BT, the only two remaining suppliers, for £12.7 billion. Fujitsu and Accenture, the other two original contractors, dropped out.

For more information online visit www.connectingforhealth.nhs.uk.

Some of the strategic bodies have been created as special health authorities responsible for specific services to the NHS or the public. Established under secondary legislation so they can only carry out functions conferred by Parliament or the Secretary of State for Health, they are subject to ministerial direction and accountable to the Secretary of State. Examples include the following.

NHS Institute for Innovation and Improvement (and Skills for Health) (NHSIII)

The Institute was set up in July 2005 from the NHS Modernisation Agency together with the NHS Leadership Centre and NHSU (NHS University). The Institute's stated aim is to take forward strategic advice and direction concerning learning in the NHS. With an annual budget of £80 million as a special health authority in England, it is based on the campus of the University of Warwick and was given the following roles:

- ○ work closely with clinicians, NHS organisations, patients, the public, academia and industry in the UK and worldwide to identify best practice
- ○ develop the NHS capability for service transformation, technology and product innovation, leadership development and learning
- ○ support the rapid adoption and spread of new ideas by providing guidance on practical change ideas and ways to facilitate local, safe implementation
- ○ promote a culture of innovation and lifelong learning for all NHS staff.

Potential areas of innovation include developing more personalised care for people with long-term conditions, the testing of new procurement models, and ensuring further value from the NHS annual £4 billion training programme for the widest possible range of staff. With the creation of the new NHS Institute, the NHS Modernisation Agency, NHSU and the NHS Leadership Centre (see above) were dissolved. All the latest information can be seen online at www.institute.nhs.uk.

NHS Business Services Authority (NHSBSA)

The three separate authorities, NHS Pensions Agency (NHSPA), Prescription Pricing Authority (PPA) and Dental Practice Board (DPB), merged to become a new payment and transactions processing body. The NHS Pensions Agency had two parts – NHS Pensions (www.nhsbsa.nhs.uk/pensions), which administers the NHS Pension Scheme, the largest centrally administered public service pension scheme in Europe, and NHS Injury Benefit Scheme (at www.nhsbsa.nhs.uk/injury), which provides an annual allowance for staff who have suffered a permanent loss of earning ability as the result of illness or injury, wholly or mainly attributable to their NHS employment. Anyone who starts working for the NHS automatically becomes a member of the NHS Pension Scheme. But membership is voluntary and you can opt not to join and can leave the Scheme at any time. The NHS Pension Scheme has undergone significant changes which became effective on 1 April 2008. If you joined the Scheme on or before 31 March 2008 you will be a member of the 1995 section of the NHS Pension Scheme. If you joined on or after 1 April 2008, you will be a member of the 2008 section of the NHS Pension Scheme.

NHS Litigation Authority (NHSLA)

Developed from Family Health Services Appeal Authority (FHSAA). The NHSLA was established as a special health authority in 1995 and made responsible for handling negligence claims made against NHS bodies in England. In addition to dealing with claims when they arise, they have an active risk-management programme to help raise standards and hence reduce the number of incidents leading to claims. They monitor human rights case law on behalf of the NHS through the Human Rights Act Information Service. Since April 2005 they have been responsible for handling family health services appeals and in August 2005 acquired the further function of co-ordinating equal pay claims on behalf of the NHS.

Up to April 2009 the NHSLA provided the administration of the FHSAA but from then the administration of the Tribunal transferred to the Tribunals Service, an executive agency of the Ministry of Justice. (See below under Tribunals, p. 32.)

In the past, NHS trusts took out commercial insurance to cover a wide range of non-clinical risks. The increasing costs of successful clinical negligence claims led to the establishment of the Clinical Negligence Scheme for Trusts (CNST), which is now administered by the NHSLA. More than 80% of NHS trusts insure their clinical risk this way.

The NHSLA handles negligence claims made against NHS bodies through five schemes. Three of these relate to clinical negligence claims (CNST, ELS and the ex-RHAs scheme), while two cover non-clinical risks, such as liability for injury to staff and visitors and property damage (LTPS and PES, known collectively as RPST). While only NHS bodies are eligible for membership of these schemes, Independent Sector Treatment Centres, treating NHS patients, may benefit from CNST cover via their referring primary care trust. For more information on these *see* Chapter 6 in Part 1 on medical negligence.

More than 98% of the NHSLA's cases are settled out of court through a variety of methods of 'alternative dispute resolution' (ADR): an analysis of all clinical claims handled by the NHSLA over the past 10 years shows that 41% were abandoned by the claimant, 41% settled out of court, 4% settled in court (mainly court approvals of negotiated settlements) and 14% remain outstanding. Fewer than 50 clinical negligence cases a year are contested in court. For the NHSLA website, go to www.nhsla.com/home.htm.

Health and Social Care Information Centre (HSCIC)

When the original NHSIA split into two to become the NPfIT, at the same time the Health and Social Care Information Centre (HSCIC) was created as a new special health authority. Set up in 2005 and situated in Leeds, its role is to make healthcare information more accessible to the public, regulators, health and social care professionals and policy-makers, leading to improvements in knowledge and efficiency.

As well as providing facts and figures to help the NHS and social services run effectively by collecting data from across the sector, analysing it, and converting it into useful information, many health-related statistics reported in the media will have originated from it; for example, statistics relating to drugs misuse, under-age drinking, 'payment by results' and general practitioner salary details. It also provides information required by MPs, often at short notice and the HSCIC's reports are often crucial in forming health policy at all levels from local right up to those made by the government. For further details go to www.ic.nhs.uk.

The National Patient Safety Agency (NPSA)

Formed from the National Clinical Assessment Authority (NCAA) and joining with National Clinical Assessment Service (NCAS) that remained as a separate division within it.

The NPSA:
○ provides confidential services to help manage concerns with the performance of practitioners
○ improves patient safety by enabling the NHS to learn from patient safety incidents
○ protects the safety and dignity of research participants by facilitating ethical research.

The NPSA (NCAS) works with health organisations and individual practitioners where there is concern about the performance of a dentist, doctor (or pharmacist from 2009) where regulatory intervention seems disproportionate. They help to clarify the concerns, understand what is leading to them and support their resolution. Their aim is to get involved early and, where possible, restore safe and valued practice. The employer, contracting body or practitioner can contact NCAS for help. NCAS covers the UK and associated administrations and both the NHS and independent sectors of healthcare. For more information go to www.ncas.npsa.nhs.uk.

National Reporting and Learning Service (NRLS)

The NRLS is a part of the NPSA, which aims to reduce risks to patients receiving NHS care and thus improve safety. They try to improve patient safety by enabling the NHS to learn from patient safety incidents. The aim is to help improve patient care with rapid response to incidents, analysis of incidents that come to them via the National Reporting and Learning System and the collaborative development of actions that can be implemented locally. At www.npsa.nhs.uk/nrls you can access Publication of Organisation Patient Safety Incident Reports, a section of the website providing details of two-page summary patient safety incident reports for individual NHS organisations in England and Wales.

National Research Ethics Service (NRES)

A further arm of the NPSA that protects the rights, safety, dignity and well-being of research participants who are part of clinical trials and other research within the NHS by facilitating ethical research which is of potential benefit to participants, science and society.

They also commission and monitor the following.

○ **National Confidential Inquiry into Suicide and Homicide by People with Mental Illness (NCI/NCISH)** which is a research project funded largely by the National Patient Safety Agency. Other funders are the Scottish Government and the Department of Health, Social Services and Public Safety in Northern Ireland. It examines all incidences of suicide and homicide by people in contact with mental health services in the UK, as well as cases of sudden death in the psychiatric inpatient population.

○ **Centre for Maternal and Child Enquiries (CMACE), which evolved from Confidential Enquiry into Maternal and Child Health (CEMACH) in July 2009.** CEMACH was set up in April 2003 as a unit within the Royal College of Obstetricians and Gynaecologists (RCOG). With the new name it also became an independent charity, reflecting significant developments since 2003. CMACE continues to work for mothers and babies but also aims to develop and expand its work on child health. The organisation has also broadened its range of activities beyond its core national confidential inquiry activity. Local review, clinical audits and research collaborations represent an increasingly important part of its work. These all support its wider mission to improve the health of mothers, babies and children.

○ **National Confidential Enquiry into Patient Outcome and Death (NCEPOD).** Its precursor was a confidential and anonymous pilot study of mortality associated with anaesthesia (Lunn and Mushin 1982). This covered inpatients from five regions in England, Wales and Scotland. Its aims were to assess perioperative information in order that the clinical practice of anaesthesia might be improved and to provide comparative figures between regions to facilitate this. A further important objective was to establish an index of contemporary standards of care to permit future comparisons. It had hoped this study might be a combined surgical and anaesthetic enterprise but this proved impossible.

In 1982 a joint venture between surgical and anaesthetic specialties named the Confidential Enquiry into Perioperative Deaths (CEPOD) was initiated. This reviewed surgical and anaesthetic practice over one year in three regions. In 1988 the National Confidential Enquiry into Perioperative Deaths (NCEPOD) was then established, supported by government funding, and its first report was published in 1990.

Since its inception NCEPOD has moved from reviewing the care of surgical patients and now covers all specialties. This is reflected in the wide range of studies being currently undertaken. They also look at near misses rather than just death and have increased the number of reports published each year.

This year NCEPOD celebrates 20 years of promoting improvements in healthcare. It has published over 20 reports derived from a vast array of information about the practical management of patients.

The distinctive feature of NCEPOD's contribution is the critical examination, by senior and appropriately chosen specialists, of what has actually happened to the patients. Recommendations have covered everything from individual clinical practice to national healthcare organisation, always with the aim of improving patient care and safety.

NCEPOD is independent of the DoH and the professional associations. It is both a charity and a company limited by guarantee. It has a board of directors that are referred to as the NCEPOD Trustees. This board oversees the charitable and corporate governance of the organisation.

In addition there is also the NCEPOD Steering Group. Members are nominated representatives of the various medical royal colleges and associations and lay representation. There are also five observers on the group from the National Patient Safety Agency, the Coroners Society, the Institute of Healthcare Management, the Scottish Audit of Surgical Mortality and The Institute for Health and Clinical Excellence. This board ensures the clinical integrity of the work that NCEPOD undertakes.

NCEPOD is mainly funded by the DoH via NPSA (about 90% of funding in 2005/06) and the Health and Social Service Executive Northern Ireland, the offshore islands and the Independent sector provide the remainder of funds.

A good start for getting more information is the NPSA at www.npsa.nhs.uk.

National Institute for Health and Clinical Excellence (NICE)

In April 2005 the National Institute for Clinical Excellence joined with the Health Development Agency (HDA) to become the new National Institute for Health and Clinical Excellence and took on their responsibilities. NICE is the independent organisation responsible for providing national guidance on the promotion of good health and the prevention and treatment of ill health.

NICE produces guidance in three areas.

o Public health – guidance on promotion of good health and prevention of ill health for those working in the NHS, local authorities and the wider public and voluntary sector.
o Health technologies – guidance on the use of new and existing medicines, treatments and procedures within the NHS.

o   Clinical practice – guidance on appropriate treatments and care of people with specific diseases and conditions within the NHS.

The booklet *NICE: our guidance sets the standard for good healthcare*, available online, explains more about NICE and the types of guidance produced. This guidance is developed using the expertise of the NHS and the wider healthcare community including NHS staff, healthcare professionals, patients and carers, industry and the academic world. Although the methods for developing the various forms of guidance differ, all the development processes are said to be underpinned by the key Institute principles of basing recommendations on the best available evidence and involving all stakeholders in a transparent and collaborative manner.

The NICE website has a 'Search NICE Guidance' facility where you can obtain its guidance on diseases and treatments. Further information can be found at www.nice.org.uk.

The National Specialised Commissioning Group (NSCG)

The NSCG was created in April 2007 to oversee national commissioning of highly specialised health services following an independent Review of Commissioning Arrangements for Specialised Services, headed by Sir David Carter (known as the Carter Review). This was commissioned by the DoH to help the NHS to plan provision for some of the most rare conditions and expensive treatments, investigate how the NHS commissions specialised services and make proposals for improvement as well as ensure the process was robust, fair, understood by all, engaged patients and offered value for money. Voting members of the NSCG are the Chair/CE NHS London and representatives from each of the 10 SCGs. Non-voting members include representatives from the medical royal colleges, SHAs and DoH. There is also a lay representative.

The National Commissioning Group (NCG)

A standing committee of the NSCG advises Ministers on which NHS services are best commissioned nationally, rather than locally. The NCG's membership is made up of leading clinical representatives including the presidents of the larger royal colleges and the Chairman of the Joint Medical Consultative Committee, as well as local commissioners, public health representatives and R&D experts. The NCG is the successor body to the National Specialised Commissioning Advisory Group (NSCAG), which was previously located in the DoH. The NCG is supported by a team of 30 officers, the National Specialised Commissioning Team (NSC Team).

In addition to the bodies described above there are 10 regionally based Specialised Commissioning Groups (SCGs) that cover the same areas as the 10 English Strategic Health Authorities. The SCGs commission services for populations of between 3 and 7 million, depending on the size of the SHA.

For more information go to www.ncg.nhs.uk.

National Treatment Agency for Substance Misuse (NTA)

The NTA was established by the government in 2001 to improve the availability, capacity and effectiveness of treatment for drug misuse in England. The agency continues to deliver the government's main drugs targets, working in partnership with national, regional and local agencies to:

- ensure the efficient use of public funding to support effective, appropriate and accessible local services
- promote evidence-based and co-ordinated practice, by distilling and disseminating best practice
- improve performance by developing standards for treatment, promoting user and carer involvement, and expanding and developing the drug treatment workforce
- monitor and develop the effectiveness of treatment.

For more information go to www.nta.nhs.uk.

Blood and Transplant Authority (BaTA)

Created from the National Blood Authority (NBA) and UK Transplant (UKT) in 2005, the authority became responsible for supporting the donation and safe use of human tissues and promoting donation. It operates as a special health authority and is the organ donor organisation for the UK, responsible for matching and allocating donated organs as well as the provision of blood supply and associated services to the NHS.

One of its key roles is to ensure that organs donated for transplant are matched and allocated to patients in a fair and unbiased way. Matching, particularly in the case of kidneys, is organised nationally, the principle being that the larger the pool, the better the likelihood of a good match.

They do not have a direct relationship with patients and do not provide 'hands on' care. However, in providing support to transplantation services across the UK, everything they do has an impact on the quality of service delivered to patients. Responsibilities include:

- managing the National Transplant Database, which includes details of all donors and patients who are waiting for, or who have received, a transplant
- providing a 24-hour service for the matching and allocation of donated organs and making the transport arrangements to get the organs to patients
- maintaining the national NHS Organ Donor Register
- contributing to the development of performance indicators, standards and protocols that guide the work of organ donation and transplantation
- acting as a central point for information on transplant matters
- providing central support to all transplant units in the UK and the Republic of Ireland
- auditing and analysing the results of all organ transplants in the UK and the Republic of Ireland to improve patient care
- improving organ donation rates by funding initiatives in the wider NHS
- raising public awareness of the importance of organ donation.

The names and history of the transplant service is complicated and best set out in chronological order of name changes.

○ 1968 National Tissue Typing and Reference Laboratory (NTTRL) established.
○ 1972 National Organ Matching and Distribution Service (MOMDS) founded.
○ 1979 NTTRL and NOMDS merge to become UK Transplant Service.
○ 1991 UK Transplant Service becomes a special health authority and is renamed United Kingdom Transplant Support Service Authority (UKTSSA).
○ 1993 UKTSSA moves to purpose-built accommodation at Bristol.
○ 2000 UK Transplant takes over from UKTSSA with new, extended remit to increase organ donation rates.
○ 2005 UK Transplant merges with the National Blood Service and Bio Products Laboratory to form NHS Blood and Transplant, an NHS special health authority responsible for optimising the supply of blood, organs, plasma and tissues and raising the quality, effectiveness and efficiency of blood and transplant services.
○ 2008 UK Transplant renamed Directorate of Organ Donation and Transplantation.

For further information go to www.uktransplant.org.uk.

There are some executive non-departmental independent public bodies performing specific national functions for NHS or the public. They have been set up under primary legislation (unlike the SHAs listed above), giving them powers independent of the Secretary of State for Health and directly accountable to Parliament. These include the following.

Monitor – Independent Regulator of NHS Foundation Trusts

Established in January 2004, this body continued unchanged in the reconfiguration of arm's length bodies as an independent organisation responsible for licensing and regulating NHS foundation trusts. It is independent of central government and is directly accountable to Parliament. There are three main strands to its work:

○ determining whether NHS trusts are ready to become NHS foundation trusts
○ ensuring that NHS foundation trusts comply with the conditions they signed up to – that they are well-led and financially robust
○ supporting NHS foundation trust development.

It is the first line of regulation in NHS foundation trusts that are asked to submit an annual plan and regular reports to monitor. The regulator board judges how well they are doing against these plans and identifies where problems might arise.

Where problems start to develop the board makes sure the trust has an action plan in place and monitors progress against the plan. Where possible it works closely with a trust to resolve a problem quickly.

The board also has powers to intervene in a foundation trust in the event of failings in its healthcare standards, or other aspects of its leadership, which result in a significant breach of its terms of authorisation. You can find out more about the Monitor's functions and powers, as detailed in the National Health Service Act 2006, at www.monitor-nhsft.gov.uk.

The Care Quality Commission (CQC)

This is the latest health and social care regulator for England, which replaced The Healthcare Commission, Commission for Social Care Inspection and the Mental Health Act Commission after the end of March 2009. It brings together independent regulation of health, mental health and adult social care whether provided by the NHS, local authorities, private companies or voluntary organisations. It also protects the rights of people detained under the Mental Health Act.

The commission ensures that essential common quality standards are being met where care is provided and works towards the improvement of care services. It has a wide range of enforcement powers to take action if services are considered unacceptably poor.

The main activities are:

○ registration of health and social care providers
○ monitoring and inspection of all health and adult social care
○ using enforcement powers, such as fines and public warnings or closures, if standards are not being met
○ improving health and social care services by undertaking regular reviews of how well those who arrange and provide services locally are performing and special reviews on particular care services, pathways of care or themes where there are particular concerns about quality
○ reporting the outcomes of their work so that people who use services have information about the quality of their local health and adult social care services.
○ helping those who arrange and provide services to see where improvement is needed and learn from each other about what works best.

The new website is at www.cqc.org.uk.

Council for Healthcare Regulatory Excellence (CHRE)

Renamed and with expanded powers, CHRE was created from the Council for the Regulation of Health Care Professionals (CRHP). It continues to oversee the various statutory professional self-regulatory bodies. CHRE was founded following the National Health Service Reform and Health Professions Act 2002, which outlined its statutory powers to investigate and report on the performance of the regulators. They also review final fitness to practise decisions, identify learning points for the regulators where they feel necessary and provide advice to the Secretary of State for Health and Ministers in Scotland, Wales and Northern Ireland on matters relating to the regulation of health professions. The CHRE is an independent body accountable directly to Parliament.

The Health and Social Care Act 2008 extended CHRE's powers to include additional responsibilities of reviewing fitness to practise cases where the health of a registrant is at issue. It also amended the governance arrangements so that the health professions regulators no longer sit on the governing council. More specific details on the appointments to and procedures of its governing council are set out in the Council for Healthcare Regulatory Excellence (Appointments, Procedures etc.) Regulations 2008.

CHRE oversees the work of nine health professions regulators who aim to protect and promote the safety of the public by setting standards of behaviour, education and ethics that health professionals must meet and deal with concerns about professionals who are unfit to practise as a result of poor health, misconduct or poor performance. Regulators register health professionals who are fit to practise in the UK and can remove professionals from the register and prevent them from practising where they consider this to be in the best interests of public safety. The regulators are as follows.

o General Chiropractic Council (GCC) regulates chiropractors.
o General Dental Council (GDC) regulates dentists, dental nurses, dental technicians, dental hygienists, dental therapists, clinical dental technicians and orthodontic therapists.
o General Medical Council (GMC) regulates doctors.
o General Optical Council (GOC) regulates optometrists, dispensing opticians, student opticians and optical businesses.
o General Osteopathic Council (GOsC) regulates osteopaths.
o Health Professions Council (HPC) regulates the members of 13 health professions: arts therapists, biomedical scientists, chiropodists/podiatrists, clinical scientists, dietitians, occupational therapists, operating department practitioners, orthoptists, paramedics, physiotherapists, prosthetists/orthotists, radiographers, speech and language therapists.
o Nursing and Midwifery Council (NMC) regulates nurses and midwives.
o Pharmaceutical Society of Northern Ireland (PSNI) regulates pharmacists in Northern Ireland.
o Royal Pharmaceutical Society of Great Britain (RPSGB) regulates pharmacists in England, Wales and Scotland.

The CHRE monitor how health professions regulators carry out their functions and every year conduct a performance review with each regulator. This review looks at how the regulators carry out their functions against agreed standards. It highlights good practice and identifies issues that might benefit from a co-ordinated approach.

They can refer cases to court where decisions are considered too lenient. When concerns about the conduct or performance of a health professional are referred to a regulator, the regulator carries out an investigation to determine whether the concerns are valid and whether the professional should continue to practise. They then look at the final-stage decisions made by the regulators on professionals' fitness to practise. If a decision is unduly lenient and fails to protect the public interest, they can refer the case to the High Court (the Court of Sessions for Scotland or the High Court of Justice for Northern Ireland).

CHRE works with the regulators to improve quality and share good practice. For example, sharing learning points arising from the scrutiny of fitness to practise cases and organising seminars to explore regulation issues. It advises health ministers, the Secretary of State and health ministers in Scotland, Wales and Northern Ireland who may request advice about the regulation of health professions.

It influences national and international policy on the regulation of health professions consulting with the UK government and governments in Wales, Scotland and Northern Ireland on the development of guidelines for the sector. In addition, it keeps abreast of international policies that may affect health regulation in the UK, particularly in Europe. It works with colleagues in the UK and abroad, ensuring that they are aware of developments and strengthening relationships with these partners.

Finally, it involves patients and the public in its work. To do this they listen to people's views and concerns and consider them when developing work. It holds public and patient consultation meetings that are attended by members of patient representation organisations, and has developed and agreed recommendations for a 'focused patient involvement plan'.

The Health Protection Agency (HPA)

The HPA is an independent UK organisation that was set up by the government in 2003 to protect the public from threats to their health from infectious diseases and environmental hazards. It does this by providing advice and information to the general public, to health professionals such as doctors and nurses, and to national and local government.

The agency identifies and responds to health hazards and emergencies caused by infectious disease, hazardous chemicals, poisons or radiation. It gives advice to the public on how to stay healthy and avoid health hazards, provides data and information to government to help inform its decision making, and advises people working in healthcare. It also makes sure the nation is ready for future threats to health that could happen naturally, accidentally or deliberately.

During the 2009 influenza pandemic (H1N1), as well as providing advice to the public it was a contemporaneous source of updated online information for health professionals with prescribing guidance on antiviral drugs and safety notices with links to further guidance on various issues such as complications of the disease.

The HPA combines public health and scientific knowledge, research and emergency planning within one organisation – and works at international, national, regional and local levels. It also supports and advises other organisations that play a part in protecting health.

The agency's advice, information and services are underpinned by evidence-based research. It also uses its research to develop new vaccines and treatments that directly help patients. Although set up by government, the agency is independent and provides whatever advice and information is necessary to protect people's health.

Local HPA services work alongside the NHS providing specialist support in communicable disease and infection control, and emergency planning. LRS (Local and Regional Services) work through nine regional offices that correspond to the Government Offices of the Regions and 28 Health Protection Units (HPUs), each covering an area broadly corresponding to a county or police boundary. There are eight Regional Microbiology Laboratories. In addition, 37 hospital microbiology laboratories participate as HPA Collaborating Laboratories. As well as a central office based in London the HPA has three major centres, as follows.

○ **The HPA Centre for Radiation, Chemical and Environmental Hazards** based at

Chilton in Oxfordshire comprises the Radiation Protection Division (formerly the National Radiological Protection Board) and the Chemical Hazards and Poisons Division.

o **The Centre for Emergency Preparedness and Response** located at Porton Down in Wiltshire plays an important role in preparing for and co-ordinating responses to potential healthcare emergencies, including possible acts of deliberate release. In addition, they undertake both basic and applied research into understanding infectious diseases and manufacture a number of healthcare products, including vaccines and therapeutics.

o **The HPA Centre for Infections (CfI)** carries out a broad spectrum of work relating to prevention of infectious disease. The remit of the CfI includes infectious disease surveillance, providing specialist and reference microbiology and microbial epidemiology, co-ordinating the investigation and cause of national and uncommon outbreaks, helping advise government on the risks posed by various infections and responding to international health alerts.

The National Radiological Protection Board (NRPB) was a non-departmental public body but joined the Health Protection Agency in 2005 so its new website is www. hpa.org.uk/radiation.

NHS Appointments Commission

Created when the Commission for Patient and Public Involvement in Health (CPPIH) was abolished and stronger arrangements put in place to provide support and advice to Patients' Forums. Responsibility for the appointment of Patients' Forum members was transferred to the NHS Appointments Commission, which also appoints chairs and members of local research ethics committees.

The NHS Appointments Commission was set up as a special health authority in 2001 following an announcement in the NHS Plan. It thus removed the need for Health Ministers to make all non-executive appointments to NHS bodies. As part of a strategy to devolve and delegate functions that did not relate to its core functions, the government had decided that the Appointments Commission would in future make all chair and non-executive appointments to NHS trusts, primary care trusts and health authorities.

There are around 4000 chairs and non-executives on NHS boards. Of these up to 1500 may be appointed annually. Recruiting and appointing people with the skills and attributes to act as advocates for their communities and provide leadership for the NHS is a crucial and challenging task.

Part of that challenge was the need to ensure that the public, the NHS and Ministers have confidence in the openness, transparency and fairness of the appointment procedures. To maintain this confidence, the Appointments Commission follows the guidance set by the Commission for Public Appointments that, building on Lord Nolan's First Report, aims to ensure that all public appointments are made on merit following a proper process.

The role of the Appointments Commission does not end once an appointment has been made. Chairs and non-executives look to the Regional Commissioners for mentoring and support and the Commission has the responsibility, with the Leadership Centre, for ensuring that chairs and non-executives receive proper induction and training in their roles. The Commission also ensures that chairs and non-executives are properly appraised in a regular and consistent way. For more information go to www.dh.gov.uk/en/Managingyourorganisation/Humanresourcesandtraining/Modernisingprofessional regulation/DH_4052361.

The Regulatory Authority for Fertility and Tissue (RAFT)

RAFT is responsible for fertility treatments and use of human tissue, and was created to encompass the work of the earlier Human Fertilisation and Embryology Authority (HFEA) and the Human Tissue Authority (HTA). See below under Advisory NDPBs for further information, or go to www.hta.gov.uk.

The HFEA was the statutory body that regulated and inspected all UK clinics providing *in vitro* fertilisation, artificial insemination or the storage of human ova, sperm or embryos and licensed and monitored all human embryo research conducted in the UK. It also carried out a policy role, advising the UK legislators of changes that it believes should be made to fertility legislation.

The Human Tissue Authority was created from the earlier Retained Organs Commission (abolished in 2004), which was set up to regulate the removal, storage, use and disposal of human bodies, organs and tissue for a number of Scheduled Purposes – such as research, transplantation, and education and training as set out in the Human Tissue Act 2004 (HT Act).

The HT Act covered England, Wales and Northern Ireland. There is separate legislation in Scotland – the Human Tissue (Scotland) Act 2006 – and the HTA performed certain tasks on behalf of the Scottish Executive (approval of living donation and licensing of establishments storing tissue for human application). The HTA was the Competent Authority under the EU Tissue and Cells Directive for regulating human application establishments. The HTA was also responsible for approving donation of solid organs and bone marrow from living donors.

For more information go to www.hta.gov.uk.

Postgraduate Medical Education and Training Board (PMETB)

Another body that remained unaffected by the reconfiguration of arm's length public bodies (ALPBs) was PMETB, the independent regulatory body responsible for postgraduate medical education and training. It ensures that postgraduate training for doctors is of the highest standard. Its vision is to achieve excellence in postgraduate medical education, training, assessment and accreditation throughout the UK to improve the knowledge, skills and experience of doctors and the health and healthcare of patients and the public by:

○ establishing and overseeing standards in postgraduate medical education and training by quality assuring training programmes and posts
○ approving specialist curricula and related management systems
○ certifying doctors for application to the specialist and GP registers, including those

applying for a Certificate of Completion of Training (CCT) and those whose skills, qualifications and experience are equivalent to a CCT

o independently leading on the content and outcomes for the future of postgraduate medical education and training.

The PMETB was established by The General and Specialist Medical Practice (Education, Training and Qualifications) Order 2003 to develop a single, unifying framework for postgraduate medical education and training, and began in September 2005 when it took over the responsibilities of the Specialist Training Authority of the medical royal colleges and the Joint Committee on Postgraduate General Practice Training; it is now accountable to Parliament and acts independently of government as the UK competent authority. For more information go to www.pmetb. org.uk.

The publication *Preparing Doctors for the Future: about PMETB* explains in more detail the role of PMETB, provides an overview of their latest work in quality and certification and outlines future work on the content and outcomes of postgraduate medical education and training (available online at www.pmetb.org.uk/fileadmin/user/ Communications/Publications/Preparing_Doctors_for_the_future_About_PMETB. pdf). At the time of writing discussion is taking place on the merger of the PMETB with the GMC. This, in addition to involving the GMC Council and PMETB Board, has drawn in groups from undergraduate and postgraduate medical education and training, the NHS and independent sector, patients and the public.

General Social Care Council (GSCC)

The GSCC was established in 2001 under the Care Standards Act 2000; it is responsible for setting standards of conduct and practice for social care workers and their employers, for regulating the workforce, and for regulating social work education and training. It is sponsored by the DoH but also works closely with the Department for Children, Schools and Families in delivering the children's and young people's care agenda. The GSCC's Council has 10 members appointed by the Appointments Commission on behalf of the Secretary of State for Health. The Council meets six times a year in a public forum. More information can be found at www.gscc.org.uk.

Next I come to some advisory non-departmental public bodies.

Expert Advisory Group on AIDS (EAGA)

An advisory non-departmental public body that was non-statutorily established in 1985 with the following terms of reference: 'To provide advice on such matters relating to HIV/AIDS as may be referred to it by the Chief Medical Officers of the Health Departments of the United Kingdom.'

Joint Committee on Vaccination and Immunisation (JCVI)

An independent expert advisory committee first set up in 1963: 'To advise the Secretaries of State for Health, Scotland, Wales and Northern Ireland on matters relating to communicable diseases, preventable and potentially preventable through immunisation.'

Tribunals

These were created by legislation and for making decisions in specialised fields of law. Examples include the following.

○ **Care Standards Tribunal** first established under The Protection of Children Act 1999. From November 2008 it formed part of the Health, Education and Social Care Chamber of the First-tier Tribunal, and deals with care standards appeals.

○ **Family Health Services Appeal Authority:** In December 2001 the Health and Social Care Act 2001 amended the National Health Service Act 1977 by replacing the NHS Tribunal with the Family Health Services Appeal Authority. But in April 2009 the National Health Service Litigation Authority that provided the administration of the FHSAA was transferred to the Tribunals Service as an executive agency of the Ministry of Justice. The Tribunal has a president, 12 legal chairs, 28 professional members and 25 lay members. The Lord Chancellor, following recommendations from the Judicial Appointments Commission, appoints all members. Appeals and applications are made to it directly.

○ **Mental Health Review Tribunal** is an independent judicial body that operates under the provisions of the Mental Health Act 1983 (as amended by the Mental Health Act 2007). The main purpose is to review cases of patients detained under the Mental Health Act and to direct the discharge of any patients where the statutory criteria for discharge have been satisfied. In some cases, they have the discretion to discharge patients who do not meet the statutory criteria.

Finally, I come to a miscellaneous collection of arm's length bodies that are hard to put into one particular classification.

NHS Professionals

One of the bodies that remained unchanged in the reconfiguration, it manages and provides temporary staff to the NHS and will eventually take on independent status. A not-for-profit organisation, it provides 'flexible staffing solutions' by supplying medical and nursing staff including doctors. Go to www.nhsprofessionals.nhs.uk.

The National Stakeholder Forum (NSF)

The NSF was formed in 2006 from The National Leadership Network for Health and Social Care (NLN). The Forum is a group of senior leaders and experts from all parts of the health and social care system that aims to provide rapid and frank feedback and early advice on emerging policy. Prior to 2007, the NLN was established as a successor to the NHS Modernisation Board in December 2004. It acts as a sounding board to ministers, permanent secretaries and director-generals.

Management at commissioning level

I now consider bodies with mainly a commissioning role and NHS Direct and NHS Choices.

Strategic health authorities and special health authorities (SHAs)

Both these authorities use the acronym SHA, but they are totally different bodies.

Strategic health authorities

Strategic health authorities are regional bodies (there are now 10) responsible for ensuring that the NHS follows DoH strategic policies bodies that purchase or commission or provide health services in England. Different organisations carry out this function in Wales and Northern Ireland and Scotland, where commissioning has been abolished. See later in this chapter on the NHS in other parts of the UK. If all NHS trusts and ultimately all PCTs acquire foundation status (see later in this chapter, p. 46), the SHAs will lose most of their function.

Created in 2002, the SHAs are a link between the DoH and NHS. There were originally 28 but in 2006, this number was reduced to 10. They are:

- East Midlands Strategic Health Authority
- East of England Strategic Health Authority
- London Strategic Health Authority
- North East Strategic Health Authority
- North West Strategic Health Authority
- South Central Strategic Health Authority
- South East Coast Strategic Health Authority
- South West Strategic Health Authority
- West Midlands Strategic Health Authority
- Yorkshire and The Humber Strategic Health Authority.

They are responsible for:

- developing plans for improving health services in their local area
- making sure local health services are of a high quality and performing well
- increasing the capacity of local health services – so they can provide more services
- making sure national priorities, e.g. programmes for improving cancer services, are integrated into local health service plans.

Strategic health authority boards

Strategic health authorities provide leadership for the improvement of health and for the development of health services in their areas. They are responsible for performance management and accountability of local NHS trusts and PCTs. They also take the lead in the development of local clinical and public health networks.

A strategic health authority board consists of:

- a non-executive chair (appointed by the Appointments Commission)
- normally, five non-executive directors (appointed by the Appointments Commission)
- up to five executive members, including the chief executive and finance director.

More information is available at www.appointments.org.uk/nhs_trust.asp and there is an excellent 76-page booklet, *Governing the NHS: a guide for trust boards*, available at www.appointments.org.uk/docs/govern.pdf. It explains the:

○ duty of NHS Boards
○ role of the Chair, non-executive directors, Chief Executive, the Professional Executive Committee (PEC)
○ various board committees
○ functions and accountability relationships
○ role of inspectorate and regulatory systems
○ role of NHS Appointment Commission
○ signposts to the future
○ plus provides 13 annexes on a number of issues.

Special health authorities

Special health authorities, of which there are now far fewer again, are bodies responsible for providing specific national services to the NHS or the public. They are established under secondary legislation and can only carry out functions conferred by parliament on the Secretary of State for Health.

Special health authorities provide a health service to the whole of England, not just to a local community; for example, the National Blood Authority. They are set up under section 11 of the NHS Act 1977. They are independent, but can be subject to ministerial direction like other NHS bodies. Each has a unique function and some have remits that extend beyond England. They are described in detail earlier in this chapter (p. 18 onwards). They are:

○ NHS Institute for Innovation and Improvement (and Skills for Health)
○ NHS Business Services Authority
○ NHS Litigation Authority
○ Health and Social Care Information Centre
○ National Patient Safety Agency
○ National Institute for Clinical Excellence
○ National Treatment Agency for Substance Misuse
○ Blood and Transplant Authority.

Boards oversee their work with both executive and non-executive members.

NHS Direct

NHS Direct was made a special health authority in 2004 but since 2008 has been part of NHS Choices. It is a 24-hour phone line, staffed by nurses, that offers quick access to healthcare advice. NHS Direct nurses will give advice and support on self-treatment or, if further help is needed, will put a patient in touch with the right service. With serious conditions or an emergency, generally the nurse will give advice on what to do and will call an ambulance if needed. You can find information and advice about NHS Direct online or by phoning NHS Direct on 0845 4647.

NHS Choices

NHS Choices is a comprehensive information service that helps patients make choices about health, from lifestyle decisions, smoking, drinking and exercise, through to the practical aspects of finding and using NHS services in England. It draws together:

o The National Library for Health (NLH)
o The Information Centre for Health and Social Care
o The Care Quality Commission
o and many other organisations.

Since the integration of the online arm of NHS Direct in 2008, NHS Choices is said to provide a single 'front door' for the public to all NHS online services and information through what is described as the country's biggest health website at www.nhs. uk/aboutnhschoices.

Next there are NHS organisations with a commissioning or purchasing role.

Primary care trusts (PCTs)

All of these primary care services are managed by primary care trusts that are statutory NHS bodies, monitored by their strategic health authority and are ultimately accountable to the Secretary of State for Health. They are freestanding NHS organisations with their own boards, staff and budgets. They work with other health and social care organisations and local authorities to make sure that the community's needs are met. PCTs provide some care directly and commission services from others, such as NHS acute trusts and private providers, with decisions on providers increasingly informed by the choices which patients make themselves.

There are about 152 primary care trusts in England, each one covering a separate local area. PCTs decide what health services a local community needs, and are responsible for providing them. They must ensure that there are enough services for people within their local area, and that the services are accessible. As well as those services mentioned above they also include NHS Direct and NHS Walk-in Centres (see later in this chapter, p. 44).

PCTs make decisions about the type of services that hospitals provide and are responsible for ensuring the quality of service. They also control funding for hospitals. Being local organisations they understand the needs of their local community. PCTs are thus responsible for:

o developing programmes for improving the health of the local community
o deciding what health services the local population needs and ensuring they are provided and are as accessible as possible; this includes hospital care, mental health services, GP practices, screening programmes, patient transport, NHS dentists, pharmacies and opticians
o bringing together health and social care, so that NHS organisations work with local authorities, social services and voluntary organisations
o ensuring the development of staff skills, capital investment in buildings, equipment

and IT, so that the NHS locally is improved and modernised and can continually deliver better services.

Every PCT aims to achieve the maximum health improvement through prevention and other interventions. This can include everything from ensuring that smoking cessation services are achieving high long-term 'quit' rates to ensuring that the primary care element of the targets of national service frameworks are met.

PCTs receive about 80% of the total NHS budget. They get most of their budget directly from the DoH and use this to purchase hospital and other services from NHS trusts and other healthcare providers. They are also responsible for making payments to independent primary care contractors such as GPs and dentists.

Teaching PCTs (TPCTs)

In 2001 the government said it would establish a number of TPCTs, as a statutory NHS body based upon the existing PCT model, in disadvantaged and underprivileged areas. It described the aim as creating new, attractive posts offering wider career development opportunities linked to part-time clinical roles and part-time teaching/learning roles. By establishing TPCTs in these disadvantaged and underprivileged areas, it was intended to attract additional high-quality staff and bring much needed capacity into areas of need. The intention was that TPCTs were not to be confined to traditional teaching activities such as postgraduate clinical training, continuing professional development and lifelong learning. The government said that TPCTs would engage in a variety of other activities that encompassed the ethos of learning, development, research, dissemination and delivery of good practice. In 2006 they were reconfigured; a DoH document about them can be downloaded at www.networks.nhs.uk/uploads/06/08/dh_policy_document_on_tpcts.pdf.

Primary care trust boards

PCT boards have responsibility to improve the health of their local community and so work closely with patients, service users, carers, GPs, other health professionals and local healthcare providers to assess local health needs and then to develop or commission suitable services.

A PCT board generally consists of:
○ a non-executive chair (appointed by the Appointments Commission)
○ at least five non-executive members (appointed by the Appointments Commission)
○ at least five executive members, including the chief executive, finance director and director of public health
○ at least two members from the PCT's Professional Executive Committee (PEC).

Clinical expertise is provided by the PEC, with representation from local GPs, nurses and other health professionals and social services. The board concentrates on the overall strategies for the trust and making sure that it meets its statutory, financial and legal responsibilities.

Commissioning

There have been a number of methods used over recent years for purchaser or commissioning bodies to purchase or commission healthcare from the providers, be they primary or secondary care providers. The latest is practice-based commissioning, described shortly. The document *Commissioning a Patient-led NHS* (2005) followed on from the publication of *Creating a Patient-led NHS* in the same year. You can see them at www.dh.gov.uk/en/Publicationsandstatistics/Publications/PublicationsPolicy AndGuidance/DH_4106506 or icn.csip.org.uk/_library/Creating_a_patient-led_ NHS.pdf; they focus on how the DoH will develop commissioning in the NHS, with some changes in function for primary care trusts and strategic health authorities.

Practice-based commissioning (PBC)

This is a massive subject and if you need to know the details of it you are recommended to read the very latest DoH guidelines. But, for a brief outline, it started with the 1998 White Paper, *The New NHS*, which stated that, 'over time, the Government expects that . . . PCTs will extend indicative budgets to individual practices for the full range of services'. *The NHS Improvement Plan* said that 'from April 2005, GP practices that wish to do so will be given indicative commissioning budgets'.

The publication of *Commissioning a Patient-led NHS* in 2005 accelerated the development of practice-led commissioning, to be in place by the end of 2006. The overall purpose of commissioning was to ensure that health needs are met through the provision of services that reduce health inequalities, promote health and improve patient care by a process of devolution. It was described as a commissioning cycle with six stages:

1   assessment of health needs of the population
2   auditing current service provision
3   agreement about the priorities
4   development of service and practice development plans with key stakeholders
5   agreements of contracts
6   evaluation of the outcomes for patients/population.

Commissioning had developed from contracting and purchasing and aimed to improve community health going beyond purchasing/contracting episodes of care provided in hospitals. Practice-led commissioning was not to be a return to GP fund-holding but, instead, attempted to reflect multidisciplinary and public involvement. Nor was it to be seen as competition for PCT-level commissioning. The DoH believed it to be consistent with greater devolution and thus enable the following.

o   Patient choice as a driver for quality and empowerment, with practices or localities able to secure a wide range of services, from which patients could choose. From 2008 the impact of free choice for elective procedures would change the dynamic further. Practices and localities could then use their commissioning abilities to identify alternative provisions, including in primary care, to give patients still greater choice.

o   Effective payment by results, by ensuring that funds follow the patient, meaning that where practices or localities were able to provide or commission services locally and as patients choose to use these services, the funds would follow.

○ Practices or localities would be able to direct funding in order to support patients with long-term conditions.

By promoting practice-level budgets for commissioning, the DoH envisaged a number of other ways in which patients would benefit:

○ a greater variety of services
○ from a greater number of providers
○ in settings that are closer to home and more convenient to patients.

Payment by Results was already a reality for foundation trusts and beginning to cover other acute trusts from 2005. Patient choice was increasing and record investment in the NHS meant that scope for innovation was enormous.

Commissioning for specialised services that are commissioned nationally and national screening programmes were not included in a practice's indicative budget. These are services provided in relatively few specialist centres to catchment populations of more than a million people covering several PCTs. This issue was covered by *Guidance on Commissioning Arrangements for Specialised Services* (2003) and the conditions are listed in the *Specialised Services National Definition Set* (www.dh.gov. uk/PolicyAndGuidance/HealthAndSocialCareTopics/SpecialisedServicesDefinition/fs/en).

Various types of care

In addition to primary and secondary care there is one other classification of care provided that you may need to be aware of. Since the last edition of this book there have been, in line perhaps with a general tendency, a relaxation and slack use of terminology. There is also a need to differentiate shared care from collaborative care that is often more general in nature, some say oriented towards relationship building and thus, perhaps, a precursor to shared care.

Then there is planned care and managed care, which are often used interchangeably with shared care. Generally, though, planned care implies the application of care pathways that aim to have the right people doing the right things, in the right order, at the right time.

Managed care, like shared care, is based on inter-professional practice, but in some views is principally focused on the provision of healthcare through service utilisation monitoring and cost containment.

Finally, some authors talk of worked team-based care that can be used interchangeably for shared care, collaborative care, planned care or managed care. So you need to establish definitions when talking about these types of care.

Community care

The NHS and Community Care Act (1990) was a piece of legislation that governed healthcare and social care. It set out how the NHS should assess and provide for patients based on their needs, requirements and circumstances. The Act introduced an internal market into the supply of healthcare, making the state the enabler rather than a supplier.

The Act states that it is a duty of local authorities to assess people for social care and support to ensure people who need community care services or other types of support get the services. Patients have their needs and circumstances assessed and the results determine whether or not care or social services will be provided. Local authority resources can be taken into account during the assessment process, but if it is deemed that services are required, those services must be provided by law and services cannot be withdrawn at a later date if resources become limited.

Community care means providing services and support to enable people to achieve maximum independence and control over their lives following an assessment of the person's needs and can include support at home, respite and day care and, for those with very high support needs, residential and nursing care.

It is a method of providing services to people who are ill or physically or mentally impaired to allow them to stay in their own homes as long as they are able, or in other settings in the community such as residential homes. This term can also incorporate a range of treatments provided in the community such as health visiting and district nursing. There are a wide range of community care services that patients may be entitled to, including a place in a care home, home care services, home helps, adaptations to the home, meals, and recreational and occupational activities.

The NHS plays an important role in providing community care services to meet the needs of the elderly, those with disabilities, the mentally ill and other frail or vulnerable members of society. Social service departments of local councils take the lead role for community care and the NHS is responsible for working with them to ensure the effective planning and delivery of community care services. This involves contributing to the assessment of people's needs for community care, liaising over hospital discharge for those requiring continuing support, as well as delivering services.

Since the introduction of community care reforms in 1993, the lead responsibility for community care has rested with social service departments. Working closely with the NHS, housing authorities and other agencies, they are responsible for planning, co-ordinating and assessing individual need for community care services. Care trusts (see above, p. 8) have been introduced in some areas across the country and are expected to develop further in the future.

The NHS makes an important contribution to meeting needs for community care. For instance, district nurses provide 2.3 million episodes of care annually, and over 1 million chiropody sessions are carried out in the home. Recent guidance has confirmed and clarified the NHS's responsibilities for meeting continuing healthcare needs and all health authorities have been required to publish local policies and eligibility criteria for continuing healthcare, giving details of local services.

There is an English Community Care Association (ECCA), the representative body for community care in England, working on behalf of the providers.

Shared care

According to the Cochrane Centre, shared care has been used in the management of many chronic conditions with the assumption that it delivers better care than either primary or specialty care alone. It has been defined as the joint participation of primary care physicians and specialty care physicians in the planned delivery of care, informed by an enhanced information exchange over and above routine discharge and referral notices. It has the potential to offer improved quality and co-ordination of care delivery across the primary–specialty care interface and to improve outcomes for patients. Reviews suggest that there is, at present, insufficient evidence to demonstrate significant benefits from shared care apart from improved prescribing. It is not within the remit of this book to discuss this further; however, I refer you to www.cochrane. org/reviews/en/ab004910.html for further reading.

While shared care is a popular term, few formal definitions exist. Of the over 50 articles consulted to establish a definition, three distinct definitions of shared care have developed.

One is a rather broad definition where shared care is an approach that uses the skills and knowledge of a range of health professionals who share joint responsibility in relation to a patient. This involves monitoring and exchanging patient data and sharing skills and knowledge between disciplines.

Another narrower approach focuses on GPs and consultants where care is jointly run by GP and specialist in care of patients with chronic conditions. There is more information exchange than just the routine discharge and referral letters.

Lastly, there is a definition from the mental health arena, a leading advocate in the development and implementation of shared care models, where there is more of an operational co-operation at local levels between different groups of clinicians.

Whatever definition you care to choose here are a few examples of shared care in practice.

Shared care in primary care:
○ GP, nurse specialist, practice nurse
○ GP, nurse specialist and a multidisciplinary team
○ mental health worker, GP and community agency/agencies
○ GP, obstetrician and midwife.

Shared care in secondary care:
○ specialist team and GP
○ hospital and specialist clinic
○ nurses in hospital where mental health and general care ward cases are jointly managed.

Shared care in the community:
○ nurse and family
○ between agencies
○ home and hospice.

So shared care is not about a relationship between one doctor and one patient. Rather, it is about multiple relationships to treat a disease or condition, involving contributions from the patient and a range of healthcare providers. The objective of healthcare is to achieve a satisfactory clinical outcome within available resources. Increasingly, healthcare professionals work as teams. Surgical and medical teams have different needs, the latter in particular may not only be multidisciplinary but also distributed between primary and secondary healthcare. Conditions that are relatively common and susceptible to timely appropriate interventions are often managed by fragmented and uncoordinated services. Such conditions tend to require primary care services, specialised secondary care services and, sometimes, highly specialised secondary care; a few require highly specialised tertiary care.

Integrated care

Integrated care has become an international healthcare buzzword and has many meanings, often used by different people to mean different things. It is most frequently equated with shared care in the UK, managed care in the US, transmural care in the Netherlands, and has other widely recognised formulations such as comprehensive care and disease management.

According to the DoH, 'integrated care is when health and social care services work together to ensure individuals get the right treatment and care they need for their health concerns'. In 2009 the DoH announced 16 Integrated Care Pilots (ICP) as part of a two-year programme, 'transforming the way people experience health and social care'. You can read all about this at www.dh.gov.uk/en/Healthcare/IntegratedCare/DH_290.

However, it is not always clear what integrated care is. Integration stems from the Latin verb *integer*, to complete, so its use is to express the bringing together of various components. Comprehensiveness overlaps with that of integration, comprehensive denoting full understanding.

In the 1970s and 80s some doctors were interested in applying systems theory to their work, reflecting a concern that rapid trends of specialisation could end up fragmenting patient care. The rise of general or family practice at the end of the 20th century grew out of the idea that medicine needs more integration. Hence calls for GPs to take a comprehensive, person-centred approach, including exercising responsibility for the co-ordination of care.

Managers were also interested in healthcare integration because policy-makers, politicians and payers in both the public and private sectors placed hope on its ability to save money or, at the very least, to ensure that healthcare resources are used more effectively. Even the WHO saw virtue in its ability to encourage a more holistic and personalised approach to multidimensional health needs.

Primary care trusts and health authorities have a responsibility for ensuring that patients within the area have a service that meets their needs. A major challenge is commissioning for a service that is met by a variety of providers in primary care, in the community, in local trusts and some in more distant regional centres. Developments in the provision of diabetic services provide a useful example of emerging approaches that include:

○ diabetes centre representatives (medical, nursing and relevant professions allied to medicine)
○ primary care representatives (medical and nursing)
○ community representatives (medical, nursing and relevant professions allied to medicine)
○ director of public health or manager
○ patient representatives
○ specialist representatives as required.

Integrated care is a logical way to approach the management of chronic diseases and models vary according to local needs and cultures.

Providers, trusts and the independent sector

Finally, I come to provider organisations.

Primary care providers

Primary care describes community-based health services that are usually the first, and often the only, point of contact that patients make with the health service. The main providers of primary care are general practitioners, dentists, opticians, pharmacists, NHS walk-in centres, NHS Direct and care trusts. They also include community and practice nurses, health visitors, district nurses, community therapists (such as physiotherapists and occupational therapists), community pharmacists, opticians, optometrists, dentists, midwives and speech therapists.

These primary care services can be accessed through a number of different ways.

○ General practitioners work with nurses and other staff to treat patients and also give health education and advice, run clinics, give vaccinations and carry out simple surgical operations. Every UK citizen has a right to register with a local doctor's surgery, and visits to surgeries are free.
○ Dentists provide check-ups, carry out treatments, and play a key role in improving dental health. Dental practices can take private and NHS patients.
○ Ophthalmic medical practitioners and optometrists provide eye services. This includes treating diseases and abnormalities of the eyes, providing eye tests and dispensing prescription glasses.
○ Pharmacists are responsible for supplying medicines for patients and the public either through a doctor's prescription or through general sale, usually from high street chemists.
○ NHS walk-in centres throughout England offer fast and free access to health advice and treatment at convenient times and locations. Their services include treatment for minor illnesses and injuries, assessment by an experienced NHS nurse, advice on how to stay healthy and information on local health services.
○ NHS minor injury units also offer treatments on a range of minor injuries and illnesses.
○ NHS Direct is a telephone line, staffed by nurses, which provides fast and free

24-hour healthcare advice, ranging from advice and support on self-treatment to details about appropriate further services.
o Care trusts combine the provision of health and social care services for different client groups through better integration. By combining both NHS and local authority health responsibilities under a single management, care trusts can increase continuity of care and simplify the administrative process.

General practice

These were and still are the main primary care providers but independent sector healthcare providers are increasingly adding to them with services from independent primary care providers in pharmacy chains, and the independent healthcare sector. Private general practice providers are winning NHS contracts to run general practices under the Alternative Provider Medical Services (APMS) contracts and are looking at the polyclinics being set up as part of Lord Darzi's review of the NHS (see below).

Polyclinics

Because they were created as an outcome of the Darzi Report, they were sometimes referred to as Darzi Centres. Originally conceived as a solution in London, they have since been more widely adopted in larger towns around England. The Darzi Report suggests a network of polyclinics, each a sort of combination of a super-sized health centre, a minor injuries unit and a small-scale outpatients department as a base for community health services. The Darzi Report did not explain the details on whether they would be run with an overall management employing staff including salaried GPs, or whether they would just operate as gigantic health centres, drawing together a large number of local GP practices under a common roof, with shared support services, which might destabilise and fragment existing GP and hospital services.

The started aims were to:
o create larger groupings of primary care professionals
o exploit economies of scale
o reduce need for patients to travel to a hospital
o integrate services
o create space for other services.

In London the proposed services in a polyclinic would include:
o general practice services
o most outpatient appointments (including antenatal and postnatal care)
o urgent care
o interactive health information services, including healthy living classes
o pharmacy
o community services
o minor procedures
o diagnostics – pathology and radiology
o proactive management of long-term conditions
o other health professionals, e.g. opticians or dentists.

Other towns then suggested adding additional services, such as:
o citizens' advice, benefits, housing etc.
o dialysis
o chemotherapy
o teaching and training
o social care
o leisure and fitness services
o cognitive behaviour therapy (CBT) and other mental health services
o patient and social groups.

Some see the polyclinic as an attempt to switch care away from hospital A&E departments as in minor injury units of the 1990s, often as a transitional step towards closing a full-scale A&E. The report seemed to propose that each polyclinic should offer supporting services including minor procedures, urgent care and diagnostics including pathology and radiology. The scale and complexity of the buildings required, with integrated X-ray and other diagnostic facilities, meant substantial capital costs. This raised questions about the sense in switching a range of outpatient clinics from their established and relatively well-resourced base in hospitals to polyclinics serving much smaller numbers.

As far as funding was concerned, each polyclinic would employ an average of around 90 medical and nursing staff, including 35 GPs and three or four consultants, be located in rented accommodation, and run on a budget of around £21 million a year. In London alone 150 polyclinics would need to enlist a total of over 5200 GPs to full-time work. There would in addition be a need for managers, experienced and qualified secretarial and clerical staff and funds for IT services.

Professor Darzi argues that 'The days of the district general hospital seeking to provide all services to a high enough standard are over' with polyclinics expected to deliver standards of treatments that until now have been provided by specialist surgical staff in hospital.

For more information se the booklet *Ideas from Darzi: polyclinics published by the NHS Confederation*, available at www.nhsconfed.org/Publications/Documents/Ideas%20from%20Darzi%20Polyclinics.pdf.

Walk-in centres (WiCs)

NHS walk-in centres, which first opened in 2000, offer access to a range of NHS services. They are managed by PCTs and there are around 93 NHS WiCs in England, dealing with minor illnesses and injuries, which they state includes:
o infection and rashes
o fractures and lacerations
o emergency contraception and advice
o stomach upsets
o cuts and bruises
o burns and strains.

WiCs are predominantly nurse-led first-contact services available to everyone, without making an appointment or requiring patients to register. Most centres are open 365 days a year and are situated in convenient locations that give patients access to services even beyond regular office hours, although some offer different opening hours during their first few months.

NHS WiCs treat around 3 million patients a year and have proved to be a successful complementary service to traditional GP and A&E services. Some NHS WiCs offer access to doctors as well as nurses. However, they are not designed for treating long-term conditions or immediately life-threatening problems. For more information go to www.nhs.uk/NHSEngland/AboutNHSservices/Emergencyandurgentcareservices/pages/Walk-incentresSummary.aspx.

Minor injuries units

There are currently 225 minor injuries units available in England offering treatments on a range of minor injuries and illnesses. MIUs are predominately nurse-led services and an appointment is not necessary. They state they can treat:

o sprains and strains
o broken bones
o wound infections
o minor burns and scalds
o minor head injuries
o insect and animal bites
o minor eye injuries
o injuries to back, shoulder and chest.

Secondary care providers

Secondary care is made up of NHS, foundation, ambulance, children's, mental health trusts and independent sector treatment centres.

o Most secondary care is provided by hospitals operating as trusts.
o Around 375 trusts manage more than 98% of all NHS hospitals and community health services.
o There are around 280 major district general hospitals in England. NHS hospitals provide acute and specialist services, treating conditions which normally cannot be dealt with by primary care specialists or which are brought in as an emergency. This covers medical treatment or surgery that patients receive in hospital following a referral from a GP.
o Independent sector treatment centres are free-standing surgical units delivering mainly elective surgical procedures which require only a very limited stay in hospital (cataracts, hip replacements, ENT etc.). They are a key part of the government's 10-year strategy for tackling waiting lists, increasing capacity in the NHS, and giving patients more choice in where they are to be treated.

Secondary care organisations seek to provide a comprehensive service and to meet the needs of patients and their GPs. At tertiary level, services focus on providing specialised service for which they alone may have the skills. Some specialist services are provided at regional and supra-regional or national level because of their complexity, cost or level of incidence.

Hospital trusts

Hospital trusts (some also known as acute trusts) run hospitals throughout England and work in partnership with the voluntary and private sector, PCTs and social care to deliver services. They are funded through the payment by results system, which offers financial rewards to trusts that continuously provide efficient and diverse services for their patients. NHS trusts provide most secondary care and specialist services in hospitals. Half of all patients treated in hospitals are emergency cases. The remainder are admissions planned either as day cases or as requiring an overnight stay.

Acute trusts employ a large part of the NHS workforce, including nurses, doctors, pharmacists, midwives and health visitors, as well as professions related to medicine – physiotherapists, radiographers, podiatrists, speech and language therapists, counsellors, occupational therapists, psychologists and healthcare scientists. There are many other non-medical staff employed by acute trusts, including receptionists, porters, cleaners, specialists in information technology, managers, engineers, caterers and domestic and security staff.

Some acute trusts are regional or national centres for more specialised care. Others are attached to universities and help to train health professionals. Acute trusts can also provide services in the community; for example, through health centres, clinics or in people's homes.

Trusts were directly accountable to the Secretary of State via the regional offices of the NHS Executive, but that was wound up in 2001 and each trust is now responsible to the local strategic health authority that monitors its performance.

NHS hospital, mental health and ambulance services are generally provided by trusts. They are managed as separate organisations and are run by a board, which includes a chief executive, a chair and non-executive directors. Non-executive directors are often people with experience of the business, public or voluntary sector who usually come from the local area.

NHS foundation trusts

NHS foundation trusts are in effect not-for-profit, public benefit corporations. They are part of the NHS and provide over half of all NHS hospital and mental health services. Often referred to as 'foundation hospitals', they were an attempt to decentralise the NHS and provide a patient-led service. They were created to devolve decision making from central government control to local organisations and communities so they are more responsive to the needs and wishes of their local people. As of May 2009 there were 120 NHS foundation trusts in operation across England, 36 of which are mental health trusts. Half of all eligible acute and mental health trusts have now achieved NHS foundation trust status. They are mainly made up of acute hospital trusts, with a few mental health trusts. The introduction of NHS foundation trusts represents a profound change in the history of the NHS and the way in which hospital services are managed and provided.

The document *A Short Guide to NHS Foundation Trusts* (2005) provides information and key points about them. They are still part of the NHS and subject to NHS standards, performance ratings and systems of inspection, and provide NHS care to NHS patients according to NHS quality standards and principles. However, NHS foundation trusts are different from existing NHS trusts in the following ways.

○ They are independent legal entities – public benefit corporations.
○ They have unique governance arrangements and are accountable to local people, who can become members and governors. Each NHS foundation trust has a duty to consult and involve a board of governors (comprising patients, staff, members of the public and partner organisations) in the strategic planning of the organisation.
○ They are set free from central government control and are no longer performance managed by health authorities. As self-standing, self-governing organisations, NHS foundation trusts are free to determine their own future.
○ They have new financial freedoms and can raise capital from both the public and private sectors within borrowing limits determined by projected cash flows and therefore based on affordability. They can retain financial surpluses to invest in the delivery of new NHS services.
○ Monitor oversees them (see earlier in this chapter, p. 25).

Care trusts

Care trusts are organisations that work in both health and social care. They may carry out a range of services, including social care, mental health services or primary care services. Care trusts are set up when NHS and local authorities agree to work closely together, usually where it is felt that a closer relationship between health and social care is needed or would benefit local care services. They were first introduced in 2002, hoping to increase continuity of care and simplify administration. At the moment there is only a small number of care trusts, mainly in England. Care trusts do not exist in Scotland, nor are there plans to introduce them.

A mixture of local councillors, health managers and patient and user representatives governs them. The first such trusts were created in Bradford, Camden and Islington, Manchester and Northumberland and later Witham, Braintree and Halstead. They can cover a local authority area, an area of more than one authority, an area covering a population which it registers or they can offer health services but not local authority services.

Mental health trusts

Mental health services can be provided through a GP, other primary care services, or through more specialist care. This includes counselling and other psychological therapies, community and family support, or general health screening. For example, people suffering bereavement, depression, stress or anxiety can get help from primary care or informal community support. If they need more involved support, they may be referred for specialist care. Specialist care is usually provided by mental health trusts or local council social services departments. Services range from psychological therapy to specialised medical and training services for people with severe mental health problems.

About two in every thousand people need specialist care for conditions such as severe anxiety problems or psychotic illness.

There are over 60 specialist mental health trusts in England. Many larger primary care trusts also provide similar mental health services to the specialist mental health trusts. The trusts work closely with local authorities and voluntary organisations to provide both short- and long-term care.

One in four people will be directly affected by a mental health problem during their lifetime. A GP can refer patients to the services provided by mental health trusts. The services that are offered vary between the different trusts, but may include those listed below.

- Counselling sessions – either on a one-to-one basis, or as part of a group.
- Courses – such as how to deal with stress, anger management, and coping with bereavement.
- Resources – such as leaflets and books about a variety of mental health issues.
- Psychotherapy – treatment that involves talking to a therapist to help identify feelings and to devise strategies for coping with problems.
- Family support – providing support to the family, friends and carers of those with a mental health problem.
- Community drug and alcohol clinics – helping people to cope with addiction.
- Community mental health houses – after a stay in hospital, these staffed houses can help patients readjust to living in the community.
- Day hospitals and drop-in centres – where people can receive informal, short-term treatment.
- For more serious mental health problems admission to hospital to receive more intensive care and treatment. On leaving hospital, mental health trusts also help with rehabilitation.

More information about Mental Health Trusts can be obtained at www.nhs.uk/service directories/Pages/MentalHealthTrustListing.aspx.

Independent sector treatment centres

ISTCs are units which provide fast, pre-booked day/short-stay surgery and diagnostic procedures in specialties which have traditionally had the longest waiting times, such as ophthalmology, orthopaedics and general surgery. These centres provide high-volume elective activity for NHS patients for a range of conditions such as hip and knee replacements, hernia repair and gallbladder and cataract removal.

This policy of commercialisation, known in England as the ISTC programme, began in 2000. The DoH has had an explicit policy of using NHS funds to contract out some elective surgery and associated clinical services to the private for-profit sector. These companies include such names as BMI Healthcare (as joint venture of equity firm Apax and South Africa's Netcare), Alliance Medical (private equity firm Bridgepoint), Atos Origin, Birkdale Clinic, Capio, Clinicentre, Interhealth Care Services, Mercury Health, Nations Healthcare Group, Netcare HealthcareUK, Partnership Healthcare Group, CareUK, UKSH, Circle, Nuffield Hospitals, Ramsey

Healthcare UK and Spire Healthcare. Some people regard them as the road to back-door privatisation. A Labour Government has actively promoted ISTCs, though many feel they have not been a success. Because of that lack of success and also probably because of embarrassment, the government has clothed the whole ISTC operation in secrecy.

The government promoted ISTCs on the premise that if there is a waiting list for, say, cataract surgery and the NHS does not have the capacity to do the necessary operations within a reasonable timescale, let private providers to do the work. A problem was that private providers said they would only set up shop if the government guaranteed them a good income even if there was no work to be done and the government agreed, plus there are other issues such as quality control and the deskilling of NHS trainee surgeons who were deprived of work experience. There were other problems too as some of the ISTCs were set up in areas where they were not needed and yet they had to be paid. According to an article in the *BMJ* by Pollock and Kirkwood (2009), in England up to £927 million was paid to ISTCs for patients who did not receive treatment.

The House of Commons reported on ISTCs three years ago and concluded:

ISTCs have not made a major direct contribution to increasing capacity, as the Department of Health has admitted. It is far from obvious that the capacity provided by the ISTCs was needed in all the areas where Phase 1 ISTCs have been built, despite claims by the Department that capacity needs were assessed locally . . . We are concerned that the Department has attempted to misrepresent the situation.

Under Freedom on Information legislation Professor Allyson Pollock, Director of the Centre for International Public Health Policy, University of Edinburgh, has been reported as saying that on the subject of the proper and productive use of public money, an indispensable element of any modern, well-managed and fully accountable democratic state, the evaluation and monitoring of a contract between the public and the private sector should be relatively straightforward – payment given for services rendered – but analysis has raised four main issues, which are supported by other commentators:

o lack of access to data
o incompleteness of data
o the contract may depart radically from normal reporting and costing
o the government's failure to release the value for money methodology means that claims often have no basis in evidence.

The government then appointed Labour peer and surgeon Lord Ara Darzi, who has published an interim review that many felt suggested a return to pre-1940s thinking and the launch of US-style healthcare – deserts of poor quality or no healthcare for the many millions (primary care polyclinics) and a few little islands of excellence for the lucky few. He signalled that Labour will continue to dismantle and privatise the NHS delivery system, its staff and services – handing taxpayers' funds to healthcare companies, and remodelling the service along the lines of US healthcare. It was all a far cry from their 1997 manifesto pledge: 'Our fundamental purpose is simple but hugely important: to restore the NHS as a public service working co-operatively for patients not a commercial business driven by competition.'

Markets do introduce new costs that do not occur in integrated public services: billing, invoicing, marketing and profits. All these divert resources and funds away from the service, creating enormous inefficiency.

For a review of ISTCs, see Pollock and Kirkwood (2009) or Pollock (2008).

For completeness it is worth mentioning two other care trusts classified by the DH as delivering secondary care.

Ambulance trusts

There are currently 12 ambulance services covering England, providing emergency access to healthcare. When a call is made for an emergency ambulance the calls are prioritised into:

○ Category A emergencies, which are immediately life-threatening, or
○ Category B or C emergencies, which are not life-threatening.

The emergency control room decides what kind of response is needed and whether an ambulance is required. For all three types of emergency, they may send a rapid-response vehicle, crewed by a paramedic and equipped to provide treatment at the scene of an incident.

The ambulance service responds to almost 5 million 999 calls a year and over the past five years the number of ambulance 999 calls has gone up by a third.

The NHS is also responsible for providing transport to get many patients to hospital for treatment. In many areas it is the ambulance trust that provides this service.

Children's trusts

In the 2004 Green Paper *Every Child Matters* the government launched the idea that key children's services (health, education and social services) could be integrated into a single organisation known as a children's trust, run by the local government, and a number of children's hospitals are now designated as such. They are accountable through local inter-agency arrangements and provide multi-agency services for children.

Later in 2008 the government published *Children's Trusts: statutory guidance on inter-agency cooperation to improve well-being of children, young people and their families,* which can be downloaded from a link at www.library.nhs.uk/CHILDHEALTH/ViewResource.aspx?resID=299833. This states the purpose of a children's trust as 'to improve the well-being of all children: improving their prospects for the future and redressing inequalities between the most disadvantaged children and their peers'.

NHS trust boards

As outlined above NHS trusts providing hospital or community health services may be a single hospital, a group of hospitals or may provide community health services to patients in clinics or their own homes, and some specialist trusts are responsible for ambulance services. Whatever their configuration the NHS requires NHS trusts, primary care trusts, strategic health authorities and NHS foundation trusts to have a board of directors that is expected to:

○ provide leadership
○ make decisions about healthcare services
○ ensure that staff, facilities and finances are managed properly
○ work as a team
○ take responsibility if things go wrong, as well as when they go well
○ plan for the future so that services improve.

A good board keeps a strategic overview of the organisation and provides a framework in which managers and clinical staff can work effectively.

Each trust has certain powers to organise its own affairs and it is the responsibility of the trust board to plan and direct the way it works. The trust board consists of:

○ a non-executive chair (appointed by the Appointments Commission)
○ normally, five non-executive directors (appointed by the Appointments Commission)
○ up to five executive members, including the chief executive, finance director and medical director recruited by open advertisement.

The trusts are not trusts in the legal sense but are in effect public sector corporations. Each trust receives most of its income through service agreements with PCTs that specify the types of treatment and services that the trust will provide. An NHS trust provides services on behalf of the NHS in England. All trust boards are required to have an audit committee consisting only of non-executive directors, on which the chair may not sit. This committee is entrusted not only with supervision of financial audit, but of systems of corporate governance within the trust.

Foundation trust boards

Foundation trusts provide hospital and community health services as part of the NHS in the same way as NHS trusts. Again they may be a single hospital, a group of hospitals or may provide community health services to patients in clinics or their own homes. But foundation trusts have more freedom than NHS trusts to manage their finances and decide how best to improve the services they provide to their patients.

They are controlled and run locally and, provided that they meet national standards, there is no intervention by the DoH. The first NHS foundation trusts were established in April 2004 and the government committed to all NHS trusts being given the opportunity to apply for foundation status at the earliest opportunity.

Foundation trusts have a board of governors who are elected from the local population, patients and staff to direct the work of the trust. They in turn appoint a chair and non-executives to a management board. This board has a similar composition of executive and non-executive members to an NHS trust board and directs the day-to-day activities of the trust.

Chairs of NHS trusts

A trust chair must have the same qualities as a non-executive director and, in addition, be able to demonstrate leadership and motivation skills, the ability to think strategically and the ability to understand complex issues. Management experience at a senior level in the public, private or voluntary sectors is seen as a desirable attribute.

Chairs and non-executive directors can speak in public on matters affecting the work of the NHS trust, but should not normally make political speeches or engage in other political activities. In cases of doubt the guidance of the Appointments Commission should be sought.

In order to avoid possible conflict of interest all NHS boards are required to adopt the Codes of Conduct and Accountability published in April 1994. The Codes require chairs and board members to declare on appointment any business interests, position of authority in a charity or voluntary body in the field of health and social care, and any connection with bodies contracting for NHS services. These must be entered into a register that is available to the public.

The NHS trust is empowered to indemnify board members against personal liability they may incur in certain circumstances while carrying out their duties.

Remuneration: Current rates for a chair's remuneration is payable in one of three bands linked to the turnover of the trust. Information about the rate payable to individual trust chairs is available locally.

○ Band 1: £23 020
○ Band 2: £20 587
○ Band 3: £18 164

Tax and National Insurance-Remuneration is taxable under Schedule E, and subject to Class I National Insurance contributions.

Allowances are permitted for both chairs and non-executive directors who are eligible to claim allowances, at rates set centrally, for travel and subsistence costs necessarily incurred on NHS care trust business. Non-executive members of NHS trust, primary care trust and strategic health authority boards are also able to reclaim expenses related to childcare responsibilities when they would not otherwise be able to undertake responsibilities incurred as a result of their board membership. However, members of DoH national bodies are able to claim for all actual carer expenses (i.e. for children or elderly or infirm relatives) incurred while absent from home on board business. The Secretary of State decided to extend the current provisions for members of NHS bodies so that they are consistent with those for members of DoH national bodies and relate to all necessary carer expenses incurred as a result of their work as a chair or non-executive.

There may be some time commitment during the working day or in the evening according to the requirements of the NHS trust but the time commitment expected of chairs is three to three and a half days per week.

There is a NED Works website for non-executive directors and chairs of NHS trusts, PCTs and arm's length public bodies at www.nedworks.net, but unless you are one you cannot access it.

Non-executive directors in the NHS

NHS boards take corporate responsibility for the strategies and actions of their organisations. The chair and non-executives are laypeople drawn from the community served by the trust or health authority. They are accountable to the local strategic health authority. They are expected to hold the executive to account and to use their skills and experience to help the board as it develops health strategies, and ensure the delivery of high-quality services to patients. These laypeople are also expected to draw from their experience in the local communities to make sure that the interests of patients remain paramount.

In practice, boards look for a balance of skills and experience from their non-executives. For example, some might have professional expertise, in accountancy or business management, which will supplement that of the executives, while others may have experience as a carer or user of the NHS, which may help the board focus its discussions on patient services. It is a particularly important part of any appointments process to ensure that this balance of skills is maintained.

The current rate of remuneration payable to non-executive directors is £6005 pa and they are normally expected to devote two and a half days a month to their responsibilities. A non-executive director who is also the Audit Committee Chair would need to spend additional time on these duties.

NHS Appointments Commission

The NHS Appointments Commission makes all non-executive directors' appointments. The interview panel consists of three people, including the chair of the organisation and an independent assessor. Selection criteria include the requirement to live or work locally, an interest in healthcare, community commitment, board level contribution, communication skills, strategic thinking and an understanding of public service values. Non-executive directors are appointed for an initial period of four years, renewable subject to satisfactory appraisal, and subscribe to the Codes of Conduct and Accountability for NHS boards.

The person specification drawn up for selection usually includes the following essential qualities:

o   live in the area served by the trust
o   have a strong personal commitment to the NHS
o   demonstrate a commitment to the needs of the local community
o   be a good communicator with plenty of common sense
o   be committed to the public service values of accountability, probity, openness and equality of opportunity
o   demonstrate ability to contribute to the work of the board
o   be available for about three days per month
o   demonstrate an interest in healthcare issues.

It is also regarded as desirable that they:
o   have experience as a carer or user of the NHS
o   have experience of serving in the voluntary sector

○ have served the local community in local government or some other capacity
○ understand or have experience of management in the public, private or voluntary sectors
○ offer specialist skills or knowledge relevant to the work of the trust.

Applications are encouraged from all sections of the community, particularly women, people from ethnic minorities and people with disabilities. Political activity should not be a consideration in selection.

Non-executive directors work with four or five other non-executives and the senior trust managers, including the medical director, as equal members of the trust board. They are expected to use their personal skills and experience of the community and the NHS to guide the trust in the following areas:
○ developing long-term plans for healthcare in the local community
○ best use of its financial resources to help patients
○ appointment of chief executive and other senior managers
○ various committees such as the: Remuneration Committee to ensure fair pay for trust executives; Audit Committee to ensure proper financial procedures; Committees to review professional conduct and staff discipline matters
○ ensuring the trust meets its commitment to the 'Standards for Better Health' and other targets
○ contributing to the relationship between the trust and the local community and media by representing the board at official occasions
○ overseeing the trust's response to complaints from the public
○ being involved in hearing appeals by patients detained under the Mental Health Act.

Clinical directorates or care divisions

A trust's management team is responsible for the operational management and the development of policy within the trust. The management team is made up of the executive directors and the clinical directors of the trust. Clinical directors, (sometimes called clinical services directors, associate directors, etc.) are usually consultant medical staff, although sometimes they may be a non-medical clinical professional. They are normally accountable to the chief executive or director of operations for the management of patient care and treatment involving clinical staff in the development and management of services. They may share leadership with an operations manager and a lead nurse.

The key elements of the clinical director's role fall under the day-to-day general management headings, and include:
○ responsibility for the directorate budget, personnel and staffing
○ clinical services including clinical audit and management
○ budget management and control
○ business and strategic planning
○ services planning, service development, strategic development, staff development, business development and clinical development of the trust.

There are usually several clinical directorates or care divisions within each trust, working alongside others to provide the services required. The number of clinical directorates and their size vary enormously from one hospital to another.

Issues for clinical directorates include the development of future patterns of service, medical staffing issues, coping with pressures (particularly in emergency admissions), reorganisations, transfers, mergers, rationalisation and waiting lists.

Clinical directors

Medicine is one of the oldest professions, with its origins dating back to ancient times. Current management strategies are a relatively new feature of the NHS, and have evolved and increased in importance quite dramatically over the last 30 years. Although doctors previously had a role in management, the creation of the clinical director post has formalised these arrangements. A Google search for 'clinical director' came up with 166 000 000 entries in just 0.36 seconds, but despite the enormous amount that has been written about this role many doctors undertaking the role believe they are poorly prepared. Clinical directors' roles and duties of course differ between organisations of different size and with different management structures, but there are issues, such as key competences, training and support, which should be relevant to all such posts.

Other topics and notes on recently published plans and reforms

A leading article in *The Times* from 26 June 2009 stated: 'The shelves of Whitehall groan under the weight of policy reviews discarded and plans never enacted.' Indeed there's something a little sad about looking back at the wreckage of grand plans. They all sounded so good at the time, all examples of what people call 'motherhood and apple pie' ideas. They seemingly all had full stakeholders' support, and user and participant buy in. Even *The Lancet* and *BMJ* usually supported the plans. And a new government had often just been elected. So this section provides a quick review in case you are asked about them at an interview. Your answer should probably be tailored to suit the questioner, but perhaps the following might help you.

The problem with the NHS, says Alan Maynard, is that it scores eight out of 10 for bright ideas and four out of 10 for implementation. One of the main reasons for its poor implementation is the constant stream of new ideas, followed quickly by a deluge of strategies. There is a feeling that there is no need to bother implementing idea A because ideas B, C and D will be along shortly, when A will be completely forgotten (or perhaps introduced as idea F some time later).

I have, within the constraints of the size of this book, been limited to considering only those papers published for the NHS in England and for that only the major ones of the last decade. The devolved parts of the NHS have published similar plans and some of these where relevant and useful to the context of highlighting differences have been mentioned elsewhere in the book when describing these services.

The NHS Plan: a plan for investment, a plan for reform (2000)

The document published by The Stationery Office in July 2000 set out how increased funding and reform aimed to redress geographical inequalities, improve service standards, and extend patient choice. We are currently still embarked on this 10-year plan but you can read it in full at www.dh.gov.uk/en/Publicationsandstatistics/ Publications/PublicationsPolicyAndGuidance/DH_4002960 and make your judgement; if critical then you'll find an interesting view at www.drrant.net/2009/04/ nhs-plan-ten-years-on.html. As a matter of interest, at the time of writing the Commons All Party Parliamentary Group on Primary Care and Public Health is running an inquiry with the title 'Was the NHS Plan really a blueprint for the NHS – 10 years on?'

Shifting the Balance of Power: the next steps (2002)

In the last edition I talked about *Shifting the Balance of Power*, the name for the programme of changes that were reforming the way the NHS works. The aim was to design a service centred on patients and put them first. It also aimed to be faster, more convenient and offer patients more choice. The main feature of the change was to give local PCTs the role of running the NHS and improving health in their areas. This also meant creating new strategic health authorities that cover larger areas and have a more strategic role. You can still read about this at www.dh.gov.uk/PublicationsAndStatistics/ Publications/PublicationsPolicyAndGuidance/DH_4008424.

The proclaimed aim of New Labour's health policy was to shift the balance of power and responsibility for services to the local level, but it is almost impossible nearly a decade after its publication to find anything written to clarify what, relevant to that document, has occurred. Certainly, there have been lots of changes, more funding and improvements, but some felt that while the government proclaimed a new decentralised NHS, doubts existed about the extent to which the reality matched the tone of policy. On the positive side, 10 years ago patients would sometimes wait over a year for treatment, and now they wait just a few weeks – and even less if cancer is suspected. Surgical patients are treated using endoscopic techniques, enabling them to leave hospital in days rather than weeks. There are more multidisciplinary approaches, meetings, clinics and changes that have meant real improvements for patients. The NHS seems to be making better achievements enabled by extra resources, by giving freedom to the frontline through foundation trusts, and by ensuring that increased funding followed patient choice. However, it is for the reader to decide how much was delivered by the dedication and hard work of NHS staff that were determined to improve services for patients and the public rather than DoH publications.

The NHS Improvement Plan: putting people at the heart of public services (2004)

The NHS Improvement Plan was published in June 2004 and set out the way in which the NHS needed to change in order to become patient-led, moving away from a centrally directed system. Claiming that the previous five years had been about building capacity and capability, it stated that the next would be about improving quality, giving best value for money and using the new capacity and capability to build a truly patient-led service. It is almost impossible to find anything written since it was published that gives a view on the success or otherwise of this plan, so I cannot offer you references and must lead you to make your own judgements on the plan. However, the part referring to the introduction of community matrons is dealt with in more detail next.

Community Matrons

The NHS Improvement Plan (2004), discussed above, described a new clinical role for nurses to be known as community matrons. The case management work of community matrons was central to the government's policy for the management of people with long-term conditions. In 2005, the Chief Nursing Officer set out how nurses would help deliver care to patients with long-term conditions by outlining a blueprint of a new role enabling them to give one-to-one support to patients with long-term conditions. Guidance set out the role of community matrons to:

- develop a personal care plan with the patient, carers, relatives and other health professionals based on a full assessment of their needs
- keep in touch and monitor the condition of the patients regularly, though home visits or telephone calls
- work in partnership with the patient's GP, sharing information and planning together.

In this type of case management, community matrons:

- use data to actively seek out patients who will benefit
- combine high-level assessment of physical, mental and social care needs
- review medication and prescribe medicines via independent and supplementary prescribing arrangements
- provide clinical care and health-promoting interventions
- co-ordinate inputs from all other agencies, ensuring all needs are met
- teach and educate patients and their carers about warning signs of complications or crisis
- provide information so patients and families can make choices about current and future care needs
- be highly visible to patients and their families and carers, and thus seen by them as being in charge of their care
- be seen by colleagues across all agencies as having the key role for patients with very high-intensity needs.

The principle of this particular model of case management is that there is one person who acts as both provider and procurer of care and takes responsibility for ensuring all health and social care needs are met, so that the patient's condition stays as stable as possible and well-being is increased. While community matrons will focus on patients with very intensive needs, other patients with long-term conditions may continue to receive case management from a range of professionals, like physiotherapists and occupational therapists, whose skills best suit their needs.

Children with long-term or life-threatening conditions can have case management from children's community nursing teams working in partnership with paediatric departments, and assertive outreach teams will provide similar care for people with long-term and enduring mental health needs.

Community matrons would thus bring the benefits of case management to a new category of patients hitherto outside its remit, and in so doing, extend the concept of case management to encompass clinical nursing interventions.

Thus case management by community matrons would:

○ help to prevent unnecessary admissions to hospital
○ reduce length of stay of necessary hospital admissions
○ improve outcomes for patients
○ integrate all elements of care
○ improve patients' ability to function and their quality of life
○ help patients and their families plan for the future
○ increase choice for patients
○ enable patients to remain in their homes and communities
○ improve end of life care.

However, a paper in the *British Journal of Community Nursing* as recently as March 2009 (Lillyman 2009) suggests that the community matrons' role in patient care is not distinguished clearly enough from that of other professions, with confusion existing over the titles used by health workers managing patients with long-term conditions. As well as community matrons, others carrying out similar work had a variety of job titles, such as 'case manager'.

The DoH website for 2007 on the subject can be viewed at www.dh.gov.uk/en/Healthcare/Longtermconditions/DH_4134132.

Choose and Book (2004)

Choose and Book is the national electronic referral service provided through NHS Connecting for Health, which gives patients a choice of place, date and time for their first outpatient appointment in a hospital or clinic. It can be accessed at www.chooseandbook.nhs.uk. It has certainly progressed since I last wrote about it as an aspiration.

There you will find a patient welcome page with links to:

○ Choose and Book
○ choose your hospital
○ book or change your appointment.

NHS staff, the media and patients are able to access the site to learn about how it allows patients to choose their hospital or clinic and book an appointment. Since summer 2004, Choose and Book has been introduced across England. Although not all hospitals are fully operational, it will eventually be available to all patients.

When a patient and GP agree the need to see a consultant they will be able to choose from at least four hospitals or clinics. They can also choose the date and time of an appointment. One section of the website provides everything you need to know about Choose and Book, what it means and how to book, change or cancel an appointment.

To choose your hospital a separate page enables a patient to choose where to go for a first consultation by comparing the hospitals. And to book or change an appointment a patient who has been referred and who has an appointment reference number (shown at the top of their appointment letter) and a password (which the GP practice gives them) can book, change or cancel an appointment online or by phone. The Appointment Line (TAL), on 0845 60 88888, is open every day from 7 a.m. to 10 p.m. For a full review of this go to www.chooseandbook.nhs.uk.

White Paper 2006: *Our Health, Our Care, Our Say: a new direction for community services*

This White Paper claimed to set a new direction for the whole health and social care system. It confirmed the vision set out in the DoH Green Paper, *Independence, Well-being and Choice*. There was to be a radical shift in the way services were delivered, ensuring that they were more personalised and fitted into 'people's busy lives'. It promised people a stronger voice so that they were the major drivers of service improvement. You can read the full document at www.dh.gov.uk/en/Publicationsandstatistics/Publications/PublicationsPolicyAndGuidance/DH_4127453. Again, there doesn't seem to be anything much written describing what it achieved, except perhaps to say that it has 'achieved small progress', so you can only review it and draw your own conclusions.

White Paper 2007: *Trust, Assurance and Safety: the regulation of health professionals*

This sets out the programme of reform to the UK's system for the regulation of health professionals, based on consultation on the two reviews of professional regulation published in July 2006: *Good Doctors, Safer Patients* by the Chief Medical Officer (CMO) for England and the DoH's *The Regulation of the Non-Medical Healthcare Professions*. It is complemented by the government's response to the recommendations of the Fifth Report of the Shipman Enquiry and recommendations in the Ayling, Neale and Kerr/Haslam Inquiries, *Safeguarding Patients*, which sets out a range of measures to improve clinical governance in the NHS. Go to www.dh.gov.uk/en/Publicationsandstatistics/Publications/PublicationsPolicyAndGuidance/DH_065946.

The paper provides a working framework for appraisal and assessment, assigning significant roles to the GMC in setting standards for revalidation, and confirms that relicensing will be based on agreed generic standards of practice set by the GMC, a revised system of NHS appraisal for doctors and any concerns known to the doctor's medical director (or responsible officer).

NHS in England: operating framework for 2008/09

This sets out the business and financial arrangement for 2008/09, describing the priorities, targets alongside national priorities, payment by results and tariff details, commissioning policies, and about engaging with staff, patients and public and delivering choice. The 2008/09 year will be the first of a three-year planning cycle, and therefore naturally this operating framework sets out in significantly greater detail our ambitions for the next three years. It also builds upon many of the themes outlined in the interim *Next Stage Review* report.

High Quality Care for All: NHS Next Stage Review final report (2008)

This is the final report of Lord Darzi's *NHS Next Stage Review 2008*. It responds to the 10 SHA strategic visions and sets out a vision for an NHS with quality at its heart. Lord Darzi stated that improvements in patient care would come about if the NHS was clinically led, more patient-centred and had greater accountability at a local level. You can download the full report or a summary from www.dh.gov.uk/en/Publications andstatistics/Publications/PublicationsPolicyAndGuidance/DH_085825. However, because it is the latest of this reviewed series of initiatives I thought it worthy of a little more detail. Essentially, Lord Darzi is stressing the need to move from quantity (i.e. more money, more clinicians, more operations) to quality, which he defines as clinically effective, personal and safe care. There is a perception that the public think it gets high-quality care now, failing to recognise the variations in outcomes around the country and even from ward to ward within a hospital. The public worries about hospital infection, but don't realise they have a more than one in 10 chance of suffering an adverse event when admitted and a one in a 100 chance of dying.

It suggests that the most difficult part of quality is the personal part. Patients may not know that they are getting clinically poor care, but they know whether or not it's personal. However, to be fair the NHS was never originally designed to deliver personal care. It was designed to get people treated, to get them 'dealt with'. Now people want more, but it's not easy to transform such a large organisation.

Darzi believes that quality care cannot be delivered from the centre; it requires the skills of frontline staff. There is an emphasis on incentives and leadership, GPs paid more to deliver the high-quality care, and hospitals rewarded for delivering not just lots of care but high-quality care. Improved quality also depends on leadership from clinicians, particularly doctors. You can't reform the health service if the doctors think your reforms are so much bureaucratic nonsense, which is roughly what they do think.

On information, Darzi hopes that a hospital or clinician seeing itself at the bottom of a league table will be spurred to action. That action might be to dispute the validity of the data. So there is a need to risk adjust, although that is not easy. Fail to adequately risk adjust for the complexity of cases and doctors are reluctant to treat them, or, as has happened in the US, over-adjusting can result in surgeons favouring the most complex cases.

Because of the importance of the report I have 'summarised the summary' but you'll need to go to the report itself for more details. It covers eight chapters within more than 80 pages, available as a pdf file from a link at www.dh.gov.uk/en/Publicationsand statistics/Publications/PublicationsPolicyAndGuidance/DH_085825.

Immediate steps identified by the Review

Immediate steps identified by the Next Stage Review were as follows.

○ Every PCT to commission comprehensive well-being and prevention services.
○ A Coalition for Better Health, with a set of voluntary agreements between govern-ment, private and third-sector organisations on actions to improve health.
○ Raised awareness of vascular risk assessment through a new 'Reduce Your Risk' campaign.
○ Support for people to stay healthy at work.
○ Support GPs to help individuals and their families stay healthy.
○ Extend choice of GP practice.
○ Introduce a new right to choice in the first NHS constitution.
○ Ensure everyone with a long-term condition has a personalised care plan.
○ Pilot personal health budgets.
○ Guarantee patients access to the most clinically and cost effective drugs and treatment.

Review: on quality
○ Getting basics right first time every time.
○ Independent quality standards and clinical priority setting with new National Quality Board and expanded NICE.
○ Systematically measure and publish information about quality of care including patients' views of quality.
○ Make funding for hospitals reflect the quality of care patients receive.
○ For senior doctors the current Clinical Excellence Awards Scheme strengthened and reinforced for quality improvement. For information, go to www.dh.gov.uk/ab/ACCEA/index.htm.
○ Easy access for NHS staff to information about high-quality care.
○ Measures to ensure continuous improvements in quality of primary and community care.
○ New best practice tariffs.
○ Clinicians' involvement in decision making.
○ Medical Directors and Quality Boards at Regional and National level.
○ Strategic plans for visions will be published by every PCT.
○ New Quality Observatory to be established in every region.
○ Introduction of new responsibilities, funds and prizes to support and reward innovation.
○ Ensuring that clinically effective and cost-effective innovation in medicine and medical technologies are adopted.
○ Creating new partnerships between the NHS, universities and industry.

Review: working in partnership with NHS staff
High Quality Care For All – NHS Next Stage Review Final Report. DoH; 2008. Go to www.ournhs.nhs.uk/wp-content/uploads/2008/06/dh-darzi-summary-report.pdf.
Responding to the claim that there is 'change fatigue' in the NHS this Review attempted to make the review primarily local and lead by clinicians and other staff working in the NHS and partner organisations (DoH 2008).

- ○ Enabling NHS staff to lead and manage the organisations in which they work.
- ○ Implementing programme to support development of successful community services.
- ○ Enhancing professionalism.
- ○ New national targets.
- ○ New pledges to staff.
- ○ Improving quality of NHS education and training.
- ○ Threefold increase in nurse and midwife preceptorships, i.e. the newly qualified to learn more from senior colleagues in first year.
- ○ Doubling investment in apprentices.
- ○ Strengthened arrangements to ensure staff have consistent and equitable opportunities to update and develop skills

The First NHS Constitution 2009

The NHS Constitution: securing the NHS today for generations to come was published on 21 January 2009. It was one of a number of recommendations in Lord Darzi's report *High Quality Care for All*, which was published on the sixtieth anniversary of the NHS and set out a 10-year plan to provide the highest quality of care and service for patients in England. The NHS Constitution brings together in one place for the first time in the history of the NHS, what staff, patients and public can expect from the NHS.

The Constitution brings together a number of rights, pledges and responsibilities for staff and patients. These rights and responsibilities were the result of extensive discussions and consultations with staff, patients and public and it reflects what matters to them.

Subject to parliamentary approval, all NHS bodies, and private and third-sector providers supplying NHS services in England will be required by law to take account of the Constitution in their decisions and actions. The government will have a legal duty to renew the Constitution every 10 years. No government will be able to change the Constitution, without the full involvement of staff, patients and the public.

Placing a duty on providers and commissioners of NHS services to have regard to the new NHS Constitution will reinforce the core purpose and values of the NHS. This legal duty is contained within the Health Bill, which was introduced into Parliament on 15 January 2009. The Health Bill also set out the procedure for reviewing and amending the NHS Constitution and handbook.

The handbook to the NHS Constitution gives NHS staff and patients all the information about the NHS Constitution in one place. It acts as a guide to:
- ○ patients' rights and pledges
- ○ responsibilities of patients and the public and staff rights and NHS pledges to its staff.

At the back of the handbook an appendix outlines the legal source for both the patient and staff rights in the NHS Constitution. Available in a dozen languages, the Constitution can be seen at www.dh.gov.uk/en/Healthcare/NHSConstitution/index.htm.

The Constitution commits the government to providing a statement of NHS accountability. This document also provides a summary of the structure and functions of the NHS.

Patient and public empowerment publications 2009

Over the last few years, the NHS has moved towards engaging people in the design and delivery of services. They are routinely asked for their views, about their experience, to contribute to staff training and to be members of NHS trusts. The DoH's Patient and Public Empowerment division tries to provide NHS organisations with the knowledge and expertise to enable them to achieve this goal. A collection of patient and public empowerment publications is available at www.dh.gov.uk/en/Managingyourorganisation/PatientAndPublicinvolvement/DH_293. There is also an NHS Centre for Involvement (NCI) that supports and encourages the NHS and other organisations to involve patients and the public in health and social care decision making; go to www.nhscentreforinvolvement.nhs.uk.

Patient and public involvement (PPI) in NHS

There have been many attempts to involve the public in decisions about the NHS and the following is a summary of a few of the organisations so involved.

The NHS Centre for Involvement

The Centre supports and encourages the NHS and other organisations to involve patients and the public in health and social care decision making. It acts as the core organisation for promoting the involvement agenda and is committed to embedding patient and public involvement into everyday practice within health and social care organisations. You can see more about it at www.nhscentreforinvolvement.nhs.uk.

Involve

Involve is a national advisory group, funded by the National Institute for Health Research (NIHR). Its role is to support and promote active public involvement in NHS, public health and social care research. It believes that involving members of the public leads to research that is more relevant to people's needs and concerns, more reliable and more likely to be used. Go to www.invo.org.uk.

NHS Evidence

This provides a patient and public involvement website (www.evidence.nhs.uk) where there is a specialist collection that aims to support the implementation of patient, user, carer and public involvement in healthcare by providing access, in one location, to the best information which is freely available on the Web. The patient and public involvement specialist collection does not contain patient information on individual medical conditions, but if you are a patient or member of the general public and have an inquiry you can telephone NHS Direct Online on 0845 4647 or visit the NHS Direct website at www.nhsdirect.nhs.uk. For more information go to www.library.nhs.uk/PPI.

Local Involvement Networks (LINks)

LINks replaced PPI Forums, which had been set up following the NHS Reform and Health Care Professions Act 2002. Their abolition was part of the Local Government and Public Involvement in Health Act 2007.

LINks aims to give citizens a stronger voice in how their health and social care services are delivered. The networks are run by local individuals and groups and independently supported. The role of LINks is to find out what people want, monitor local services and to use their powers to hold them to account. LINks were established in most areas by the end of 2008. Each local authority (that provides social services) has been given funding and is under a legal duty to make contractual arrangements that enable LINk activities to take place.

The introduction of LINks was part of a wider process to help a community have a stronger local voice. Its role is to:

o ask local people what they think about local healthcare services
o provide a chance to suggest ideas to help improve services
o investigate specific issues of concern to the community
o use its powers to hold services to account and get results
o ask for information and get an answer in a specified amount of time
o be able to carry out spot-checks to see if services are working well
o make reports and recommendations and receive a response
o refer issues to the local 'Overview and Scrutiny Committee'.

To read more about them go to www.dh.gov.uk/en/Managingyourorganisation/PatientAndPublicinvolvement/DH_076366.

NHS Networks

NHS Networks (www.networks.nhs.uk) is a means of promoting and connecting networks which exist throughout the NHS and encouraging the formation of new ones. They encourage networks to use their website for communication, including discussion forums and submission of news stories. NHS Networks is also developing roles in the areas of accreditation, and helping the DoH with consultations. There are administrative offices in Leicester, and associates working around the country. They have a weekly email newsletter highlighting what is new on their website, including links to initiatives, information about individual networks, and resources within their specialist themes. NHS Networks is governed by a board that holds regular meetings.

Patient Advice and Liaison Service (PALS)

A patient, relative or carer who needs to turn to someone for on-the-spot help, advice or support can access the Patient Advice and Liaison Service. They are also at the time of writing launching a PALS for Children and Young People service. The PALS website is at www.pals.nhs.uk.

They provide a confidential one-stop service, helping patients, relatives or carers to sort out any concerns they have about the care a trust provides. They will guide them through the different services available from the NHS and where necessary steer them towards the complaints process. Most trusts have their own specific website.

There is a separate service in Wales working on patient and public involvement in the NHS in Wales that aims to improve access to information about PPI in Wales. The Welsh Assembly has produced a number of documents to provide information and advice to all NHS bodies in Wales about how to develop public and patient involvement in order to achieve the 10-year vision outlined in *Designed for Life*. All the important publications produced by the Welsh Assembly on PPI are available on this site. They facilitate the sharing of information by local health boards, NHS trusts and other organisations. Fore more information go to www.wales.nhs.uk/sites3/home.cfm?OrgID=420.

National PALS Network (NPN)

The National PALS Network is a membership organisation for PALS staff and volunteers. Membership is also open to organisations and individuals wishing to support and participate in the network.

NPN is a registered charity and a not-for-profit company that brings together the Patient Advice and Liaison Services of the NHS. It aims to ensure that people have ready access to high-quality PALS. Working together, and with the support of others, NPN aims to:

o empower and support colleagues throughout the service to deliver high-quality, accessible and consistent services for patients, carers and the public
o raise the profile of PALS and promote the service effectively
o act as a focal point for stakeholder involvement and a national voice for PALS
o provide leadership and influence policy and public debate.

You can access it through a link on the PALS website (www.pals.nhs.uk).

Healthcare in other parts of the UK

o The NHS in England
o The NHS in Scotland
o The NHS in Wales
o The NHS in Northern Ireland
o NHS Isle of Man
o The Isle of Man Government
o States of Guernsey Government
o States of Jersey Government.

Although funded centrally from national taxation, NHS services in England, Scotland, Wales and Northern Ireland are managed separately.

The NHS in England

The NHS in England is far and away the biggest part of the system, catering to a population of 50 million and employing more than 1.43 million people. Devolution

has had significant implications for the structure and provision of health services across the UK as Wales and Scotland have assumed responsibility for a wide range of services. Westminster has retained UK-wide power only over the following:
○ abortion
○ human fertilisation
○ human genetics
○ xenotransplantation
○ regulation of medicines.

In England, in contrast to the devolved countries, greater freedoms for foundation trusts and local commissioners have shifted power away from the centre in England. Unlike Scotland, Northern Ireland and Wales, the focus of the English service has changed frequently to concentrate on at first standards, then targets and governance, followed by competition and choice, with the focus now being on the patient experience and quality.

It has been suggested by one author that the NHS in England is now about contestability driving improvement and greater choice, while Scotland's system is 'collectivist', with very little competition. The key feature of the system in Northern Ireland meanwhile is greater integration between health and social care, while Wales is widely believed to enjoy a better working relationship between health and local authorities than is commonly the case in much of the UK.

But there is, however, one common thread between the health services in the three devolved countries: a reluctance to comment on how well they think they are doing. Scotland, Wales and Northern Ireland are much smaller countries than England and two are in the middle of reorganisations that may explain the reluctance. Even external observers with a view are difficult to find. Perhaps with the alternatives still evolving, it is too early to say which systems, and which parts of those systems, work best. Perhaps it will only be after time that a judgement can be made.

Other parts of the UK

Although devolution began in 1997 when the newly elected Labour Government produced its promised White Paper on the subject it was not until two years later that the Scottish Parliament and Welsh and Northern Ireland Assemblies assumed control of their NHS, whereupon they were quick to use their new powers to restructure their health systems. In 1999 Scotland, Wales and Northern Ireland assumed new powers and they have now run their own NHS for nearly 10 years. The devolved health systems all have unique features, although there is reluctance to comment on how they compare. The Scottish system has moved away from market-oriented models, and the reorganisations in Northern Ireland and Wales have cut the number of health bodies and both are working more closely with local authorities and social services. Northern Ireland's political situation meant devolution was initially short-lived and then enormously complex, while the government's intention to pursue English devolution was rejected in the North East in 2004.

The NHS in Scotland has a budget of £14 billion and Wales £7 billion. Scotland also has tax varying powers, although Wales has not. Scotland spends 30% more per capita and Wales 15% more than England.

The NHS in Scotland

There have always been differences between the English and Scottish health services. The devolved Government for Scotland (known as the Scottish Executive when it was established in 1999 following the first elections to the Scottish Parliament) is responsible for most of the issues of day-to-day concern including health as well as education, justice, rural affairs and transport. A First Minister who is nominated by the Parliament and who in turn appoints the other Scottish Ministers who make up the Cabinet leads the Scottish Government. Civil servants in Scotland are accountable to Scottish Ministers, who are themselves accountable to the Scottish Parliament.

The Scottish Government Health Directorate is responsible both for NHS in Scotland and for the development and implementation of health and community care policy.

The Chief Executive of NHS Scotland leads the central management of the NHS and is accountable to ministers, and also heads the Health Department, which oversees the work of NHS boards responsible for planning health services for people in their area.

The Scottish Government Health Directorate also has responsibility for the following.

- The Scottish Ambulance Service, which serves all of Scotland and is a Special NHS Board funded directly by the Scottish Government Health Directorate.
- NHS 24, which provides 24-hour telephone access to medical advice from clinical professionals.
- The State Hospital situated at Carstairs, which cares for patients who require treatment under conditions of special security.
- NHS Health Scotland, which promotes positive attitudes to health and encourages healthy lifestyles.
- NHS Quality Improvement Scotland, which sets and monitors clinical standards.
- The department is also responsible for social work policy and in particular for community care and voluntary issues.

In 2006, the NHS in Scotland had around 158 000 staff including more than 47 500 nurses, midwives and health visitors and over 3800 consultants. There are also more than 12 000 doctors, family practitioners and allied health professionals, including dentists, opticians and community pharmacists, who are independent contractors providing a range of services within the NHS in return for various fees and allowances.

Health services are delivered through 14 regional NHS boards. These boards provide strategic leadership and performance management for the entire local NHS system in their areas and ensure that services are delivered effectively and efficiently. NHS boards are responsible for the provision and management of the whole range of health services in an area including hospitals and general practice.

Scotland has in addition a further eight Special Boards, as follows.

o The NHS National Services Scotland (formerly known as the Common Services Agency) provides a number of important specialist services ranging from provision of health statistics through blood transfusion services, national surveillance of communicable diseases, national screening programmes to managing payments for primary care practitioners.

o The Scottish Ambulance Service provides an A&E service that responds to 999 calls as well as a Non-Emergency service that performs an essential role in getting patients to and from health services.

o NHS24 is a telephone health advice and information service that provides 24-hour access to medical advice from clinical professionals.

o The State Hospital is one of four high-security hospitals in the UK – the only one of its kind within Scotland and located at Carstairs.

o NHS Health Scotland provides a national focus for improving health and reducing inequalities in health in Scotland.

o NHS Quality Improvement Scotland is concerned with improving the quality of healthcare in Scotland, working with NHS professionals and the public to produce, put into practice and monitor national standards for care.

o NHS Education for Scotland is the training organisation of NHS Scotland and exists to ensure that the staff of NHS Scotland can continue to develop and enhance their skills to deliver the best standards in patient care.

o National Waiting Times Centre Board (The Golden Jubilee National Hospital) provides a dedicated elective facility in key specialties for patients throughout Scotland to assist in reducing waiting times).

Scotland's centrally controlled NHS has been criticised as not providing value for money. It has been suggested handing the commissioning role to health boards again and making hospitals and other care providers independent of the boards to reintroduce the purchaser–provider split. Immediately after devolution, the Scottish White Paper *Designed to Care* softened some of the market dynamics in the NHS there, reducing the number of trusts and introducing managed clinical networks. In 2003, 15 NHS boards were introduced, now reduced to 14.

This reorganisation reduced the purchaser–provider split. The NHS Reform Bill 2004 abolished trusts, absorbing them into the health boards. The Scottish government was aiming for partnership within the NHS. At the same time, it unveiled popular initiatives, such as its intention to abolish prescription charges by 2011 while parking charges at hospitals have also been scrapped, except at private finance initiative hospitals.

The Scottish health secretary said the aim was to run the Scottish NHS as a 'mutual', in which patients and the public are 'co-owners'. The Scottish government's 2007 strategy document *Better Health, Better Care* develops this model, outlining how health boards and community health partnerships would work more closely with local authorities, thus 'distancing NHS Scotland still further from market oriented models'.

The Scottish Government regards hitting a series of targets as the Scottish health service's biggest success since devolution, comparing waiting lists as better than in England, although also stating that comparisons between the different systems would become increasingly difficult to make as they diverge further. They claimed a focus on shifting the balance of care towards outpatient, primary and community care meant more patients in Scotland could be treated for less complex procedures without an acute setting and nearer to home, thus impacting on average length. They also acknowledged that several of their rural communities needed different types of hospitals.

The lack of a purchaser–provider split, with unified health boards planning, commissioning and providing the range of healthcare in Scotland, is the biggest obvious structural difference between the health services in England and Scotland.

For more information go to www.show.scot.nhs.uk.

Also, at www.show.scot.nhs.uk/elibrary you can access a large resource (delivered by the Knowledge Services Group in NHS Scotland) known as the e-Library, a national online knowledge service, providing high-quality knowledge support. The e-Library provides access to a wealth of resources including electronic books and journals, guidelines, policy documents, patient information, evaluated web resources and interactive learning opportunities. It also provides tools to enable users to keep up to date and to share resources and experience. A single username and password, available via online registration, provides access to these resources. It provides access to over 4000 full text electronic journals, over 20 major databases, 200 electronic textbooks and over 1500 free quality health information websites, so it caters for the work, research, education and personal development needs of the full range of NHS staff.

In addition to the main e-Library, the Knowledge Services Group provides a wide range of portals providing special collections of services and resources on particular topics and audiences. Portals are available for clinical practice (such as Cancer, Diabetes and Midwifery), clinical and non-clinical staff groups (such as General Practitioners, Community Pharmacy and Estates and Facilities). A recent development is delivery of Social Services Knowledge Scotland (www.ssks.org.uk) in partnership with the Institute for Research and Innovation in Social Services – an e-Library for the social services sector. The Virtual Learning Centre (www.learningcentre.scot.nhs.uk), created in partnership with Learn Direct Scotland, enables users to identify their learning needs and preferred learning styles, find learning resources mapped to the Knowledge and Skills Framework, and contact local learning centres.

The NHS Shared Learning Portal (www.sharedlearning.scot.nhs.uk) enables users to create, contribute, find and share learning resources. It enables distribution of learning objects across virtual learning environments and learning management systems.

NHS Education for Scotland Knowledge Services delivers a wide range of information and learning services, including: NHS Shared Learning, the NHS Scotland e-Library, the Shared Space service, My Community Space and others.

Many of these resources and services are available for everyone to use, whether or not you register for a username and password. Freely available resources provided by NHS Shared Learning comprise a wide range of quality-assured health and social care e-Learning resources, including images, videos, webcasts, audio tracks, IMS content packages and much more. Any user can also access the Virtual Learning Centre, which provides online learning resources for IT, management, core skills and life skills, including many provided by LearnDirect Scotland.

NHS Scotland staff and partners can register for an NHS Scotland ATHENS username and password. This provides access to password-protected content and services within the NHS Scotland e-Library, NHS Shared Learning, and the other services provided by NHS Education for Scotland Knowledge Services. An ATHENS password also enables you to create your own personal web space (My Community Space), where you can save and share resources and subject interests with others and establish collaborative workspaces to work and learn together with colleagues. You can also keep up to date with news and new research journals through newsfeeds and alerting services.

The following are eligible to apply for an NHS Scotland ATHENS username and password.

o Staff of NHS Scotland (including general practitioner staff, community pharmacy staff, dental surgery staff).
o Undergraduate or postgraduate students working or training with NHS Scotland
o Social services, public library staff and other local authority staff.
o Other partners of NHS Scotland (including staff in higher and further education, Scottish Government staff, voluntary sector organisations, nursing homes, the armed services and patient/public representatives on NHS groups).
o Others may also be eligible. If you are unsure which group you fit into, or feel you need access and don't belong to one of these groups, you can inquire by email or phone 0141 352 2892.

Special access is available to members of the public via libraries in the NHS and wider community.

Registering for e-Library services for other users may still be possible by registering for a restricted e-Library password if you don't belong to the above groups, but you won't get access to the full text of journals, books and databases. You will, however, get access to My Community Space. If in doubt you can check first with the Managed Knowledge Networks team on eligibility to register for these services.

The NHS in Wales

Founded by Welshman Aneurin Bevan, the NHS is as close to Welsh hearts as rugby union and close harmony singing. The NHS in Wales employs 71 000 people. During 1999, all the health responsibilities of the Welsh Office passed to the National Assembly for Wales. A big post-devolution structural change was prompted by the 2001 publication of *Improving Health in Wales'*, which replaced health authorities in 2003 with 22 local health boards.

Intended as a blueprint for shifting care into the community, a 2005 publication of a 10-year strategy *Designed for Life* led in 2008 to the Welsh Health Minister announcing proposals for major change in the structure of the NHS in Wales, saying they were intended to reduce bureaucracy and improve patient care. Proposals were unveiled to wipe out the internal market completely.

Instead, the NHS in Wales would now be run through seven autonomous local health boards. A National Advisory Board, chaired by the health minister, and a performance monitoring delivery board would be created. There would be a 'unified public health organisation' with executive responsibility for public health through the local health boards.

The new structure followed the signing by the coalition Labour/Plaid Cymru Government of the *One Wales* document that contained a commitment to abolish the internal market in the Welsh NHS. Prior to the change there had been two distinct NHS bodies in Wales: the local health board as the commissioner of services; and the trust as the provider of those services. This it was felt involved two separate teams often working on the same issues but from a different perspective that was seen to be an unnecessary duplication and wasteful. There were also transactional costs of a market structure, although these bodies were not operating as market-run systems. In early 2009 the seven new local health boards (LHBs) commenced operation.

One Wales had committed the Welsh Assembly Government to 'move to end the internal market' in order to improve services. Separating purchasers and providers was always likely in Wales, because of its small size, and the Welsh Assembly moved quickly to eliminate the market from its NHS. The end of the internal market in health was also part of a wider Welsh Assembly Government determination to make co-operation, rather than competition, the bedrock of public service delivery in Wales. The local health boards model was chosen over the trust model to emphasise partnership working. Seven new LHBs were called upon to focus on changing behaviour not structures, collaboration not confrontation, planning rather than commissioning, whole systems not hospitals, clinical engagement, partnership working and wellness not illness. In addition to these main changes there were plans to create a Public Health Trust to bring together the National Public Health Service and the Wales Centre for Health. By reducing the numbers of NHS bodies, they were slimming down structures, with one NHS body responsible for what were previously two functions and the total number of organisations reducing from 31 to nine.

The new NHS Trust, to be known as Public Health Wales, was introduced, incorporating National Public Health Service for Wales, The Wales Centre for Health, The Welsh Cancer Intelligence and Surveillance Unit and Screening Services Wales. The Board of Public Health Wales comprises seven non-executive directors and five executive directors. The new Director of Public Health posts will be employed by the local health boards and will be an integral part of the public health system.

Community health councils (CHCs) in Wales are the statutory, independent voice of all citizens within the NHS. They are engaged in a dialogue through their communities and are one of the major conduits for gathering and cascading information from and to local communities. The confidential, independent complaints advocacy service offered to the public by CHCs provides the NHS with trends in patient/public experiences of services; it includes the performance of primary and secondary care practitioners. The NHS in Wales has been going through such change it was felt essential that the CHCs hold the NHS to account, and have their powers of scrutiny strengthened by the Minister for Health and Social Services.

The Director of Postgraduate Education for General Practice in Wales and a GMC Council member has developed single systems of practice-based clinical governance assessment (an electronic toolkit), a single system of performance management and a single web-based system of appraisal for all GPs in Wales. In addition the Medical Performers List in Wales now encompasses the Medical List and the Supplementary List. GPs cannot practise in Wales unless they have been accepted onto the Medical Performers List, except GPs who are currently included on a PCT list. These GPs have two months to be able to work in Wales while their application is being processed. Once accepted onto the list, GPs will be registered with the LHB in the area in which they are working and they will need to inform the Business Services Centre if they intend to move LHB area. The GP will then need to complete a new application for inclusion on the new LHBs list. In the case of locum GPs, they are able to practise anywhere in Wales, but need to be registered with the LHB in the area where they predominantly work.

Healthcare Inspectorate Wales (www.hiw.org.uk) has responsibility to undertake reviews and investigations into the provision of NHS-funded care either by or for Welsh NHS organisations in order to provide independent assurance about and to support the continuous improvement in the quality and safety of Welsh NHS-funded care. HIW is also responsible for undertaking reviews and investigations into independent healthcare settings which include acute hospitals, mental health establishments, dental anaesthesia settings, hospices, private medical practices and specialised clinics. In addition HIW has responsibility for the statutory supervision of midwives and has entered an agreement with the Nursing and Midwifery Council (NMC) to conduct annual monitoring of higher education institutions in Wales which offer approved NMC programmes.

As elsewhere in the UK there have been cycles of changes in the NHS in Wales and as elsewhere sometimes these changes reflect political rather than purely operational motives. Free prescriptions were introduced in 2007, and free hospital parking promised in 2011.

For more information on the NHS in Wales including statistics go to www.wales. nhs.uk.

The NHS in Northern Ireland

The NHS in Northern Ireland employs 67000 people. Funding for health and social services in Northern Ireland amounts to 40% of the devolved government's budget, making it a big player in the country's politics. As in Wales, the Assembly minister has taken an increasingly hands-on role, while a recent reorganisation meant a number of senior managers lost their jobs.

A Review of Public Administration (RPA) in Northern Ireland was launched by the Northern Ireland Executive in 2002, and the final outcome was published in 2005. The reorganisation announced later that year reduced the number of health and social services trusts from 19 to six, including a national ambulance service.

In 2009 its four health and social services boards were replaced with a single Health and Social Care Board for Northern Ireland, responsible for commissioning and performance. It includes five local commissioning groups that mirror the five regional trusts. The overhaul also introduced a new Public Health Agency and Business Service Organisation as follows.

o Health and Social Care Board replacing the four existing Health and Social Care Boards, focusing on commissioning, resource management and performance management and improvement. Its role is to identify and meet the needs of the local population through its five Local Commissioning Groups that will cover the same geographical area as the HSC trusts. It has a chair and chief executive.

o Public Health Agency incorporating and building on the work of the Health Promotion Agency, but having a much wider responsibility for health protection and screening and health improvement and development to improve overall public health and address existing health inequalities. It also has a chair and chief executive.

o Business Services Organisation providing a range of support functions for the whole of the health and social care system. The Central Services Agency was dissolved and the majority of its services, along with other functions, have been undertaken by the new organisation. Again there is a chair and chief executive.

o The Patient and Client Council replacing four Health and Social Services Councils, with five local offices operating in the same geographical areas as the existing trusts, providing a voice for patients, clients and carers. Once again, there is a chair and chief executive.

There are plans to ensure that there is adequate and equitable representation for allied health professionals at a strategic level. More information can be found on the Department of Health, Social Services and Public Safety website; go to www.dhsspsni. gov.uk/index/hss/rpa-home or visit www.hscni.net.

NHS Isle of Man

The provision of the National Health Service on the Island is set out in the NHS Act 2001. A copy can be seen at www.gov.im/infocentre. Section 1 of the Act places a duty on the IoM Government Department of Health and Social Security to provide a National Health Service to promote a comprehensive health services designed to secure improvement in the physical and mental health of the people of the Island, the prevention, diagnosis and treatment of illness, and for that purpose provide or secure the effective provision of services in accordance with the provisions of this Act. The services provided under this Act are to be free of charge.

As part of the requirements of the NHS Act 2001, the department has set up a number of related Committees, Health Services Consultative Committee, Research Ethics Committee, and Independent Review Body (Complaints).

The NHS Act 2001 also provides powers for the department to introduce legislation modifying the regulation of healthcare professionals.

These regulations also:

o provide for a scheme whereby the department can pay in certain circumstances the travel expenses and an accommodation allowance to persons referred by the department for NHS treatment in the UK

○ establish the procedures by which the department can appoint consultant medical practitioners
○ establish a Complaints Procedure for the NHS.

For further information go to www.gov.im/dhss/health/centraladmin/nhs_acts.xml.

States of Guernsey Government

The States of Guernsey Health and Social Services Department is responsible for promoting, protecting and improving the health and social well-being of the people of Guernsey and Alderney. It has a wide mandate, delivering a range of services including preventing, diagnosing and treating people with illnesses and disease and caring for them in its hospital services and supporting people in the community, including people with disabilities.

Guernsey's Health and Social Services Department is the largest employer on the island with over 2100 people employed including clinical and non-clinical staff, and an annual budget of £84 million. The Corporate Management Team in charge of the day-to-day operations of Health and Social Services is made up of the Chief Officer and six directors who are responsible for the services.

A change in healthcare arrangements by the UK government means that most Guernsey and Alderney residents needing medical treatment while visiting the UK will now have to pay. Treatment in a UK A&E department, and for a number of specified illnesses, remain free but operations, outpatient appointments, treatment on a hospital ward and any other health services needed as a result of an accident or illness will be charged.

Guernsey and Alderney residents were therefore advised to have insurance cover for healthcare treatment when visiting the UK, just as they would when travelling to other countries on business or holiday. Charges are still not made if patients are referred for treatment in the UK.

The changes also affect people visiting Guernsey and Alderney from the UK. Visitors will now have to pay for all health services while in Guernsey and Alderney. For further information go to www.gov.gg/ccm/navigation/health---social-services.

States of Jersey Government

The Jersey Department of Health and Social Services promotes health and social well-being for the whole community, providing services to all. It provides acute hospital treatment, prevention and education, investigative procedures, long-term nursing care and works closely with centres in the UK.

There used to be a reciprocal agreement for the healthcare costs when islanders visited the UK but this was abolished in April 2009. Jersey residents having an accident or falling ill while visiting the UK will receive free treatment at A&E, and for a number of specified illnesses, but will now have to pay for operations, outpatient appointments, treatment on a hospital ward and any other health services, including repatriation. Henceforth Jersey residents were strongly advised to take out travel insurance to cover possible medical costs. If they live in Jersey and are referred for treatment in the UK, they still do not have to pay as the Health and Social Services Department already fund this.

People visiting Jersey from the UK are also affected. Visitors will get free treatment at A&E but will have to pay for all other health services while in Jersey. For more information go to www.gov.je/HealthWell.

A brief historical review of UK healthcare

Just in case you find references in the literature to old structures I include a very brief historical review.

The Ministry of Health was established in 1919 to bring together the medical and public health functions of central government and to co-ordinate and supervise local health services in England and Wales. It published its first White Paper in 1928. The co-ordinated emergency hospital service set up during the Second World War provided a blueprint for the National Health Service.

The right to medical treatment for everyone under a new national health service was first proposed in 1942 as part of the Social Insurance and Allied Services Report. These proposals were followed by the publication of the National Health Service Act in 1946. The NHS was founded on 5 July 1948, bringing together hospitals, GPs, opticians, dentists and other services into an integrated and organised healthcare service. Aneurin Bevan was the Health Minister in 1948 who established the NHS as a free, comprehensive healthcare service, available to the entire population.

The following decade saw the introduction of patient prescription and standard dental treatment charges, as well as the publication of the Guillebaud Committee Report in 1953, which called for better information and analytical services to resolve financial difficulties in the NHS.

Since the 1960s, the Department of Health has ensured that England's social services offer a range of support to protect vulnerable children and help adults to carry on in their daily lives.

In 1965, the Seebohm Committee reviewed the provision of personal social services in England, and published a report in 1968 on Local Authority and Allied Personal Social Services. The report recommended the creation of local authority departments to manage social services and provide professionally trained generic social workers.

Throughout its history, the DoH has evolved, taking on new areas of responsibility, and transferring parts of the department to other departments or new bodies that are better placed to provide services.

The first major reorganisation took place in 1968 when the Ministry of Health merged with the Ministry of Social Security to form the Department of Health and Social Security. The department underwent further restructuring in 1974, following the NHS's own reorganisation.

The DoH created the Social Services Inspectorate (SSI) in 1985 to improve quality and set standards for personal social services. The SSI was replaced in 2004 by the Commission for Social Care Inspection (CSCI), an independent body that works alongside the DoH.

Landmarks in social care legislation have included the Mental Health Act 1983, which has helped improve the care of detained patients, and the Children Act 1989's framework for making children's welfare a health policy priority.

The department split again in 1988 to form the Department of Health and the Department of Social Security. It then began to devolve power to newly created arm's length bodies in 1989, with the creation of the Medicines Control Agency.

In 1989 a Conservative Government introduced the White Paper *Working for Patients*, a fundamental review of the NHS which proposed major reforms with two main aims: to give patients greater choice among services available and to give greater satisfaction and rewards for those working in the NHS who successfully responded to local needs and preferences. It did not address any question of perceived underfunding but concentrated on the need to make the NHS more efficient. To do this it planned the following.

o Delegated responsibility for the delivery of healthcare to local level: regional health authorities, health authorities and hospitals through the introduction of the internal market.
o Created NHS trusts with more control over their affairs.
o Through the internal market, money would follow the patient and hopefully allow purchasers to make better use of the funds available.
o The introduction of general practitioner fundholders (GPFH) allowing GPs to hold budgets with which to purchase services for patients.
o Reforms to the regional health authorities (RHA), district health authorities (DHA) and family practitioner committees (to be known as family health services authorities – FHSA) by reducing membership and removing representation of local authorities, the new authorities having both executive and non-executive directors. The family health services authorities were to have general managers and were to be directly accountable to regional health authorities. Community health councils would continue to represent the interests of the patient.
o At a national level, the Supervisory Board within the DoH was to be replaced with a Policy Board, and the Management Board became the NHS Management Executive (NHSME).
o There were to be improved audit arrangements and the Audit Commission (*see* Chapter 2, p. 96) would in future be responsible for auditing the financial accounts of health authorities.
o Medical audit was to be extended throughout the NHS.

While the language was that of the market, the reality of the relationship between trusts as providers of services and health authorities as purchasers was, in effect, that of a managed market. As Professor Klein put it, 'purchasers became commissioners: a recognition that monogamy, rather than polygamy, characterised the internal market, with most purchasers and providers locked into permanent relationships in which each partner sought to modify the other'.

The NHS went through its next major change when New Labour entered government in 1997. Changes were set out in the next White Paper of that year, *The*

New NHS: modern, dependable, and accompanied by papers for Scotland, Wales and Northern Ireland. The main commitment was to replace the internal market with a system based on co-operation and partnership. In England this meant essentially two key factors: retaining separation between health authorities and trusts and replacing GP fundholding with commissioning through primary care trusts. The 1990s included the introduction of the NHS Chief Executive post.

The New NHS was to be based on six principles:
○ a national service
○ delivery against national standards, and local responsibility
○ characterised by partnership, not competition
○ efficiency through a rigorous approach to performance and cutting bureaucracy
○ moving the focus on to excellence and quality
○ rebuilding public confidence in the NHS.

Although co-operation and partnership were stressed, competition did not disappear entirely, as PCTs were still able to choose which NHS trust provides care for their patients. Data published about performance seeks to ensure that competition is by comparative results.

The NHS marked the turn of the millennium with the publication of *The NHS Plan in 2000*, setting out a 10-year modernisation programme of investment and reform. In 2003, the DoH was made smaller with six ministers, 2245 staff and three executive agencies.

Responsibility and accountability

The DoH was responsible for:
○ supporting ministers in accounting to the public and Parliament
○ looking after and allocating public money to the NHS and adult social care services
○ explaining to the public how their money is spent, and what is being achieved as a result.

The work on accounting to Parliament and the public includes:
○ answering parliamentary questions – both written and oral and dealing with other parliamentary business, debates and inquiries
○ responding to letters, emails and phone calls from the public and members of Parliament
○ communicating to the public through the media and through visits and speeches.

The NHS Improvement Plan followed in 2004.

The 2005 'Your Health, Your Care, Your Say' listening events asked the public, service users, and professionals how local NHS services could be improved. These views helped shape the policies within the 2006 White Paper, *Our Health, Our Care, Our Say: a new direction for community services.*

A founding principle of the NHS was that it should improve health and prevent disease, and not just provide treatment for those who are ill. Much of the DoH's work on public health has been shaped through the publication of White Papers, health education initiatives and advertising campaigns.

The Health Education Council and the Department of Health and Social Security began to launch national campaigns in the late 1960s. Landmark campaigns have included the first no-smoking campaign in 1974 and the first AIDS and HIV awareness campaign in 1986.

Three White Papers, published between 1977 and 2004, represent the DoH's ongoing commitment to public health. The White Paper *Prevention and Health* led to a single focus for the department on preventative work. The 1991 White Paper, *Health of the Nation*, identified coronary heart disease (CHD), cancer, mental health, AIDS, HIV and sexual health, and accidents as five key areas for improvement. The White Paper *Choosing Health* outlined the DoH's strategies for improving public health and tackling health inequalities in 21st-century England.

In recent years, The 2006 White Paper *Our Health, Our Care, Our Say: a new direction for community services* set out ways to provide improved social services in local communities. This is described in more detail in the section above on the NHS structure (p. 59).

Related reading

Beware when reading anything about the NHS structure. Things change so frequently and anything more than a year old is very likely to be out of date. I have therefore not generally recommended any textbooks, papers or articles in this edition. My best advice for further information is to visit the websites I have indicated, or carry out Internet searches and even then with any source, always check the date of writing.

DoH. www.dh.gov.uk/en/Publicationsandstatistics/Statistics/Performancedataandstatistics/AccidentandEmergency/DH_077485

DoH. *High Quality Care For All – NHS Next Stage Review Final Report*. London: Department of Health; 2008. Available online at www.ournhs.nhs.uk/wp-content/uploads/2008/06/dh-darzi-summary-report.pdf

HES. www.hesonline.nhs.uk/Ease/servlet/ContentServer;jsessionid=dchk4fgry1?siteID=1937&categoryID=1117

Lillyman S. Community matrons' role still undefined. *Br J Comm Nurs.* 2009; **14**: 70–3.

Lunn JN, Mushin WW. *Mortality Associated with Anaesthesia*. Oxford: Nuffield Provincial Hospitals Trust; 1982.

Pollock AM. Farewell to a free NHS. *Guardian*, 1 July 2008. Available online at www.guardian.co.uk

Pollock AM, Kirkwood G. Independent sector treatment centres: learning from a Scottish case study. *BMJ.* 2009; **338**: 1421. Available online at www.bmj.com/cgi/content/full/338/apr30_2/b1421

Clinical governance and quality

This chapter aims to develop an understanding of the role of clinical governance in delivering quality in healthcare services. It also explores risk management, clinical audit, evidence-based practice and some of the NHS quality initiatives.

In essence, clinical governance is the method by which a systemic approach to the maintenance and improvement of a quality service and patient care is managed. The most widely cited formal definition describes it as:

> A framework through which NHS organisations are accountable for continually improving the quality of their services and safeguarding high standards of care by creating an environment in which excellence in clinical care will flourish. (Scally and Donaldson 1998)

This definition is intended to embody three main attributes: recognisably high standards of care; transparent responsibility and accountability for those standards; and a constant dynamic pathway to improvement.

Clinical governance should consist of a framework which pulls together all the initiatives within a healthcare provider associated with quality assurance. It is easy to over-complicate the definition of clinical governance in the attempt to explain the phrase in words, for the precise characterisation of quality is elusive both as a concept and within the day-to-day workings of healthcare provision. In its simplest form it can be described as 'doing the **right thing** at the **right time** to the **right person** in the **right way**. It is 'doing anything and everything required to maximise quality'. There also has to be a balance between cost-effectiveness and quality, because there can be a tendency to throw money at quality in the attempt to be seen to be taking it seriously but not to adequately measure the outcomes. In short, the concept of governance and quality is tricky to quantify and hence several national systems have been put in place to ensure its presence within all hospitals and other healthcare providers, with its ultimate goal to make certain the culture of healthcare provision contains quality improvement as a routine element of clinical practice. Governance and quality are synonymous and good governance evidences a quality service.

The NHS Act (1999) placed a duty of quality on NHS organisations. The Act introduced corporate accountability for clinical quality and performance. Clinical governance also means that healthcare providers have a statutory duty to:

> Continually improve the overall standard of clinical care, whilst reducing variation in outcomes of, and access to, services as well as ensuring that clinical decisions are based on the most up-to-date evidence of what is known to be effective. (NHSE 1999: 5)

As an intrinsic part of the above, there has to be an increased focus on risk management, which can be defined as a means of reducing the risks of adverse events in organisations by systematically assessing, reviewing and identifying possible risks in processes, environments, staff roles and so on, and then seeking ways to prevent their occurrence (adapted from NHSE 1999).

Prior to 1999 trust boards had no statutory duty to ensure any particular level of quality. Their principal statutory responsibilities were to ensure proper financial management of the organisation and an acceptable level of patient safety. Maintaining and improving the quality of care was understood to be the responsibility of the clinical professions. This changed from 1999 when trust boards assumed the legal responsibility for quality of care in equal measure to their other statutory duties. Clinical governance is the mechanism by which this responsibility is discharged.

The elements of clinical governance

Clinical governance includes the following elements.

○ **Risk management** – as well as the definition above, risk management describes the systems used to understand, monitor and minimise the risks to patients and staff, and to learn from mistakes. Risk management has to consider risks to patients (compliance with statutory regulations, critical event learning), and risks to practitioners (ensuring that clinicians are immunised against infectious diseases and work in a safe environment). Systems can include risk registers, risk assessments and incident reporting. Risk management also has to include the identification of business risk and risks to the organisation, risks from the environment or from pandemic illness, from catastrophic events, from personnel management and HR. The appropriate response to complaints, then learning from them, can be a key element in risk management. These are a few examples within a very wide field of potential risk. (There is more information about risk management later in the chapter.)

○ **Clinical effectiveness** – the extent to which clinical interventions maintain and improve health and secure the greatest possible health gain from available sources.

This may include the implementation of NICE guidelines, clinical audit and staff reviews.

○ **Education, training and continuing professional development (CPD)** – often referred to as Life Long Learning – this covers the support available to enable staff to be competent in doing their jobs as well as developing their skills. It reflects the importance of staff having up-to-date skills and knowledge through continuous learning and development.

○ **Use of information** – describes the systems in place to collect and interpret clinical information and use it to monitor, plan and improve the quality of patient care. This should also stress the importance of **openness** – open proceedings and discussion about clinical governance issues should be a feature of the framework. Information which can be open to public scrutiny, while respecting individual patient and practitioner confidentiality, is again essential to quality assurance.

○ **Staffing and staff management** – the recruitment, management and development of staff, promoting good working conditions, family-friendly policies, effective methods of working, absence management, annual leave allocations and so on – elements of this section can also be referred to as workforce planning.

○ **Clinical audit** – systematic and critical analysis of clinical performance and the measurement of performance against agreed standards. This includes the procedures for diagnosis, treatment and care, the associated use of resources and the resulting outcomes in respect of quality of life for patients. It also encompasses the refining of clinical practice from results from audit – and results in a cyclical process for the improvement of patient care.

○ **Patient/service user and public involvement** – patient/user satisfaction surveys, patient organisations – these describe how patients and users can have a say in their own treatment and how services are provided.

○ **Research and development, research-based management and evidence-based practice** – good professional practice has always sought to change in the light of evidence from research. The time lag between obtaining research-based information and introducing the required change from this can be very long, so a governance framework needs to include emphasis not only on carrying out research but also on using and implementing the results of such research. Techniques such as critical appraisal of literature, project management and the development of protocols and guidelines are all tools for promoting the implementation of research practice. There is further explanation of evidence-based practice later in this chapter (*see* p. 89).

Clinical governance requires change and innovation at three levels: by individual healthcare professionals; by teams; and by organisations. Individual healthcare workers have to look at what needs changing by thinking about what they do and placing patient need at the centre of their thinking. Teams need to become true multidisciplinary groups. Understanding roles, sharing information and knowledge, and supporting each other should be part of everyday practice. General practices and primary care trusts need to have systems and local arrangements to support the teams and to ensure the provision of good-quality care. Commitment and leadership from the PCTs and from general practices is crucial to the development of quality improvements.

In the 1950s and 1960s it was often assumed that more spending on healthcare would lead to better health. Increased awareness of other determinants of health, such as housing, employment, family, education and social class positioning, has resulted in a more political approach. Other factors such as the oil crisis of the 1970s, the emergence of previously non-industrial countries as key players in the world economy, the increasing availability of new health technologies and the ever growing proportion of the aged population have led to increased pressure to contain costs. In addition, the advent of the Internet has led to the population being increasingly aware of treatment options, leading to higher expectations from the medical profession and the ability to 'check things out'. Health professionals can no longer expect the population to accept what is told them with out questioning, and often have done their research before seeing a doctor. The creation of the NHS internal market as part of the reforms in the late 1980s and 1990s was accompanied by a plethora of initiatives aimed at improving quality. Quality then became focused on the twin concepts of clinical effectiveness and evidence-based medicine. Quality, and evidencing ongoing improvement, was the focus of Lord Darzi's High Quality Care for All published in 2008 (Darzi 2008), the final report in his series of NHS Next Stage Review documents, which responded to the 10 SHAs' strategic visions and set out the holistic vision for an NHS with quality at its heart.

In addition, there is considerable information out in the public domain giving comparative data about the way healthcare organisations perform. Access to websites such as the Doctor Foster Hospital Guide and the fact that patients can get into these types of sites on their telephones while sitting in a waiting room waiting to see a doctor has to be considered. Doctors have to be prepared for the patients asking far more questions based on being extremely well informed. Also, it has to be remembered that whereas patients may be able to obtain all this data, it does not necessarily mean that they understand it.

The service provided by a healthcare organisation may be excellent but will not be considered successful unless valued by the patient. The delivery process also has to be excellent. This is difficult in a health service where the expectations and requirements of the diverse numbers of parties involved may be very different. The first real acceptance of this ethos was in 1989 when the White Paper *Working for Patients* was published (DoH 1989). This proposed a set of seven patient-focused factors:

○ appropriateness of treatment and care
○ achievement of optimum clinical outcome
○ clinical-recognised procedures to minimise complications and similar preventable events
○ attitude which treats patients with dignity and as individuals
○ environment conducive to patients' safety, reassurance and contentment
○ speed of response to patients' needs and at minimum inconvenience to them (and their relatives or carers)
○ involvement of patients in their own care.

These factors still provide a relevant way of determining a quality service for patients and you can see how the elements of clinical governance structures and the contribution of the nationwide organisations (see later) all contribute to these ideals.

There have been many methodologies introduced over the past 20 years or so pertaining to the management of quality and if you undertook a search on a website there are a large number of 'buzzwords' associated with quality in healthcare organisations. However, if quality initiatives are driven based on the elements of clinical governance, this will result in a quality-led organisation which can categorically evidence patient-focused care, which in turn is reviewed in line with patient, staff and doctors' feedback. Woe betide a management team that neglects to take notice of these latter three key parties. Quality and governance has to be embedded in the culture of the organisation and it calls for commitment at all levels.

Implementing clinical governance

The following systems and mechanisms contribute to clinical governance:
- clinical audit
- risk management
- health needs assessment
- evidence-based clinical practice
- patient feedback
- continuing professional development
- accreditation of healthcare organisations or providers
- development of clinical leadership skills
- effective management of poorly performing colleagues
- systems to ensure critical incidents are openly investigated and lessons learnt are implemented.

The requirements placed on healthcare organisations include:
- developing leadership skills among clinicians
- developing mechanisms to ensure that change in clinical practice occurs as a result of audit, risk management and complaints findings thus closing the 'audit loop'
- developing appropriate accountability structures
- working more collaboratively and effectively between primary and secondary care
- developing more effective multidisciplinary working
- building continuing medical education and continuing professional development into quality improvement programmes
- improving the information infrastructure of the NHS.

Thus, at trust level, the main principles of clinical governance are:
- clear lines of responsibility and accountability for the overall quality of clinical care
- a comprehensive programme of quality improvement systems (including clinical

audit, supporting and applying evidence-based practice, implementing clinical standards and guidelines, workforce planning and development)
○ educational and training plans
○ clear policies aimed at managing risk
○ integrated procedures for all professional groups to identify and remedy poor performance.

Trust chief executives are ultimately responsible to their boards for assuring the quality of services provided. Trusts usually have clinical governance committees, chaired by a clinical professional. Monthly reports are presented to trust boards and they are obliged to publish annual clinical governance reports. The **Clinical Governance Support Team** (www.cgsupport.nhs.uk) is a body which supports clinical governance developments.

An action list may be used to check that clinical governance is an active element within a healthcare provider.
○ Are there quality improvement programmes (e.g. clinical audit)?
○ Are leadership skills developed at clinical team level?
○ Is evidence-based practice in everyday use?
○ Is good practice and innovation disseminated within and outside the organisation?
○ Are there clinical risk-reduction programmes?
○ Are adverse events detected, openly investigated and lessons learned applied?
○ Are lessons learned from complaints made by patients?
○ Are problems of poor clinical performance recognised early and dealt with to prevent harm to patients?
○ Do all professional development programmes reflect the principles of clinical governance?
○ Is the quality of data collected to monitor clinical care consistently of a high standard?

Benchmarking

The NHS Benchmarking Network was established in 1996 in order that NHS organisations could contribute to a structure which would enable them to share best practice and to learn from each other. Subscribers come from primary care trusts, strategic health authorities and NHS trusts in England plus other equivalent organisations within healthcare systems in the UK.

The vision statement on the website www.nhsbenchmarking.nhs.uk explains that the network's purpose is: 'Supporting NHS organisations to improve the effectiveness, patient experience, productivity and value for money of services by using benchmarking and knowledge exchange to identify, share and promote excellent and innovative practice.'

Its objectives, again quoted from the site, are to:
○ promote the use of benchmarking among members
○ act as a network hub and learning zone for members in a safe and protected environment

o test out new ideas
o carry out excellent benchmarking projects with members which achieve results that can be implemented
o identify and share good practice in a 'practical' form, e.g. use of matrices, reports
o help members implement change.

Risk management

The New NHS (DoH 1997) and *Clinical Governance: quality in the new NHS* (DoH 1999) placed clinical risk management as a key component of clinical governance. This was further elaborated on when Lord Darzi (2008) defined quality of care as clinically effective, personal and safe. This means protecting patient safety by eradicating such avoidable problems such as healthcare-acquired infections and foreseeable accidents. Clear policies aimed at managing risk and supporting staff in identifying and tackling poor performance must therefore be in place.

Effective risk management at trust level demands clear unequivocal systems that are embedded in each area of healthcare provision. Most healthcare providers have committee structures with lines of responsibility for defined areas of risk, such as clinical risk, infection control and medicines management. Named individuals are given the task to facilitate risk management throughout the organisation. There is usually a multidisciplinary group given the autonomy to drive the process – a Quality and Risk Management Committee.

Risk assessment is an integral element. Risk assessments are normally undertaken using a risk rating scale/score. First, the risk is identified and the likelihood of it occurring is assessed on a scale of 1 to 5, 1 being rare and 5 being almost certain. Second, the consequences or impact of the risk occurring is assessed on a scale of 1 to 5, 1 being negligible and 5 being extreme. The scores are multiplied, giving a risk rating number between 1 and 25 – and responses can be determined based on the calculated rating. Many models for risk assessment are available and these can be viewed on the web.

An element of any risk-management process is the reporting mechanism for adverse incidents, which are completed by any member of staff. These are usually entered into a software tool developed to provide reports broken down into types of incident, grading the severity of impact, the incidence of harm to patients or identification of 'near miss' scenarios. The detection of trends is vital so that interventions can be initiated to prevent recurrence. These of course do not necessarily have to be clinical issues, but also include non-clinical such as manual handling, bullying and stress claims.

Trusts are normally insured against risk through the Clinical Negligence Scheme for Trusts. This scheme rewards trusts for compliance with its standards by discounting fees. The scheme is administered by the NHS Litigation Authority (www.nhsla.com), an authority with the responsibility for handling negligence claims made against NHS bodies in England. The NHSLA manage their risk-management programme by providing a range of NHSLA standards and assessments. Healthcare organisations are regularly assessed against these risk-management standards, which have been specifically developed to reflect issues that have arisen in negligence claims reported

to the NHSLA. There is a set of standards for each type of healthcare organisation incorporating organisational, clinical, and health and safety risks:
o NHSLA Acute, PCT and Independent Sector Standards 2009/10
o NHSLA Mental Health and Learning Disability Standards 2009/10
o NHSLA Ambulance Standards 2009/10.

In addition, there is a separate set of clinical risk management standards for NHS maternity standards:
o NHSLA Maternity Standards 2009/10.

All the standards are divided into three levels of compliance. Organisations that are graded at level 1 receive a 10% discount on their CNST contributions, at level 2: 20% and at level 3: 30%.

Organisations that achieve level 1 are assessed against the relevant standards once every two years, but the frequency of assessment can reduce at higher levels to at least once in any three-year period. If an organisation fails to comply, they have to be assessed on an annual basis until they have achieved compliance. Assessments take place over two days and are carried out by an external company who are responsible for much of the day-to-day administration of the risk-management processes.

In order to facilitate the assessments, evidence templates have been produced which must be completed and submitted. Self-assessments may be conducted using the templates and these may be used by assessors to record their scores and findings, which in turn enable the organisation to prepare an action plan.

Clinical audit

Medical audit was formally introduced into the NHS in 1989, changing its name to clinical audit in 1993 to reflect a more multidisciplinary approach. Clinical audit is a quality-improvement service that seeks to improve patient care and outcomes through systematic review of care against explicit criteria and the implementation of change. Indicated changes are implemented at an individual, team or service level and further monitoring is conducted to confirm improvement in healthcare delivery (NICE 2002).

Types of audit may include standards-based audit, adverse occurrence screening and critical incident monitoring, peer review or patient surveys and focus groups, obtaining users views about the quality of the care they have received.

The audit process

In all types of audit, the audit process applies Figure 2.1. It is a cyclical movement, each cycle aspiring to a higher level of quality.
1 Identify a problem or issue (centre of the circle).
2 Set the criteria and the standards against which to audit.
3 Observe practice/collect the data.
4 Compare performance with criteria and standards.
5 Implement change.

6 Re-audit in order to sustain change, reset the criteria and return to Stage 2 in the audit cycle.

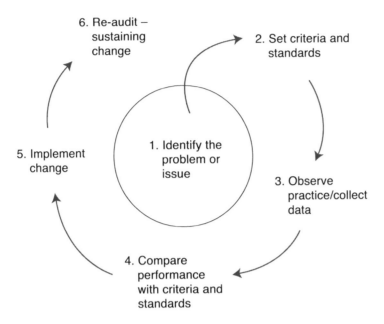

FIGURE 2.1 The audit process

Stage 1: Identifying the problem or issue

This is likely to involve comparison with healthcare processes that have been shown to produce best outcomes for patients – and can be influenced by factors including a search for national standards or examples of clinical practice, problems that have been encountered in practice, problems raised by colleagues, patients or relatives, potential for improving service delivery or recommendations by national bodies such as the CQC or NICE.

Stage 2: Criteria

Criteria are explicit statements that define what is being measured and that can be measured objectively. They cannot include statements which rely on personal opinions or values.

A criterion is a measurable outcome of care, aspect of practice or capacity.

A standard is the threshold of the expected compliance for each criterion (these may be expressed as a percentage).

Stage 3: Data collection

Details of what is to be audited must be established from the outset. These include the user group to be included with any exceptions noted, the healthcare professionals involved in the care, and the period over which the criteria apply.

Consideration must be given to what data will be collected and how (electronic or manual), where it will be found and who will collect it.

Ethical issues must also be considered – data must relate only to the objectives of the audit. Staff and patient confidentially must be respected, and identifiable information must never be used. Any potentially sensitive topics should be discussed with the local research ethics committee.

Stage 4: Comparison of performance with criteria and standards

The final stage of analysis is to conclude how well the standards were met, and identify the reasons for failure to meet them. Where a standard is not met, there may be the potential for improvement in care. However, if it is very close to being met, it may be decided to leave this particular event as it is and concentrate on something that needs further attention. In life and death situations it would be crucial to achieve 100% in an audit, but in other circumstances a lower score would be acceptable.

Stage 5: Implementing change

Once the results have been published and discussed then agreement must be reached about the recommendations for change. An action plan can be created, recording who is going to do what and by when.

Stage 6: Re-audit and sustaining improvement

This is often termed 'closing the loop'. Re-audit should demonstrate any impact created by the changes. This stage is critical to the successful outcome of an audit process as it verifies whether the changes implemented had an effect and whether further improvements are required to achieve the standards set in Stage 2.

The differences between clinical research and audit are as follows.

o Research is often deductive and concerned with critical testing.
o Research is more likely to use control groups and validating measures.
o The scope of research is likely to be wider and will reach a greater audience in terms of publication of results in journals, etc.
o Research can provide answers in areas that audit could not tackle, and will challenge the efficacy of a particular therapy.
o Research raises questions about purposes – and the means of achieving them.
o Audit is often concerned with small-scale problems requiring local solutions.
o Audit evaluates what exists and takes purposes for granted.
o Audit ascertains whether the inputs and processes achieve the outcome desired.
o Audit can give rise to research questions – if the outcomes of audit are not what was intended or raise unexpected queries, research can ask why.
o Audit and research can feed into each other.

Research is finding the right thing to do . . . and audit is about ensuring you are doing the right thing right!

Clinical audit, education and professional development

Clinical audit is a professional development activity that highlights education needs through audit methods and data analysis. By generating new knowledge, clinical audit can contribute to the postgraduate and undergraduate curricula in the healthcare professions. The providers of education can use this new knowledge to modify curricula, while providing healthcare professionals with advice on research methods.

Clinical audit can be seen as a means to broaden the team by the development of reflective practice. The potential for learning that takes place through participation in the audit process can be recognised and accredited as part of an individual's continuing professional development. Records can be kept in a revalidation folder as evidence of involvement in continuing learning.

Evidence-based clinical practice

'Evidenced-based clinical practice is an approach to decision making in which the clinician uses the best evidence available, in consultation with the patient, to decide upon the option which suits that patient best' (Muir Gray 1997). However, a true quality service exists when this is combined with the doctor's education and experience and their insight into and knowledge of a patient. It is the opposite of conjecture-based decision making. There are many organisations, journals, Internet sites and electronic databases which are dedicated to the pursuit of evidenced-based clinical practice and encouraging its growth within all healthcare professions in the NHS and other healthcare providers. A few of these are described below.

PubMed

PubMed is a service of the United States National Library of Medicine and it includes multi-million citations for MEDLINE and other life science journals for biomedical articles back to the 1950s. PubMed includes links to full-text articles and to other related resources. The website address is www.ncbi.nlm.gov/pubmed.

The Cochrane Library

This site contains high-quality, independent evidence to inform healthcare decision making. It includes reliable evidence from Cochrane and other systematic reviews, clinical trials and more. Cochrane reviews bring the combined results of the world's best medical research studies and are recognised as the gold standard in evidence-based healthcare.

The website address is www.wiley.com/Cochrane.

The UK Cochrane Centre was established at the end of 1992 by the NHS Research and Development Programme and is part of the National Institute for Health Research. The website address is www.cochrane.co.uk.

Bandolier

The first issue of *Bandolier*, an independent journal of evidenced-based healthcare written by Oxford scientists, was published in February 1994. It has appeared monthly ever since and have become the most recognised source of evidence-based healthcare information in the UK and worldwide for all healthcare professionals and consumers. The paper version was discontinued in 2007, but the Internet version is updated at more or less regular intervals.

The website address is www.medicine.ox.ac.uk/bandolier.

Ovid's evidenced-based medicine reviews

Ovid is a definitive resource for electronic information which combines seven of the most trusted evidenced-based medicine resources into a single database that is easily searchable. The website address is www.ovid.com/site/catalog/DataBase/904.jsp.

Department of Primary Health Care

This is based at Oxford University. Together with the Department of Public Health the Division of Public Health and Primary Health Care is part of the university's Medical Science Division. The Division aims for excellence in teaching and research and the department is one of the five founding members of the National Institute for Health Research School for Primary Care Research. Primary research focus is based on the prevention, early diagnosis and management of common illnesses in general practice.

UCL Institute of Child Health

This institute is based at Great Ormond Street Hospital for Children NHS Trust and together they form an international centre of excellence for treating sick children and teaching and training children's specialists. It is the largest centre of research into childhood illness outside the US and promotes evidenced-based medicine in relation to children.

The website address is www.ich.ucl.ac.uk.

Institute of Public Health

Based at Cambridge University, this institute aims to improve the health of the population by understanding the cause and natural history of disease, and to identify and evaluate new possibilities for both primary and secondary care intervention and prevention. The website address is www.iph.cam.ac.uk.

Centres for Evidenced Based Mental Health

The Centres for Evidenced Based Mental Health and the Department of Psychiatry at Oxford University provide information, and promote and support evidence-based healthcare in mental healthcare. The website addresses are www.cebmh.com and www.psych.ox.ac.uk.

NHS quality initiatives

The following organisations and initiatives exist to contribute to the maintenance and improvement of quality in healthcare. They are numerous and diverse, each providing a specific function within the structure of quality and governance.

Care Quality Commission

The Care Quality Commission is the independent regulator of health and social care in England. The aim is to make sure that better care is provided for everyone whether in hospital, in care homes, in people's own homes or elsewhere. The CQC regulates health and adult social care services whether provided by the NHS, local authorities, private companies or voluntary organisations. It also protects the rights of people detained under the Mental Health Act. The website address is www.cqc.org.uk.

Until March 2009 regulation of health and social adult care was carried out by the Healthcare Commission and the Commission for Social Care Inspectorate. The Mental Health Act Commission had monitoring functions with regard to the operation of the Mental Health Act 1983. The Health and Social Care Act 2008 established a single, integrated regulator of health and adult social care – The Care Quality Commission which replaced the three previous bodies.

The Act set the CQC's functions in terms of assuring safety and quality, assessing the performance of commissioners and providers, monitoring the operation of the Mental Health Act and ensuring that regulation and inspection activity across health and adult social care is managed and co-ordinated effectively. This joined-up approach should help to ensure better outcomes for the people who use the service.

All providers of health and social care – including, for the first time, NHS providers – will be required to register with CQC. Regulation requirements are consistent across all groups, and the regulatory system provides clear expectations of the requirements needed to provide services. It is a risk-based approach which means that regulation activity is targeted where action is required.

The CQC has a wide range of enforcement powers along with flexibility as to how and when to use them. The regulator will have greater powers to achieve compliance with registration requirements. In order to be granted registration, care providers will have to demonstrate that they can meet, or are already meeting, the requirements; and to maintain registration, they will need to demonstrate an ongoing ability to continue to comply with requirements.

NHS providers will have to achieve registration by the end of April 2010 and independent sector providers by October 2010. For the NHS, the registration criteria will replace Standards for Better Health.

Assessment of providers will be based on completion of a self-assessment process which will require the submission of verifiable evidence pertaining to each stated requirement.

In Scotland and Wales regulation of healthcare comes under different legislative bodies. The Scottish Commission for the Regulation of Care website is www.care commission.com and information regarding the Health Care Inspectorate in Wales can be found at www.hiw.org.uk. Scotland and Wales have specific areas on the NHS website: www.scotland.nhs.uk and www.wales.nhs.uk.

Quality indicators

The Department of Health and the NHS Information Centre published a set of National Indicators for Quality Improvement. NHS clinical teams are able to view a list of more than 230 existing quality indicators on the NHS Information Centre website. The Indicators for Quality Improvement will allow clinical teams to measure the quality of care they deliver to patients against local and national benchmarks. They will also support providers and commissioners of NHS services.

The National Patient Safety Agency

The NPSA has a wide-ranging quality role within the NHS. It has been estimated that around 10% of patients admitted to the NHS each year are unintentionally harmed in some way and that half of these incidents may be preventable (Vincent *et al.* 2001). Since April 2005 the NPSA has been responsible for the co-ordination of organisations and individuals in healthcare to investigate and learn from patient safety incidents occurring within healthcare providers. The website address is www.npsa. nhs.uk.

The NPSA also encompasses work within the safety aspects of hospital design, cleanliness and food and nutrition. It ensures that research work is carried out safely and ethically through its responsibility for the Central Office for Research Ethics Committees (COREC).

The NPSA manages the contracts with the three confidential inquirers: the National Confidential Enquiry into Patient Outcome and Death (NCEPOD), the Confidential Enquiry into Maternal and Child Health (CEMACH) and the National Confidential Inquiry into Suicide and Homicide by People with Mental Illness (NCISH).

The NPSA seeks to ensure that all incidents are reported, and promotes an open and fair culture in hospitals and across health services. Doctors and staff are encouraged to report incidents and 'near misses'. It is vital to encourage staff to report incidents without fear of personal reprimand. It is not responsible for investigation of complaints or issues concerning individuals.

The NPSA has set up a national reporting structure, which is aimed at collecting and analysing information from all staff and patients, and it produces publications including case studies with expert advice.

The National Clinical Assessment Service

The NPSA incorporates the National Clinical Assessment Service (www.ncas.nhs. uk). This was set up to promote public confidence in doctors and dentists by giving confidential advice and support to NHS organisations on how to manage doctors and dentists whose performance was giving cause for concern. Contact to NCAS can be made by an employer, contracting body or a single practitioner. The aim of NCAS is to work with all parties to clarify the concerns and make recommendations, with the ultimate aim being to help the practitioner deliver a high-quality and safe service for patients. It is an advisory body and the referrer retains responsibility for handling the case throughout the process.

NCAS also helps NHS organisations improve local management of performance concerns so that difficulties are recognised and addressed before they become serious.

NCAS has working arrangements with a number of partners including the General Medical Council (GMC), the General Dental Council, the Care Quality Commission and the Academy of Medical Royal Colleges.

The Institute for Innovation and Improvement

This was created in 2005 and it superseded the Modernisation Agency, the NHSU and the NHS Leadership Centre. Its mission is to support the NHS in accelerating the delivery of world-class healthcare for patients and public by encouraging innovation and developing capability at the frontline. The website address is www.institute.nhs.uk.

The institute has expertise in service transformation, technology and product innovation and incorporates the National Innovation Centre, which is based at the University of Warwick. This provides an entry point for industry and the NHS to explore and adopt new concepts, and to develop specific products for particular needs.

The institute seeks to lead and commission development and research to build an evidence base of new and best practice in service transformation.

It also works to promote a culture of lifelong learning for all NHS staff by working with NHS organisations to develop learning systems to accelerate organisational growth and individual core learning materials to enhance personal development. Many of the learning programmes and outputs of the previous organisations are still available (www.nhsu.nhs.uk and www.wise.nhs.uk) – the series of Improvement Leaders' Guides represent the best known in NHS improvement practice.

The National Confidential Enquiry into Patient Outcome and Death (NCEPOD)

NCEPOD was originally the Confidential Enquiry into Perioperative Deaths but expanded its remit to cover a far greater number of studies than just death within 30 days of surgery. Its purpose now is to assist in improving the standards of medical and surgical care by reviewing the management of patients by undertaking confidential surveys and research into a varied number of conditions and patient groups – a recent example of this in 2009 being death within seven days of surgery in the patient aged over 80. The results of the surveys are published; its work does not involve new treatments or therapies, but a review of outcomes of current practice. Individuals or organisations may initiate studies by submitting a proposal to NCEPOD that should be relevant to the current clinical environment.

NCEPOD staff may be invited to visit hospitals and give presentations as part of multidisciplinary meetings such as audit days. NCEPOD also holds conferences where they present the results of their surveys.

The website address is www.ncepod.org.uk.

National Institute for Health and Clinical Excellence

NICE's role was identified in the White Paper *Choosing Health: making healthier choices easier* (DoH 2004). Within this the government set out key principles for informing people so that they may make healthier and more informed choices about their health, and the DoH required NICE to bring together knowledge and guidance of ways of promoting good health and treating ill health.

NICE is an independent organisation, and produces national guidance in three areas of health, as follows.

○ Public health – guidance on the promotion of good health and the prevention of ill health for those working in the NMHD, local authorities and the wider public and voluntary sector.
○ Health technologies – guidance on the use of new and existing medicines, treatments and procedures within the NHS.
○ Clinical practice – guidance on the appropriate treatment and care of people with specific diseases and conditions within the NHS.

Each guidance area is the responsibility of one of the three centres of excellence.

○ The Centre for Public Health Excellence.
○ The Centre for Health Technology Evaluation – technology appraisals are recommendations for the use of new and existing medicines and treatments within the NHS. Interventional procedure guidance evaluates the safety and efficacy of the procedures where they are used for diagnosis or for treatment
○ The Centre for Clinical Practice which develops and produces clinical guidelines – these are recommendations on the treatment of people with specific diseases and illnesses based on the best available evidence.

NICE has staff based in London and Manchester who deliver the institute's work. The guidance is developed by a number of independent advisory groups who consist of health professionals, staff from the NHS, patients, their relatives or carers and the public. There is a Board and Senior Management team who set the strategic direction and oversee the delivery, provide stewardship and ensure corporate governance. In addition NICE produces a wide range of resources to help practitioners implement the guidance into their practice. Details of these can be found on the website at www. nice.org.uk.

Once NICE guidelines are available, organisations who employ health professionals as well as the healthcare professionals themselves are expected to take them into account when deciding which treatments to give to patients. However, the guidance does not replace the skills or knowledge of the individual professionals – treatment still remains their ultimate decision about particular patients, always in consultation with the patient themselves and relatives/carers.

What health professionals are expected to do depends on the type of NICE guidance.

○ *Public health guidance:* Take into account when developing local area agreements.
○ *Clinical guidelines:* Review the current management of the conditions then consider the resources and time needed to implement the guidelines.

○ *Technology appraisals:* Fund and resource medicines and treatments recommended. Three months is the usual time between guidance and implementation.
○ *Interventional procedures:* Practitioners should always check whether NICE has issued guidance before carrying out a new procedure. If there is no guidance, a practitioner must seek approval from their NHS trust clinical governance committee – and ensure that the patient has given informed consent before carrying it out.

Medicines and Healthcare Products Regulatory Agency

This government agency is responsible for ensuring that medicines and medical devices work and are acceptably safe. It acknowledges that no product is risk free – but robust and fact-based judgements are gathered to ensure that the benefits to patients and the public justify the risks. The MHRA observe medicines and devices and take any necessary action very promptly to protect the public if there is a problem. MHRA Alerts are issued to all healthcare providers and it should be an active part of the governance structure that prompt action is taken to disseminate the alerts throughout the healthcare organisation, and that relevant action is identified, implemented and documented. As much information as is possible is made publicly available. The MHRA encourages everyone – the public, healthcare professionals as well as industry – to report problems with a medicine or a medical device. Investigation is prompt and necessary action is communicated through the alert system.

National Service Frameworks (NSFs)

These are policies set by the NHS in the UK to define standards of care for major medical conditions such as cancer, coronary heart disease, mental health and diabetes. Frameworks are also defined for some patient groups including children and older people. The main purposes of NSFs are:
○ to set defined quality requirements for care based on best available evidence of what treatments and services work most effectively for patients
○ to offer strategies and support to help organisations achieve these.

One of the main strengths of each NSF is that they are inclusive, in that they have been constructed in partnership with health professionals, health service managers, patients, carers, voluntary agencies and other experts as relevant to each one. They are intended to be long term; they set national standards with measurable goals within set time frames. Individual frameworks can be reviewed on the website at www.nhs.uk/nhsengland/NSF/pages/Nationalserviceframeworks.aspx.

Critical Appraisals Skills Programme (CASP)

Since its birth in 1993, the Critical Appraisal Skills Programme has helped to develop an evidence-based approach in health and social care, working with local, national and international groups. It is a programme within learning and development at the Public Health Resource Unit.

CASP aims to enable individuals to develop the skills to find and make sense of research evidence, and helps them to put knowledge into practice.

The website address is www.phru.nhs.uk/pages/PHD/CASP.htm.

The NHS Information Centre (NHS IMC)

This centre is a central and authorative source of health and social care information. Information is sourced to aid local decision makers to improve the quality and efficiency of frontline care. The Information Centre acts as a hub for high-quality, national and comparative data.

The website address is www.ic.nhs.uk.

The National Audit Office (NAO)

This body scrutinises public spending on behalf of Parliament. Currently a review is taking place of the implementation of clinical governance in PCTs – recommendations are published upon the completion of their reports.

The website address is www.nao.org.uk.

The Audit Commission (AC)

This is another independent public body responsible for ensuring that public money is spent economically, efficiently and effectively in health and other areas. Their mission is to be a driving force in the improvement of public services, promoting good practice and helping to achieve better outcomes.

The website address is www.audit-commission.gov.uk.

Good Medical Practice guide

The General Medical Council regularly reviews their *Good Medical Practice* guide, the latest being November 2006 (GMC 2006). The booklet is designed to strengthen the process of professional self-regulation. Its forms the basis of the GMC's medical appraisal scheme and provides advice on how to maintain good practice and what to do in cases of poor practice, the procedures involved and whom to contact.

The website address is www.gmc.co.uk.

Continuing medical education (CME) and continuing professional development (CPD)

Lifelong learning and continuing education is a component part of the maintenance of professional registration. CPD has to be evidenced at performance review and as part of a revalidation programme. NHS organisations are expected to provide programmes for education and training, personnel and organisations, particularly around clinical governance.

Safeguarding Patients

The document *Safeguarding Patients: lessons from the past, proposals for the future*, published in February 2007 (DoH 2007), brings together all the initiatives in this area that have occurred in the last decade. The government published *Safeguarding Patients* as a response to the recommendations of the Shipman Enquiry's fifth report and to the recommendations of the Ayling, Neale and Kerr/Haslam Inquiries in February 2007. (Dr Harold Shipman, a GP from Hyde, murdered around 250 of his patients over a 20-year period). Each of the five inquiries made recommendations to balance the need for additional safeguards for patients with the need to avoid placing unnecessary obstacles in the way of the normal processes of patient care. The embedding of clinical governance within the NHS to promote continuous quality improvement has been driven since the publication of the Shipman Reports, for it is widely accepted that had the systems that have now been introduced been in place at the time of Shipman's crimes, then it would have been highly unlikely that those abuses could have continued for such a long period of time.

The fifth inquiry report recognises that the NHS and the context in which it operates have changed radically since Shipman's crimes came to light.

The overall quality strategy, *A First Class Service* (DoH 1998) was set out in 1998 with explicit standards to be monitored by the then Healthcare Commission. This was preceded by *The New NHS: modern, dependable* in 1997 (DoH 1997). Developments in the regulations of healthcare organisations have continued to evolve, and the central role of clinical governance in assuring quality and promoting quality improvement has been totally embedded within the management structures of healthcare providers. New approaches to the handling of disciplinary and performance issues including the role of the NCAS in both primary and secondary care have been introduced. The patient safety agenda was further launched by *An Organisation with a Memory* in 2000 (DoH 2000).

Increasing recognition has been given to the role of patients' experience and involvement in shaping services, and providing feedback to improve service quality. There has been an increasing movement towards 'a patient-led NHS' and the wider health reform programme.

Recruitment and screening processes for employees in health organisations are now robust, following guidance issued by NHS Employers, a part of the NHS Confederation.

The White Paper from the Department of Health, *Our Health, Our Care, Our Say* (DoH 2006), launched a review of the complaints system. It has been recognised that complaints from patients or their representatives and concerns raised by fellow professionals can provide vital information in identifying potential risks to patient safety.

The safer management of controlled drugs was introduced in 2004, and *Good Doctors, Safer Patients* was published in July 2006 by the Department of Health (DoH 2006).

Licences issued to doctors by the GMC (*see* also Chapter 2, Part 1 – on Licensing and Revalidation) are the beginning of a process to establish 'revalidation and recertification' initiated by the CMO's (DoH 2006) report mentioned above, *Good Doctors, Safer Patients*; followed by the White Paper *Trust, Assurance and Safety*, in February 2007 (DoH 2007); and the CMO's second report, *Medical Revalidations: principles and next steps*, in July 2008 (DoH 2008).

All doctors on the GMC register have been asked to declare whether or not they wish to have a Licence to Practice. In the future, all doctors who wish to perform the clinical functions of a medical practitioner, to write prescriptions, sign death certificates etc., now require a licence. Licences were due to be issued on 16 November 2009. When revalidation and recertification processes commence in 2010 there will be a process of review of appraisals, feedback, patient outcomes and the like by a designated 'Responsible officer', and if approved the doctor will have the licence renewed for a period of five years. The document, *Safeguarding Patients*, published in February 2007 (DoH 2007) brings together all the initiatives that have occurred in the last decade.

High Quality Care for All

In 2008 Lord Darzi published *High Quality Care for All* (Darzi 2008), co-produced with the NHS during a year-long process involving more than 2000 clinicians and 60 000 staff from the NHS, patients, members of the public and other stakeholders. In June 2009 Lord Darzi published a second report: High Quality Care for All: our journey so far (Darzi 2009). These are both available on the Department of Health website www.dh.gov.uk.

Over the last 10 years, the NHS providers have focused on the provision of capacity. This has needed a significant investment in resources (in 1996/7, the budget for the NHS in England was £33 billion and in 2008/09 it is £96 billion) and it is timely therefore to align the system to support the delivery of high-quality care by frontline staff. Care has to be effective, from the start of the intervention, to the clinical procedure the patient receives to their quality of life after their treatment. High-quality care is also about the patient's opinion of the entire experience of the NHS, including their need to be treated with compassion, dignity and respect in a clean, safe and well-managed environment.

The Quality Framework will support local clinical teams to improve the quality of care by:

o bringing clarity to quality – making it easy to access evidence about best practice by asking NICE to develop quality standards
o supporting clinicians to measure quality to support improvement
o requiring quality information to be published, making it available to the public and making it as important to NHS chief executives as it has always been for NHS staff
o rewarding the delivery of high-quality care
o safeguarding basic standards through a new independent regulator, the Care Quality Commission
o staying ahead by ensuring that innovation in medical advances and service design is fostered and promoted
o recognising the role of clinicians as leaders and giving them the freedom to drive improvements in quality of care.

A workforce strategy has been created to support Lord Darzi's report – many of the features described in the report already existed in the NHS but not in any definitive systems – this explains why freeing up staff is such a big theme within the workforce proposals – as it is by unlocking the talents of NHS staff that the *High Quality Care for All* visions can be provided across the board.

However, greater freedom will come with a new and enhanced accountability – for the expectation is to be far more open about the quality of outcomes that are achieved for patients. The workforce strategy also states that there will be strong leadership.

Staff pledges, underpinned by core NHS values and an NHS Constitution, will help to ensure the high-quality workplaces which will be required to deliver the high-quality services. Both the values and the constitution will stretch the system or promote greater engagement with staff and excellence in education and training – all supported by transparent funding and structured career pathways.

The workforce strategy expresses the importance of being responsive to what staff need to succeed in a very important part of getting services to patients right. Workforce systems, including quality-assured, aligned workforce planning and education commissioning plus an increased transparency of reporting will help develop the system as a whole so it is fit to deliver all that is required. All the greater freedoms and accountabilities need to be translated into meaningful and significant outcomes for patients.

Related reading

Darzi A. *High Quality Care for All: NHS Next Stage Review final report*. London: Department of Health, HMSO; 2008. Available online at www.dh.gov.uk/en/publicationsandstatistics/publications/publicationspolicyandguidance/DH_085825

Darzi A. *A Year of Progress towards High Quality Care for All*. London: Department of Health, HMSO; 2009. Available online at www.dh.gov.uk/en/Publicationsandstatistics/Publications/PublicationsPolicyAndGuidance/DH_101670

DoH. *Working for Patients*. London: Department of Health, HMSO; 1989.

DoH. *The New NHS: modern, dependable*. London: Department of Health, HMSO; 1997. Available online at www.dh.gov.uk/en/Publicationsandstatistics/Publications/PublicationsPolicyAndGuidance/DH_4008869

DoH. *A First Class Service: quality in the new NHS*. London: Department of Health, HMSO; 1998. Available online at www.dh.gov.uk/en/publicationsandstatistics/publications/publicationspolicyandguidance/dh_4006902

DoH. *Clinical Governance: quality in the new NHS*. London: Department of Health, HMSO; 1999. Available online at www.dh.gov.uk/en/Publicationsandstatistics/Lettersandcirculars/Healthservicecirculars/DH_4004883

DoH. *An Organisation with a Memory*. London: Department of Health, HMSO; 2000. Available online at www.dh.gov.uk/en/Publicationsandstatistics/Publications/PublicationsPolicyAndGuidance/DH_4065083

DoH. *Choosing Health: making healthy choices easier*. London: Department of Health, HMSO; 2004. Available online at www.dh.gov.uk/en/Publicationsandstatistics/Publications/PublicationsPolicyAndGuidance/DH_4094550

DoH. *Good Doctors, Safer Patients: proposals to strengthen the system to assure and improve the performance of doctors and to protect the safety of patients*. London: Department of Health, HMSO;

2006. Available online at www.dh.gov.uk/en/Publicationsandstatistics/Publications/PublicationsPolicyAndGuidance/DH_4137232

DoH. *Our Health, Our Care, Our Say.* London: Department of Health, HMSO; 2006. Available online at www.dh.gov.uk/en/Healthcare/ourhealthourcareoursay/index.htm

DoH. *Professional Standards Programme: responses to the Shipman Inquiries, including Kerr/Haslam, Neale and Ayling Inquiries.* London: Department of Health, HMSO; 2007. Available online at www.dh.gov.uk/en/Managingyourorganisation/Humanresourcesandtraining/Modernisingprofessionalregulation/DH_085914

DoH. *Safeguarding Patients: lessons from the past, proposals for the future.* London: Department of Health, HMSO; 2007. Available online at www.dh.gov.uk/en/Publicationsandstatistics/Publications/PublicationsPolicyAndGuidance/DH_065953

DoH. *Trust, Assurance and Safety: the regulation of health professionals.* London: Department of Health, HMSO; 2007. Available online at www.dh.gov.uk/en/Publicationsandstatistics/Publications/PublicationsPolicyAndGuidance/DH_065946

DoH. *Medical Revalidation: principles and next steps: the Report of the Chief Medical Officer for England's Working Group.* London: Department of Health. HMSO; 2008. Available online at www.dh.gov.uk/en/Publicationsandstatistics/Publications/PublicationsPolicyAndGuidance/DH_086430

GMC. *Good Medical Practice.* London: General Medical Council; 2006.

Health Act 1999. Available online at www.opsi.gov.uk/acts/acts1999/ukpga_19990008_en_1

Muir Gray JA. *Evidence-based Healthcare: how to make health policy and management decisions.* London: Churchill Livingstone; 1997.

NHSE. *Clinical Governance: quality in the new NHS.* (HSC 1999/0065). London. HMSO; 1999.

NICE. *Handbook to Help NHS Staff Improve Standards Following the Bristol Royal Inquiry.* London: NICE & CHI; 2002. Available online at www.nice.org.uk/newsroom/pressreleases/pressreleasearchive/pressreleases2002/2002_014_nice__chi_launch_handbook_to_help_nhs_staff_improve_standards_following_the_bristol_royal_inquiry.jsp

Scally G, Donaldson LJ. Clinical governance and the drive for quality improvement in the new NHS in England. *BMJ.* 1998; **317**: 61–5.

Vincent C, Neale G, Woloshynowych M. Adverse events in British hospitals: preliminary retrospective record review. *BMJ.* 2001; **322**: 517–19.

The future

In this chapter I split our survey of the future into consideration of the NHS and healthcare systems in general, particularly with regards to structures and resources and how those resources are found and managed. Then I consider the hospitals and their future roles separately from new technology. Finally, I consider the changes facing the profession.

One of the most common questions asked at workshops I have run and attended is along the lines of 'What is going to happen in the future?' I have no crystal ball, but I have had the opportunity to do a little research for you into this question. In earlier editions I dealt with this question in a small section in Chapter 1. In this edition I give it a separate chapter because of the concern around it and because so much is now being written about it whether from governments, the DoH, academics or just interested observers. In the previous chapter I have already set out some of the immediate developments that are being introduced now. Here I concentrate on what may happen next. And don't forget that with every new Secretary of State for Health there will always be new initiatives and change.

If you feel that change is a new issue, you need look no further than *The Principles and Practice of Medicine* by William Osler (1895) who wrote over 100 years ago, 'Everywhere the old order changes and happy those who change with it.' And indeed change in medicine as elsewhere is older even than that. Hippocrates (c. 460–377 BC) is generally credited with the foundation of modern medicine when he developed a new approach to medicine by refusing to use gods to explain illnesses and disease. This changed medicine radically in that it came to be seen as a science rather than a religion. In effect he managed a major change 2400 years ago.

In 1999 a paper in the *BMJ* said: 'Research into the running and planning of hospital services has been neglected, surprising given the importance of hospitals for the public, politicians, and healthcare.' Since then I have detected a large rise in papers and discussion of the future of hospitals and medicine.

Healthcare is generally accepted to be complex and interlinked, but some services are completely unrelated. Thus facilities need to be decentralised but adjacent. This is a gross oversimplification of course, but it's like the advice for your desk or work station: if you use it every day keep it within arm's reach; if you use it monthly put it in a file; and if you use the same group of things together only once a month put them all in a box in your drawer.

Changing cultures and expectations

Cultural shift caused by societal, individual, political or professional change has tended to try to decentralise power and influence, and increase user involvement, leading in policy-making to different expectations of healthcare. Social changes must be taken into account in both the domestic and working environment. Increasing patient expectations and patient autonomy, together with the information revolution that allows individuals greater access to global information, are drivers for change in the responsiveness of professionals. There is also rising demand due to ageing and medical advances.

The NHS has plans for reform and outlined visions of a health service designed around the patient that covers:

- a new delivery system for the NHS
- changes between health and social services
- changes for NHS doctors, nurses, midwives, therapists and other NHS staff
- changes for patients
- changes in the relationship between the NHS and the private sector.

NHS resources

If you read *The New NHS* (Talbot-Smith and Pollock 2006) or the White Paper *Our Health, Our Care* (DoH 2006) it appears at first glance that the government intends to contract out commissioning functions and budgets of PCTs to the private sector through practiced-based commissioning (*see* Chapter 1, p. 37), where providers of GP services will hold the budget and commission all medical services, including primary care, community health services and hospital care. This would mean the private sector commissioning secondary care services for patients, although possibly the emphasis would be on the private sector taking over the community services, not all the budgets.

The DoH is already working with a number of organisations and PCTs are already contracting with private companies such as United Health Europe and Kaiser Permanente to operate GP practices and provide community health services through practice-based commissioning so that they will become healthcare commissioners for the patients in their care. Indeed the Mid Surrey PCT provided an example of the first management buyout of community health services by NHS staff.

The future of general practice

It is important to stress here that this chapter is not the author's views of the future but a distillation of the literature on the subject. Much is written about the future of general practice and it seems that the future of general practice is clearer than other areas of medicine. Governments will always want to cut costs and they could try to 'flood the market' with new GPs by increasing GP training numbers and medical student output so that unemployment will eventually drive doctors into salaried posts with alternate provider medical services (APMS). Or they could even get physician assistants to compete with doctors for such work.

Primary care trusts could then put practices out to tender and offer contracts to the cheapest APMS who may turn them into polyclinics staffed with cheaper salaried doctors, physicians' assistants, medical care practitioners or advanced nurse practitioners. Nurse practitioners are already employed in general practice. It seems that all 152 PCTs in the UK have already received instructions to set up such polyclinics.

The other thing of note is that Darzi polyclinics are not being built in remote, under-serviced areas but amid areas of heavily populated existing surgeries, and as Professor Pollock (2006) said, 'Of most concern is the fact that no standards for quality of care are laid down for APMS providers. Their regulation will be through the contract that may never even see the light of day if deemed to be commercially confidential.'

So the future could see the end of the generalist and the rise of salaried doctors working for APMS polyclinics run by managers. The US is said to be 20 years ahead of the UK in this and so provides a window into the future of medicine. Patients in the US are not registered with a family physician; they see a paediatrician for children with upper respiratory infections for example, an obstetrician and gynaecologist for antenatal care, smear tests etc., and an endocrinologist for diabetes. The family doctor is an employee of an APMS and works much like a junior working for a mini hospital/polyclinic covering their own admissions, doing rounds on their patients, running morning and afternoon clinics and being on call.

The future of general hospitals

Already acute services privatised by transfers to private providers account for 15% of elective surgery and further transfers will include pathology and radiology. The NHS may well become a mere funder of healthcare with control over resource allocation devolved to the private or voluntary sector. Whether they are for-profit or not-for-profit organisations the logic may be that they will concentrate on profitable treatments and services and avoid the least profitable and attempts may be made to restrict access or cap prices. There may be a move away from services related to needs and universal access.

Further, there may be a move from free at point of delivery to provide additional resources by introducing user fees such as hotel costs, and enhanced services with top-up fees, superior packages, with perhaps MRI scans and dermatology by passing waiting lists and going privately. A scheme might then involve vouchers for use in funding basic care, allowing people to pay extra for additional care. So by the introduction of top-up fees, choice may come to mean choice of level of care.

Some authorities write of their belief that even the future of district general hospitals (DGHs) (Ham 2005), the traditional historic backbone of NHS hospital care, are at risk under the government's healthcare reforms. The threat is perceived to come from independent providers together with the public's increasing promise and expectations of choice. It is possible that with pressure from limited budgets some services may become uneconomical in hospitals struggling to achieve financial balance, particularly with future Private Finance Initiative (PFI) and Public Private Partnership (PPP) 'mortgage' commitments.

A range of strategies seems likely for dealing with this. Hospitals could compete aggressively for their market share, but this might not be financially sustainable. An alternative would be to reduce some services and focus on better productivity in areas of competitive advantage. More complex arrangements for the commissioning of care through independent networks of doctors and other professionals seems likely to follow. Another strategy might be for some hospitals to diversify their services; for example, into only sub-acute and primary care. Some writers already see this beginning to happen.

What seems certain, however, is that district general hospitals will have to compete with other NHS hospitals, NHS treatment centres, independent sector treatment centres, and established private hospitals. This could destabilise the NHS and will need careful management, although the problem might be whether all this has been fully thought through. Even Professor Darzi in his report *High Quality Care for All* (2008) argued that 'The days of the district general hospital seeking to provide all services to a high enough standard are over' with polyclinics now expected to deliver standards of treatments that until now have been provided by specialist surgical staff in hospital.

Discussions about the hospital of the future often tend to revolve around technology, things such as:

o genomics (areas of biological investigation related to the development and application of cutting-edge technology, related not only to cancer treatments but other diseases)
o robotic surgery
o integrated patient records.

It seems inevitable that advanced technology will make future improvements possible, but our research suggests that experts on the subject think the hospital of the future will be based on improvements to care rather than technology. Indeed, this focus will result in changes to a hospital's physical space, staffing strategies and patient care models.

Resource developments in primary care will also create further pressure for change in the structure of hospital provision. So looking at examples of hospitals that have already moved in that direction, what might future hospitals look like? I have identified a number of headings, some interrelated, that appear in papers, reviews and reports, as follows.

Hospital roles

Healthcare systems across the world face a challenging problem, for in order for healthcare to meet changing needs and to improve health, the traditional district general hospital needs to change. The Institute for Public Policy Research (IPPR) have published a report, *The Future Hospital: the politics of change* (Farrington-Douglas and Brooks 2007) and is one attempt to discuss this subject; further reading is available at sources listed in the related reading list at the end of this chapter.

The IPPR report explains that healthcare needs to adapt as health needs change and as the technologies and techniques of delivering modern care develop. Healthcare provision needs to change, with wide-ranging effects on the location and functions of district hospitals. They argue that changes to health services should be driven by progressive objectives. In particular, changes should aim to:

o   improve safety
o   improve access
o   increase efficiency
o   prevent ill health
o   raise responsiveness
o   reduce inequity and inequalities.

However, the progressive changes that IPPR advocates are, they say, hampered by a damaging and dysfunctional politics associated with changes to hospitals. At present, the best outcomes from the health system are not being achieved, nor are they achieving public engagement and confidence in the NHS. The public do not trust the process of hospital change.

The Future Hospital project at IPPR aims to develop a new process and politics of change through which changes to the health system provide safe, equitable, efficient and accessible care, while engaging the public and maintaining confidence in the NHS.

Everybody seems agreed that healthcare is changing and hospitals need to adapt. But hospitals tend to be popular local institutions, so making changes can be difficult politically. The IPPR feel that even the role of hospitals is not a simple one, as differing stakeholders have varying priorities while the public values a range of roles for their hospitals.

One other issue that has been raised is that while hospitals may contribute to improving health and even reducing inequalities, their impact on public health is limited. They could be described as providing a health 'rescue' function for life-threatening conditions and improving outcomes by concentrating technology and expertise. So for that role hospitals will continue to have an important place.

Current thinking is that the NHS should do more to prevent ill health, by being proactive and helping people avoid the need for hospital treatment. Thus what is seen and described as a preventative, equitable NHS would prioritise towards primary and community care, with the hospital sector providing more complex treatment at a safe and efficient level of specialisation.

But this introduces another paradox. The public probably assumes their local hospital will provide a full range of services, all safe, where more can be done for patients with what were previously disabling or life-threatening conditions. In order to provide this complex healthcare safely, however, teams need to see sufficient numbers of particular conditions, so it is probable that all treatments cannot be provided at all DGHs because there will not be enough patients for teams to maintain their skills. Based on this assumption, it is no longer sustainable to maintain some services in all DGHs. And this before any account is taken of hospitals perhaps using locum staff or doctors working long hours and the results of the European Working Time Directive (EWTD). So the argument goes that more lives could be saved if some services were centralised in specialist hospitals.

However, to return to the theme of healthcare moving priorities towards health rather than illness, while some services will need to be more centralised and some other services will need to continue to be provided at the DGH much more could be provided more locally in community hospitals or GP surgeries. Outpatient diagnostic and routine surgery could be provided more locally. So although life-saving emergency care would still be centralised, minor injuries and health problems that it is said make up the majority of A&E cases could be provided locally.

A further factor in considering such a system moving towards health rather than illness care is that when people are living longer more patients are likely to be living with long-term health needs. These are not thought to be well met by hospitals focused on short-term acute treatment. So providing ongoing support and management of long-term conditions in the community and at home is a better approach than waiting for acute flare-ups and regular emergency readmission. Hence the shifting of resources from hospitals to community services it is felt will ensure that the NHS can care better for the future patient, preventing the need for hospital care and improving well-being.

So the thinking progresses to consider that more important than local access to hospitals is ensuring that primary care is more easily accessible, particularly for disadvantaged groups. More care provided in the community or at home. People should only be kept in hospital for the minimum time necessary for their treatment. More patients should be seen as day cases, rather than being admitted the day before or staying in hospital after their operation. The aim is to 'improve efficiency and productivity' but is likely to lead to and require reductions in hospital bed numbers.

Hence the stress (Darzi 2008) on improving the accessibility of primary care, with polyclinics, especially in deprived areas, particularly out of hours, so that people do not go to hospital unnecessarily, seen as a key success factor. In order to shift from an acute to a primary and community-led health service, the current reliance on hospitals needs to be reversed. And accepting that not all community facilities are in the right place or the right buildings, everyone needs to be able to see improvements in community services to justify accepting changes to their DGH.

While the present choices available to patients have not so far resulted in enough patients choosing alternative hospitals to have much impact, in the future Darzi (2008) foresees that some hospitals will need to expand or contract, depending on the movement of patients around the healthcare system. Even where patients do not significantly switch between hospitals or where patient choice is more restricted in

Wales, Scotland and Northern Ireland, hospitals will still need to respond to changing needs and to challenges to hospital configuration.

When considering efficiency, effectiveness, responsiveness and quality it is often suggested that some competition in healthcare may improve these factors. But it is stressed as important that competition does not prevent the collaboration that is required to achieve the progressive and useful change, a further dilemma considered elsewhere in this chapter.

In the past hospitals traditionally set up their services on the basis that most service is dominated by inpatient and outpatient care, but authorities claim that strategy has never received critical attention. Outpatient care developments are suggested to be uncoordinated. Evidence suggests that currently outpatient care will grow much faster than inpatient care and certain outpatient services will grow extra fast; for example, radiology, some surgical procedures and oncology will increase dramatically.

A two-day stay may become the norm with two-day discharges perhaps tripling in 10 years. These changes will require hospitals to organise staffing, work flow and dedicated units solely for the two-day patient.

The vision you will find reflected in the Darzi Report is that hospitals already offer compassionate care as a given, but tomorrow's patients will want much more. Keeping patients safe and offering the latest treatment options will also be taken as a given and will increasingly be demanded in a transparent, competitive healthcare world. So hospitals will no longer be expected to just diagnose, prescribe and undertake surgeries, but will be expected to become part of wellness centres, part hospital, part investigative centre, part hospice, part nursing school, part medical school and part group medical centre. In short, patients and their families will find integrated features from across the provider spectrum.

Hospital technology

There exist technological forces for change, such as minimally invasive therapies, diagnostic scanning techniques, microchip technology, advances in biotechnical diagnostic testing, more finely targeted drugs, together with new drug delivery systems and, perhaps, routine genetic therapy.

One such advance was 'telemedicine' where the patient consults the doctor from home via a video link, which incorporates special sensors to relay vital signs. There are now cases of robotic surgeons controlled by experts on the other side of the world successfully operating on patients.

The telephone has long been used to monitor the heart, and patients are now able to send a 30-second recording for analysis by a doctor. Follow-up telephone consultations at pre-agreed times to discuss progress mean that patients don't have to journey to the outpatients and the results have already been published. Certain specialties such as rheumatology, dermatology and neurology are more suited to this approach, and many centres already carry out post-op follow-ups, particularly for day surgery patients.

Technology is also being used to make changes to reduce workload and reduce staff levels. Hospital beds, operating tables and trolleys could be wheeled around the corridors by robots as a universal piece of equipment. A sophisticated life support and transport unit (designed for use under battlefield conditions and commercialised after the turn of the century) was the forerunner of this mobile bed. The apparatus combines aerospace materials, information processing and systems integration technologies in a unit that is capable of autonomous function. With embedded sensors, it monitors vital signs and blood chemistries, and is equipped to provide mechanical, sensor-controlled ventilation, suction, IV infusion and cardiac defibrillation. It is used for surgery and then, after a change of linen, is moved to a recovery area, all the time providing continuous monitoring by smart sensors that can respond by activating a programmed countermeasure. A central ICU is no longer needed for monitoring acutely ill and postoperative patients, reducing the threat of cross infection.

The cardiac catheter laboratory has entered the age of molecular cardiology, drugs, having reduced the incidence of atherosclerosis, can also dissolve plaques and clots, and the number of patients requiring coronary angioplasty has dwindled. Instead, sensor-directed catheters are used to deliver angiogenesis factors and cultivated myocardial cells to ischaemic and damaged heart muscle. A few patients have been treated with recently developed sensor-based micromachines that can remove plaque from within clogged coronaries.

Hospital economics

By economics I mean the need for increasing efficiency and reducing costs because of the high costs and diversity of new procedures and complications. A recent paper suggesting that hospitals must respond in new ways to meet the increasing complexity of patient care and to address rising healthcare costs caused some observers to comment that consideration of both together was a recent new phenomenon.

Hospital patient-centred care

While patient-centred care may be thought of as philosophically at the core of any relationship between patient, hospital and doctor, it will become increasingly more common to involve patients in decisions. It is said that hospitals' most innovative qualities will be ones of process and culture. Take admitting as an example. There will be no admissions office, admitting desk or place or information desk. People entering the hospital are greeted and escorted or directed to their destination depending on whether they are a patient or visitor. A patient checking in will have a greeter to escort them directly to the inpatient room where an admitting nurse will check them in. All registration in the building is done at point of service.

Hospital staffing

All hospitals currently tend to suffer staff shortages, which causes more work for the existing staff, and longer waits for patients. Scientists think that the future lies in the hands of robotics. (See also above under technology.) Prototypes have already been used in hospitals, but the technology community sees robotics taking an even stronger hand, with robotic nurses. In the US an IWARD project goal is to have three working prototypes available of different robots designated to different nursing responsibilities by 2010. These 'nurbots', as they like to call them, 'will be able to mop floors, talk to patients, and guide visitors to rooms'.

Eventually, the plan would be to have a fully integrated information system with guide points, producing an intelligence system that would make the entire hospital an interactive part of the system. Fortunately, these nurbots are not designed to take the place of nurses, but to let the staff spend more time with the patient.

Hospital design

I'm not sure you will be particularly interested to know much about this. Suffice to say that writers envisage that hospital entrances will be bright, open, spacious places and patient rooms will be more private and large enough to accommodate patient families around the clock, and it is suggested that the layout of each room should be identical and standardised to 'decrease inefficiency and reduce errors'. However, in the writings about this no mention is ever made of the need for cost cutting in the straitened circumstances the economy is now in.

Hospitals move to outpatient treatments

I've already mentioned the move to outpatient treatments, particularly related to new technologies. Here are some of the examples I have read about.

- Outpatients provided with smart pacemakers, artificial retinas, and chemical sensors seen in local primary care clinics. The doctor or nurse obtains online information about any patient's blood chemistries, electrocardiograms, blood pressure and temperature.
- A diabetic patient freed from diabetes-related medical problems after having a smart glucose sensor and insulin reservoir system implanted.
- A healthy-looking patient with transfusion-related AIDS managed by a smart viral count sensor integrated with an implanted reservoir containing medication.
- A smart sensor and drug reservoir system has been equally effective in the management of a patient whose dysfunctional manic-depressive illness is now modulated by chemical sensors that catch the beginning of chemical imbalance and actuate the injection of appropriate drugs.
- Home healthcare telemedicine and sensor technologies have moved the outpatient laboratory and the GP surgery into the living room. Interactive video conferencing, educational programmes and a broad range of sensors now provide healthcare at a distance.
- Ambulatory treatment with smart blood pressure sensors manage the medication for patients with hypertension and send an immediate alert to the central monitoring unit when integrated sensors for cardiac function and vital signs indicate an unexpected problem.
- A 'gut program' detects the start of episodes of diarrhoea in a patient with irritable bowel syndrome, allowing him or her to terminate them abruptly by pressing a subcutaneous reservoir of drugs.

The future of doctors

In the US, it is said that some 20 conditions account for 80% of healthcare expenditure and 70% of personal healthcare expenditure is used on those with chronic conditions, so this has implications for clinical practice and therefore the NHS. It has therefore been suggested that healthcare provision needs to be organised around the needs of those with chronic disabilities, perhaps with more integration of primary, secondary and social care. Sir Cyril Chantler in the 2002 Harveian Oration (a lecture at the Royal college of Physicians, London) asked if the traditional divide between GPs and hospital consultants was still helpful in an age of teamwork and flexibility in the NHS, and suggested that maybe the time has come to discard the term 'consultant' in favour of the word 'specialist'.

Sir Cyril went on to identify three paradoxes at the heart of modern medical practice:

o doctors have never before been able to do so much for patients, yet not since the advent of the NHS have we been so criticised and perhaps so unhappy
o we spend massive amounts on the NHS but continue to be short of resources
o in spite of such spending and the successes of modern medicine, the prevalence of disability and illness continues to rise.

Some of these paradoxes stem from the benefits of medicine itself – people are living with disability whereas before they would have died, the achievements of medicine are leading to greater expectations and the plethora of new drugs and treatments puts more pressure on budgets. Sir Cyril also draws out the need for doctors to take a lead in their organisation of care, while continuing to conduct research, not only in the biomedical field but on how better to deliver care to patients.

He concluded:

> We shall need help. Doctors in the NHS are under great pressure, we need more understanding and less criticism, more trust and less regulation. Perhaps the public, government and profession need, as has been suggested, a new concordat that sets out the rights and responsibilities of each and maybe explicitly recognises the limits of what the NHS can provide and what modern medicine can achieve.

There is also a change occurring with the people going into medicine, according to a recent study published in the *JAMA*. It found that an increasing number were picking their specialty based on the lifestyle it permitted, including more time to spend with the family, rather than on such traditional factors as pay and prestige. It was not the number of hours or the intensity of the work, but the ability to go home at the end of the day and be away from any professional responsibilities.

This trend may represent the increasing number of women in the profession, who seek a closer balance between family and professional duties. But the findings point to potential shortages of doctors in specialties, such as surgery and obstetrics, as newly qualified doctors shun fields where they are required to be on call for many hours. These critical shortages may begin to appear in as little as 10 years in some areas.

Previous studies had detected this trend, with students more inclined to select specialties with fewer work hours per week and fewer nights on call. This study showed that 55% of students' choices related to lifestyle factors, compared to 9% basing their decisions on potential income. As well as the increasing number of women doctors it also foresaw that a loss of decision making to insurance companies and treatment protocols were likely to exacerbate the trend.

There has been particular interest recently, perhaps as a response to cultural changes or professional anxiety, in several reviews of the role of and future of the doctor. There have been reports and statements on 'the role of the doctor', 'medical professionalism' and 'the future doctor'. Certainly, I have found many doctors are unhappy, feel disempowered, alienated from the system in which they work, and often yearning after a lost age when things were different.

Many health managers see doctors as part of the healthcare problem rather than part of the solution, doctors as barriers to change rather than drivers of change. These problems are true everywhere and not just a British phenomenon and perhaps as Smith (2009) put it, must 'stem in part from a gap between what doctors are trained for and the world they inhabit'.

Interestingly, nearly all articles title doctor in the singular person and thus there is a danger of thinking of the need for one kind of future doctor. Doctors do many different things, and the skills needed to be successful in public health are quite different from those needed by a neurosurgeon. Indeed a past Dean of St Mary's used to argue that medical students should be randomly picked from those reaching a minimum academic standard so that a wide range of skills and attitudes were selected, a process that avoided a row of elderly male doctors picking students in their own image.

We may also see a continuing move away from professional self-regulation towards more direct accountability. Indeed, since the previous edition there have been dramatic changes in the GMC's role and the introduction of revalidation for continued registration of all doctors (*see* Chapter 2 in Part 1). The careers of consultants will change, as the position may no longer represent the pinnacle for hospital doctors. Having reached consultant level they will have various branches to follow: towards clinical director in service work, teaching, research or management; medical director and even chief executive.

There is one final issue that is still being resolved: the move from a consultant-led to a consultant-delivered service and what kind of doctor should deliver care in the NHS. Clearly, the policy is now defined that care should be consultant-delivered. However, this does not necessarily mean that consultants should carry out every assessment or procedure. Care should be delivered by fully trained specialists (called consultants in the UK) and by those training to be consultants, a model found in most first-world countries. What NHS employers want and understand may be different as they are also concerned about the cost of a consultant-delivered service. It is possibly the responsibility of the medical profession to show that a consultant/trainee-only service will not only provide the requisite high standards but will also be cost-effective.

GMC and *Tomorrow's Doctors*

In September 2009 the General Medical Council released its publication *Tomorrow's Doctors: outcomes and standards for undergraduate medical education*. This specifies the duties of a doctor registered with the GMC. It updates the 2003 version and sets out some new GMC requirements to ensure medical students have more opportunity to apply their knowledge and skills in hospitals and surgeries before graduation. It introduces new, more rigorous standards for the delivery of medical education with a stronger emphasis on equality and diversity, involving employers and patients, the professional development of teaching staff, and ensuring that students derive maximum benefit from their clinical placements. It also places emphasis on NHS employing organisations that provided input into the earlier consultation leading to publication, emphasising service and patient requirements for the doctors of the future.

The new GMC standards have implications for resources and priorities, both for medical schools and for the NHS. It introduces student assistantships undertaken before a graduate student enters year FT1. Designed to help students become more familiar with work in a hospital or community setting and to understand practical tasks such as filling in a prescription form or ordering a blood sample, the standards will assist a junior doctor become familiar with the workplace and undertake supervised procedures. The publication can be read or downloaded at www.gmc-uk.org/education/documents/GMC_TD_2009.pdf.

Attributes for future doctors

By taking information from a wide range of sources I have tried to put together a list of attributes that are currently considered essential for modern doctors.

- **Comfortable with the collection, analysis and interpretation of data:** No longer does a doctor rely on what has been described as the 'magic' or 'art' of healing, where the power of the doctor is all, because although that was once all doctors had in their armoury there is now often a range of effective treatments. So you must have an understanding of evidence, not just of hierarchies of evidence and randomised controlled trials but of how to combine many different sorts of evidence, weighting them effectively. This is hard, and most doctors still need help, so you will need to understand the questions to ask and that you may still need help.
- **Comfort with technology:** Linked to the above and particularly with information technology and a recognition that you plus technology will be much more effective than you alone. Patients increasingly use the Internet to access information and are confronted by a maze of sometimes conflicting information. Future doctors may not be telling patients what to do but helping them navigate through the maze of information. In the past doctors have stressed 'diagnosis, diagnosis, diagnosis' as a key task. Although still true, it will be a much more complex diagnosis on multiple levels, with the help of machines and computers that will also contribute to treatment and action plans.
- **Patient-centred:** Truly and even to a point that may be uncomfortable. Patients will make choices that seem wrong and even stupid to doctors. Doctors will need to accept the authority and autonomy of patients and families in a wholly new

concept of dominance and knowledge. As one writer put it, 'doctors are guests in patients' lives not priests in a cathedral of technology'. There must be a willingness to trade privilege for reliability, providing not just your best but the world's best.

o **Communication skills:** Listening more than telling because of the above. Not developed further here as it is the subject of the first four chapters in Part 1.

o **Health adviser and well-being coach:** No longer just using science to treat people's diseases but being experts on helping people to live healthier lives and adapt to the chronic disease that will be their lot as they age.

o **Teamwork:** Not dominating teams but being part of them and understanding what makes effective teams – because many teams are ineffective; doctors will no longer be lone actors but important players in increasingly complex systems. Future doctors will need to understand the complex systems and know how to work with and improve them. A lot of this is not part of the current trend towards touchy-feely skills but a set of highly technical skills that can be learned and taught. It will involve both leadership and followership skills and these can both be taught, and most doctors will need to be leaders and followers at different times. This will demand a love of diversity and enjoying working with people from different backgrounds and of different views and skills, and recognising that together we are stronger.

o **Technically aware:** Because although it is unlikely that in the near future robots will perform procedures alone, doctors probably will be aided by robots.

o **A capacity to change:** Will be vital as it is certain that healthcare in, say, 30–40 years from now, when many current medical students and junior doctors will still be practising, is going to be very different. Future doctors will probably need more than a capacity for change; they will need an enthusiasm for change.

o **Profound ethical understanding:** Including recognition of the omnipresence and increasing importance of ethical issues and involving a capacity to think ethically.

o **Enthusiasm for lifelong learning:** But we must not only continue to learn, we must love to learn.

o **Doctors as managers:** Will be responsible for much more than the care of individual patients and will need to be aware of and maybe manage resources and staff. Doctors' roles in management will continue to develop, as interested parties demand that doctors fulfil their roles with skill. As Plato said, quoting Protagoras in the fifth century: 'Of all things the measure is man: of things that are, that they are, and of things that are not, that they are not.'

Staffing will remain the key, for even with the most sophisticated technical advances there will always be the need for human contact. There will be staffing changes and there are already shortages of both nurses and doctors. Adequate staffing levels may, however, be interpreted and reacted to differently by governments, patients and healthcare professionals.

Doctors will need to understand quality assurance in order to contribute to improving systems. This could make practising more rather than less fulfilling. There will be access to more effective treatments than there is now.

There will be a need to enhance and maybe develop new competencies, co-operation, teamwork, inquiry and communication, skills described as less to know answers than to find answers in a world of rapid expansion of new knowledge displacing the old.

Standing Medical Advisory Committee (SMAC)

SMAC was a statutory advisory NDPB (now abolished) established in 1949 as one of nine separate bodies to advise the Minister and the (then) Central Health Services Committee on matters relating to services provided under the National Health Service Act 1946. In 2001 the DoH published *Doctors for the Future: advice by the SMAC*, which it felt would enable doctors to have satisfying careers in the future and outline what changes might be necessary in the ways they work, bearing in mind the apparent shortage of doctors to implement the NHS Plan. Although SMAC is now abolished, I thought it worthwhile giving some space to the findings from this document as feedback at workshops has shown that one issue that often dominates questions is 'the future', and its finding serves to reiterate and reinforce some of the research into the future plans outlined above and show that some of the issues raised are not new.

The background to the document was an apparent shortage of doctors, threatening implementation of the NHS Plan. Further shortening of hours for both career doctors and trainees makes the outlook bleak, but with major innovative changes in recruiting, retention and support for doctors who will be working in more flexible ways, the decline can be prevented.

It recognised that the great majority of doctors are committed to the NHS and it is their commitment and out-of-hours work that is one of the major factors that has enabled the NHS to reach its present state of development.

However, at the time of the report there were many unfilled consultant posts and although it has been estimated that 10 000 new GPs would be needed to implement the plan, only 110 had been recruited over the previous year. Even more worrying is the fact that 20–30% of GPs intend to retire before the age of 60 and many consultants are retiring around the age of 60 instead of 65. The loss of expertise and experience is profound. Doctors are enthusiastic about change and flexibility once they are convinced it really will enhance patient care rather than divert doctors' skills and time into apparently unproductive avenues.

In order to avert a crisis and improve the health service, the SMAC identified five areas for doctors' careers that needed to be addressed urgently:
1 the role of doctors in the future
2 recruitment of medical students
3 undergraduate and postgraduate training
4 flexibility in career path
5 retention of older doctors.

Doctors' role in the future

It was the part on doctors' roles in the future that is pertinent to this section and that I summarise here. Doctors are trained to understand, in depth, the aetiology, pathology, natural history and epidemiology of disease as well as the diagnosis and treatment of sick patients. This is so that they can manage the huge areas of uncertainty in diagnosis and discuss treatments with patients who present with symptoms, when the number of treatment options is progressively increasing. Doctors need to understand what patients want to achieve from treatment.

Doctors have no monopoly of caring and are part of an interdisciplinary team but their main role has been the differential diagnosis of disease and the planning of care pathways in collaboration with the patient.

Patients want someone to be in overall charge of their illness even if that person is not delivering all or most of that care. Doctors also are strongly committed to 'continuity of care', but continuity of care is not the same as continuous care, which will be completely impossible under the EWTD; doctors must find new methods of ensuring continuity as well as continuing to assume legal responsibility.

This may mean doctors focusing on the role and skills they can best provide, leaving other aspects of care to those who might be better qualified to deliver it.

The papers discussed what would give doctors satisfying careers and what would encourage doctors to continue working, particularly for the NHS. Also how the career structure for doctors might change and become more flexible and how the roles of doctors will and could change.

Recruitment

The SMAC publication asked, 'Who are we recruiting for medicine?' It stated that the applications for medical school were falling and their nature changing:

o the younger generation's attitude to work is different
o younger people in general want more regular hours
o more applicants are now women, so we have to make careers appropriate for them.

It felt that because there is a range of specialties in medicine that a range of people with differing talents (not necessarily all with 4 A* levels) and interests could contribute to medicine in a variety of ways. Special access schemes could be used more widely. These schemes might even become the main way to enter medicine in the future.

More effort could be made to attract students trained and developed from other backgrounds without poaching professionals in other specialties (e.g. nurses) and cause shortages there. The selection procedures could select for more variety in types with characteristics suited to the different specialties.

Undergraduate and postgraduate training

The SMAC discussed postgraduate training, recommending a sea change with regard to flexible and part-time training.

They defined what the training is for values and ethics as well as science. On the subject of ethics there was an interesting study in the *International Journal of Health Services* in 2007 that suggested that in addition to doctors being taught military medical ethics the broader problem of dual loyalty needs to be addressed when doctors' advocacy for the patient conflicts with other institutional or societal objectives. In other words, as medical students they should be taught how they can and should stand up to health plans, the military, HMOs, drug makers, the government or any other entity that asks doctors to violate medical ethics. Indeed the American Medical Association supported comprehensive medical education that keeps pace with the ethical challenges facing doctors. It was felt that medical students should graduate with enough ethical education to stiffen their resolve when institutions ask them to do the wrong thing.

Doctors are currently judged as competent at the end of their training largely on the basis of theoretical knowledge and technical ability. SMAC believes the current lengthy training period may reduce flexibility, harm teamwork, create rigidity in attitudes and has a deleterious effect on staffing in the NHS. In other words, there is a need to train for jobs that are doable and not for jobs which one might eventually be asked to do (when further training could be arranged and indeed should be available through lifelong learning).

Mentoring was a model that a number of members of SMAC had used or were using. SMAC recommended its more widespread use, not just for problems but for the whole of people's careers.

Information technology has a vital way of supporting clinical practice, and becoming familiar with the possibilities and technology will ultimately support doctors.

Flexibility in career path

SMAC considered how doctors make career choices, an important topic affecting recruitment into specialties. Aspirations tend to be traditional, with most doctors wanting to be GPs, surgeons or physicians. It highlighted difficulties in recruiting into some specialties, some not known or experienced by undergraduates, while others (e.g. psychiatry) are known but are perceived as more arduous or less attractive. It suggested that undergraduates need to know what different specialties involve at some stage of their undergraduate training and have some experience of all different branches of medicine.

On the issue of what makes for interesting careers for doctors, SMAC feels strongly that quality of care relates to values, commitment and enthusiasm. It is vital to take careers seriously and be proactive about managing careers. A good career is not necessarily one that relies on rising up the career hierarchy – increasing satisfaction can be achieved by lateral moves. The work–life balance is important and not something which all doctors are good at.

Retention of older doctors

Retention of specialists and GPs was identified as becoming an increasing problem. Whereas once doctors retired at the usual retirement age of 65, now they are seeking to retire earlier, so it is important to create interesting jobs throughout doctors' careers.

Doctors might also be encouraged to stay by the prospect of more flexible working patterns, improved staffing levels, preservation of pension rights for part-time working, fewer NHS administrative changes and greater professional freedom. Experience was recognised as a very important aspect of medicine and the years between 50 and 65 are particularly important in many ways to the service. The SMAC thought it important to focus on the needs of those doctors of 55 plus as their requirements of jobs may change at that stage of their careers and accommodating to their changing needs may be one way to retain them.

Doctors are faced with high demand but little ability to control their workloads and are thus liable to burn out or disengage. They do need greater control over their workload and to feel valued. The UK Medical Careers Research Group findings support GPs' expressed views. One way of enabling doctors to feel valued is to create the right type of appraisal system that enhances medical practice rather than makes doctors feel overburdened by it. One way of reducing a burden might be to consider ways of reducing time spent on less challenging, more routine activities and promote career opportunities for people approaching retirement.

SMAC felt that increasing bureaucracy might in part be due to the gap between decision makers and doctors providing the service. So it is inevitable that service providers should think of it as part of their job to become more involved in policy setting and decision making. However, the effect on clinicians of taking on managerial roles can all too often result in deskilling clinicians who are regarded as neither clinicians nor professional managers. SMAC points out the need for excellent clinical leadership, with the right level of support to enable clinical leaders to do excellent jobs.

Doctors' work is skewed by a huge number of targets they have to achieve, including those arising from the cancer plan. Targets are more easily applied to clear-cut treatments like minor surgery or time to be seen in A&E, but a large proportion of medicine is far less quantifiable and is far more complicated. Simplistic targets can easily introduce perverse incentives that disrupt the equitable provision of healthcare according to need. The government was advised to consider prioritising targets and better understanding their knock-on effects. Alternatively, the government might concentrate on standards. This is particularly important as the EWTD already affects the career grade of doctor, reducing their available working hours, and could affect all doctors when next reviewed.

Doctors are professionals whose main role is to judge possibilities and deal with undifferentiated illness. Differential diagnoses are generally the responsibility of doctors. SMAC feels that it would be difficult to transfer these responsibilities to other professionals such as nurses and that there was some evidence and experience that nurses generally did not always wish to have this responsibility. This is an issue SMAC wanted to discuss with the Standing Nursing and Midwifery Advisory Committee (SNMAC). Doctors need their role accepted, which implies a more subtle performance management approach than blunt targets.

SMAC was keen to discuss how to achieve better collaborative working and cross-over roles with other professionals, which is likely to benefit patients and also allow professionals to deliver a better service.

The popularity of salaried GP contracts (Primary Medical Services Contract – PMS) suggests jobs for GPs involving controllable hours and agreed objectives. Targets tend to be set more realistically and doctors have more face-to-face contact with patients, which is what primary care doctors generally train to achieve.

Dealing with change

On the one hand, some doctors feel overburdened by change. On the other hand, some specialties, such as public health, are more familiar with change. The lesson learned is that doctors have to engage with change in as constructive a way as possible. Doctors ought increasingly to be able to describe what they do and acquire new competencies and skills, which will enable them to make the moves they want. For instance, 'laddering across' is a concept that needs to be investigated. The idea is that doctors could become specialists in one specialty but that that specialty should not constrain their practice too rigidly. In the spirit of lifelong learning, ideally doctors should be able to acquire new skills and practise new aspects of specialism, without necessarily changing the whole specialty. Medical colleges may be able to facilitate this. It is crucial that standards of care are high and monitored. Further work needs to be done to explore how laddering across might be enabled, while standards are safeguarded. Modular training may be one way of training and formal appraisal may be one way of safeguarding standards, limiting practice to areas that have been appraised. Also, continuity of care for patients must be maintained.

They understood that colleges were looking at this and urged that they pursue this seriously. While SMAC would recommend generally shorter training, with certification of particular expertise after that, one college is currently lengthening training by one year. However, the possibility of doctors working for a time overseas, either in developed or developing countries, as part of their training or for career development, is worth fostering so that it becomes commonly accepted.

The British Association of Medical Managers (BAMM) has also published a paper, *Consultant Careers: times of change* (2001) that deals with many of these issues (but it does not seem to be available online).

Continuity of care

How doctors spend their time is an important factor, as is the extent to which they can see their contribution to patient treatment and can have some form of continuity of care, which is important to maintaining job satisfaction. The trend recently, particularly since the EWTD, in hospitals and for the out-of-hours arrangements in primary care, has been away from continuity of care.

SMAC recommended urgent consideration of how more continuity of care could be maintained, which SMAC thinks would benefit patients and improve job satisfaction of clinicians. The electronic patient record would enhance continuity of records and care.

Supporting and valuing doctors

There would be some benefit to doctors to have multidisciplinary team training with other professionals. In general, SMAC recommends that more emphasis should be given to supportive development of doctors to balance the current emphasis on appraisal, regulation, clinical governance and revalidation. They welcomed the publication of *Improving Working Lives for Doctors* (DoH 2001) and recommend its urgent implementation, stressing the need to support and value doctors so that they can in turn support and look after their patients. They recognised the need to allow doctors' careers to evolve over time and make use of their interest and enthusiasms, otherwise they may lose that interest and enthusiasm.

Interestingly, SMAC was abolished in 2005 as part of an ongoing regular review process for NDPBs. The review findings were that while SMAC and SNMAC had been a unique source of advice, providing authoritative and respected guidance to DoH and Ministers, an increasing number of other and emerging advisory mechanisms with professional medical, nursing and midwifery representation now existed, and so it recommended abolition.

The development of paramedical personnel

Medical care practitioners (MCP)

An MCP has been defined as 'someone who is a new healthcare professional who, while not a qualified doctor, works to the medical model, with the attitudes, skills and knowledge base to deliver holistic care and treatment within the general medical and/ or general practice team under defined levels of supervision'. In 2005 the government began steps to introduce this new breed of medical practitioner with nurses and other professionals including science graduates being retrained as medical care practitioners. These practitioners would be able to undertake many of the tasks undertaken by GPs and would be regulated by the Health Professions Council. In 2006 a health minister said: 'By introducing new roles we are able to offer patients skilled practitioners who are able to manage the care of patients in primary and secondary care.' They will work in hospitals and primary care diagnosing patients and prescribing drugs, but not have the same medical qualifications as doctors. The role is already well established in the US, where it is known as a physician assistant (PA).

The move was part of an upheaval of who does what in the NHS, which was said at the time of introduction of this role to be in debt and short of staff, particularly after the introduction of the EWTD. The NHS said that it wanted to use each type of worker to the peak of their skills, which meant doctors becoming more specialised, nurses doing some jobs once restricted to doctors, and some traditional nursing roles being given to healthcare assistants.

The new role would fit in somewhere between a nurse and a doctor. Canada and the Netherlands were bringing in physician assistant roles into their civilian healthcare systems, and Liberia, South Africa, Australia, New Zealand and Guyana were among several other countries showing interest. Physician assistants are generalists and basically do the jobs of a junior doctor.

In the US, they diagnose and treat illnesses, order and interpret investigations, and prescribe drugs. They practise autonomously but not independently. There is a newly established UK Association of Physician Assistants. There is a good summary article in the *Medical Journal of Australia* detailing their development and work in the UK, which can be read at www.mja.com.au/public/issues/185_01_030706/par10411_fm.html.

The Competence and Curriculum Framework for the Medical Care Practitioner (DoH 2006) outlined the proposed national educational and practice standards and proposed a regulatory framework that future healthcare workers will need to meet before being able to treat patients as an MCP. Once qualified and registered, it is proposed that an MCP will be able to:

o obtain full medical histories and perform appropriate physical examination
o diagnose, manage (including prescribing) and treat illness within their competence
o request diagnostic tests and interpret the results
o provide patient education and preventative healthcare advice regarding medication, common problems and disease management issues
o decide on appropriate referral to, and liaison with, other professionals.

The 2006 document also sets out the proposals for the framework that describes the standards required of a robust and rigorous training programme, assessment, validation and revalidation. MCPs will practise under the supervision of a physician and the supervising physician will continue to be responsible for the medical care the patient receives.

The consultation document was developed at the request of the National Practitioner Programme (previously part of the Modernisation Agency, Changing Workforce Programme) and has been jointly led by the Royal College of Physicians and the Royal College of General Practitioners.

The document states that the MCP role builds upon an extensive evidence base of similar successful roles such as the physician assistant in the US and the recognition that the global labour market requires the UK to have a process in place that recognises the talent of this international workforce and can exploit the skills and experience these workers have should they wish to work in the UK in accordance with migration and work permit legislation. The document can be read at www.dh.gov.uk/en/Consultations/Closedconsultations/DH_4127837 or www.library.nhs.uk/health management/ViewResource.aspx?resID=112754.

Advanced nurse practitioner (ANP)

ANPs are nurses designated as having a higher level of expertise in a particular field. The RCN defines an advanced nurse practitioner as a registered nurse who has undertaken a specific course of study of at least first degree (Honours) level and who:

o makes professionally autonomous decisions, for which they are accountable
o receives patients with undifferentiated and undiagnosed problems and makes an assessment of their healthcare needs, based on highly developed nursing knowledge and skills, including skills not usually exercised by nurses, e.g. physical examination

o   screens patients for disease risk factors and early signs of illness
o   makes differential diagnosis using decision-making and problem-solving skills
o   develops with the patient an ongoing nursing care plan for health, with an emphasis on preventative measures
o   orders necessary investigations, and provides treatment and care individually, as part of a team and through referral to other agencies
o   has a supportive role in helping people to manage and live with illness
o   provides counselling and health education
o   has the authority to admit or discharge patients from their caseload, and refer patients to other healthcare providers as appropriate
o   works collaboratively with other healthcare professionals and disciplines
o   provides a leadership and consultancy function as required.

The RCN has published a guide to the advanced nurse practitioner role, competencies and programme accreditation, available online at www.rcn.org.uk/__data/assets/pdf_file/0003/146478/003207.pdf. Another interesting discussion paper that gives a summary of the emerging issues about proposals to modernise the nursing workforce is available from a link at www.nhsemployers.org/Aboutus/Publications/Pages/TheRoleOfTheNurse.aspx.

The role of ward sister

In 2009 the RCN published a report, *The Ward Sister and Charge Nurse Role: key to quality patient care*, which concluded that 'the role of the ward sister remains central and absolutely critical to the organisation and delivery of hospital nursing and high standards of patient care'.

Research by the RCN has demonstrated that although the majority of ward sisters enjoy their work and find nursing worthwhile, they felt that the standard of care on their wards has fallen. Ever since the Salmon Report (1966), the sister role has been devalued, it is no longer regarded as the 'career grade' in nursing, with management and specialist nursing offering shorter hours and better pay. The responsibility remained but the authority has been eroded. Then the 'management revolution' occurred following the Griffiths Report (1983), and ward-cleaning staff for example no longer worked directly for the ward sister. Formerly, if something was dirty, sister would make sure it was cleaned immediately. Now the sister must contact the domestic services manager, ask for a job number and await assistance.

This new report concluded that 'the role of the ward sister remains central and absolutely critical to the organisation and delivery of hospital nursing and high standards of patient care'. Among its recommendations is that all ward sisters become supervisory to shifts and that directors of nursing review the remit of their ward sisters to ensure they have appropriate authority over key areas such as nutrition and cleanliness. It further showed that where ward sisters already have authority and the resources to make their wards run as well as they possibly can, patients felt the benefits.

The full report can be seen at www.rcn.org.uk/aboutus/wales/empowering_ward_sisters.

Related reading

Berwick DM. The epitaph of profession. *Br J Gen Pract*. 25 Nov 2008. Available online at www.rcgp.org.uk/pdf/bjgp_08_JohnHuntLecture_Berwick_AOP.pdf or www.ihi.org/NR/rdonlyres/B3933FEC-CF14–482B-9B4A-A699AAC8FEFD/0/BerwickHuntLecture_BJGPNov08.pdf

BAMM. *Consultant Careers: times of change*. Stockport: British Association of Medical Managers; 2001.

Darzi A. *High Quality Care for All: NHS Next Stage Review final report*. London: Department of Health, HMSO; 2008. Available online at www.dh.gov.uk/en/publicationsandstatistics/publications/publicationspolicyandguidance/DH_085825

DoH. *Doctors for the Future: advice by the SMAC*. London: Department of Health; 2001.

DoH. *Improving Working Lives for Doctors*. London: Department of Health; 2001.

DoH. *Our Health, Our Care*. London: Department of Health; 2006.

DoH. *The Competence and Curriculum Framework for the Medical Care Practitioner*. London: Department of Health; 2006.

Farrington-Douglas J, Brooks R. *The Future Hospital: the politics of change*. The Institute of Public Policy Research; 2007. Available online as pdf file at www.ippr.org

GMC. *Tomorrow's Doctors: outcomes and standards for undergraduate medical education*. London: General Medical Council; 2009. Available online at www.gmc-uk.org/education/documents/GMC_TD_2009.pdf

Griffiths Report. *National Health Service Management Inquiry Report*. London: DHSS; 1983.

Ham C. Does the district general hospital have a future? *BMJ*. 2005; **331**: 1331–3.

IPPR. *The Future Hospital: the progressive case for change*. The Institute of Public Policy Research; 2007. Available online at www.ippr.org

MSC. *The Consensus Statement on the Role of the Doctor*. London: Medical Schools Council; 2008. Available online at www.medschools.ac.uk/news.htm

Morrison I. The future of physicians' time. *Ann Int Med*. 2000; **132**: 80–4. Available online at members.rsm.ac.uk/login.php?url=http://jrsm.rsmjournals.com/cgi/ijlink?linkType=ABST&journalCode=annintmed&resid=132/1/80 but you need to be a member to log in.

Pollock A. Privatising primary care. *Br J Gen Pract*. 2006; **56**(529): 565–6.

RCN. *Breaking down Barriers, Driving up Standards: the role of the ward sister and charge nurse*. London: Royal College of Nursing; 2009.

RCN. *The Ward Sister and Charge Nurse Role: key to quality patient care*. London: Royal College of Nursing; 2009.

RCP. *Doctors in Society: medical professionalism in a changing world*. London: Royal College of Physicians; 2005.

Salmon Report. *Report of the Committee on Senior Nursing Staff Structure*. London: HMSO; 1966.

Smith R. Thoughts on future doctors. *J R Soc Med*. 2009; **102**: 89–91.

Talbot-Smith A, Pollock AM. *The New NHS*. Abingdon: Routledge; 2006.

Tooke J. *Final Report of the Independent Inquiry into Modernising Medical Careers*. London: MMC Inquiry; 2008.

Ward C, Eccles S. *So You Want to be a Brain Surgeon? A medical careers guide*. Oxford: Oxford University Press; 1997.

Funding and the NHS

The aim of this chapter is to inform you about national and local NHS funding structures. There are two major differences in this latest edition. First, it has expanded, as funding is now more complex; second, some of the figures given below cannot be guaranteed because not only do different authorities sometimes give different figures but you occasionally find contradictory figures quoted on official DoH websites.

Since its launch 60 years ago, the NHS has grown to become the world's largest publicly funded health service. It is also one of the most efficient, most egalitarian and most comprehensive. The system was born out of an ideal that healthcare should be free and available to all. With the exception of charges for some prescriptions and optical and dental services, it remains free at the point of use for everyone who is resident in the UK – more than 60 million people. The money to pay for the NHS comes directly from taxation that, according to independent bodies such as the King's Fund, remains the 'cheapest and fairest' way of funding healthcare when compared with other systems.

Early funding policies of the NHS were concerned with cost control but lacked processes to achieve equity and efficiency in funding. Governments of the 1980s sought to add efficiency through budgetary squeezes that culminated in funding problems in the late 1980s. The result was an NHS internal market that promised efficiency by introducing a purchaser–provider split and a system of provider competition in which money would follow the patient.

In updating this chapter the writers found an increasing problem not only in finding figures that are consistent but because the various parts of the UK are now devolved you need to be aware as to whether the gross and percentage figures for GDP relate to England or the UK in total.

According to OECD Health Data published in 2005, in 2002–03 the total expenditure was 7.7% of GDP. Although some claim that by 2006 NHS UK as a percentage of GDP had risen to 9.4%, compared to 7.1% in 2001, other authorities claim it was nearer 8.4% of GDP. There is an increasing tendency for 'official' figures to talk in terms of percentage increases rather than in absolute terms of budget size. Politicians and political parties in particular skew the argument by not stating whether they are talking in absolute terms or after adjusting for inflation. To give a further example of current difficulties, I found the figures for 2007–8 of the total NHS cost from three reputable sources (including Hansard and DoH) were £105.6 billion, £104 billion and £105 billion with surplus of £1.8 billion (i.e. £103.2 billion).

One other key consideration is the fact that all budgets are reduced by a percentage each year to reflect the national minimum requirement for Cash Releasing Efficiency Savings (CRES). All NHS Service Level Agreements are automatically reduced by this percentage, thus delivering 'savings'. The figure is currently 3% and it is always important to identify, although usually difficult to ascertain, whether a budget takes into account this 'efficiency saving'.

By 2010, total expenditure was planned to be 10.5–11.0% of GDP, which would be well above the European average and more than 50% higher than the GDP shares of Scandinavia and New Zealand. But the credit crisis of 2009 may alter that.

It has been suggested that future problems may arise from funding the Private Finance Initiative (PFI) and Public Private Partnership (PPP) outcomes, changes and developments in primary care, preferential contracts to private providers, reintroduction of the internal market, and inflation in medical technology and drug costs. All these issues put pressure on traditional large hospitals, including foundation hospitals.

As well as additional funding, the government reintroduced a system of provider competition in which money is intended to follow the patient. In 2002, the Wanless Report stated that the NHS would face ever-growing financial pressure in the following 10 to 20 years. However, Wanless argued that continuing to fund the health service through general taxation was the most cost-effective and fair system for the future. The pdf file of the full report is available at www.hm-treasury.gov.uk/consult_wanless_final.htm.

The finances of the NHS

In **2003–04** the Department of Health achieved financial balance overall across the 600 local NHS bodies and most individual NHS bodies also achieved financial balance, although the proportion failing to achieve financial balance increased from 12 to 18%.

The position deteriorated in **2004–05** when the DoH estimated that overall the NHS incurred a small deficit figure quoted from £251 million to £594 million. The number of individual parts with significant deficits also increased. At least 12 strategic health authorities ended 2004–05 with a deficit compared with seven the previous year. At that time an Audit Commission report concluded that the basics of financial management at most NHS bodies were sound, but that greater control was needed. It stated that nearly half of all acute trusts and primary care trusts suffered from either 'weak' or 'fairly weak' financial planning. It also said that the current financial management of most PCTs was inadequate to meet the challenges, and all board members, executives and non-executives needed to have greater knowledge and skills to discharge their responsibilities effectively.

It is difficult to assess how long the NHS had been overspending as deficits were hidden in the past. Deficits came to light when policy changed and increased transparency, in particular the switch in accounting procedures associated with the introduction of the Resource Accounting and Budgeting (RAB) regime. As a result it was no longer possible to underspend on capital and use the money to subsidise current spending. In addition, RAB led to the double-deficit problem whereby a trust's income in the current year has both to pay for that year's provision and pay back the previous year's deficits.

2005–06 was another deficit year of between £547million and £1.2 billion, with 174 organisations in deficit. As a result of the introduction of RAB the deficit for 2005/06 was claimed to have been exaggerated by £117 million. The figure would also have been higher but for a growth in SHA surpluses.

So while there have long been underlying deficits, their size increased and the Secretary of State promised that the NHS as a whole would be in balance by March 2007 and would take personal responsibility for that. The government then started to tackle the problem in earnest, not an easy task.

2006–07 was to be another deficit year; the number of PCTs and trusts in deficit was rising again with the total number of organisations reporting a deficit of 22%. The House of Commons Report on Health Deficits 2006–07 (which can be seen at www. publications.parliament.uk/pa/cm200607/cmselect/cmhealth/73/73i.pdf) blamed poor local management, and said it had a good deal of evidence of poor financial management. Nevertheless, poor financial management was not just caused by local managers and boards, the government had also contributed, by repeated changes and the emphasis on meeting targets at short notice.

By **2007–08** the government forecast a surplus of £916 million but said that the NHS had at the end of that year a surplus of between £1.67 and £1.8 billion (depending on the source of data). It also pledged to find another £15 billion of savings over the following three years. Only 3% of the organisations in NHS reported deficits.

2008–09 was to be the first year of a new three-year planning cycle. The other item of note was that the Treasury announced its intention of adopting the International Financial Reporting Standards (IFRS) for the public sector in 2008/09 so that NHS trusts would no longer have income adjustments caused by the RAB regime (see above). The effect of this is that any underspend or overspend by an NHS trust would affect the balance sheet of that trust, but will not result in a carry forward of surpluses or a carry forward of deficit into the following year in the form of an RAB adjustment. The RAB rules continue to apply to PCTs and SHAs. It is too early to determine what was spent during this financial year as at the time of writing a reliable figure is not available.

For **2009–10** the size of the budget cannot be ascertained with any accuracy, as at the time of writing it is still not decided whether the surplus from the previous year will be carried forward, used as a contingency fund or removed to assist in the repayment of government debt. A parliamentary answer quoted in Hansard gives a figure of £102.6 billion. It is impossible to obtain figures for future years' NHS budgets, because of the enormous financial debt of the UK. The influential King's Fund think tank has said: 'No matter who is in power from 2011 the NHS will have to manage with very low or no growth in its funding.' So it seems that with little or no cash increase from 2011/12 the NHS has to prepare itself for real reductions in what it can afford to do. At the time of writing estimates by DoH place the 2010–11 figure at about £110 billion.

Unfortunately, in the middle of 2009 the NHS chief executive gave a warning to finance directors referring to the need for between £15 billion and £20 billion worth of savings from 2011 and by 2014. The NHS Confederation had already warned of a £15 billion shortfall facing the NHS by 2016. This sum was to be delivered by £15–20 billion of efficiency savings, although a study by McKinsey & Company (2009) recommended more drastic measures such as cutting the NHS workforce by 10% over five years; this was rejected by the government. For details go to www.nhshistory.net/mckinsey2009.html.

Mr Micawber in David Copperfield said with 'annual income twenty pounds, annual expenditure nineteen six, result happiness. When annual income twenty pounds, annual expenditure twenty pounds ought and six, result misery.' But as we have seen the NHS appears not quite to follow the same rules because it is difficult to indentify both income and expenditure precisely and at the same time there can be simultaneous talk of increasing and decreasing budgets and expenditure!

At the start of Chapter 1 there is a statistical picture of the NHS. The following data, which is much of a summary of the foregoing paragraphs, may be added to that list to complete the financial picture of the NHS.

The figures quoted are for NHS in England, as the NHS in Scotland, Northern Ireland, Wales, The Isle of Man and the Channel Islands have their own independent health service structures.

When the NHS began in 1948 (and included Scotland, Wales and Northern Ireland) it cost £437 million per year (that's roughly £9 billion at today's prices).

○ By 2002–03 the NHS cost £65.4 bn, although some sources say £57.2 bn.
○ By 2003–04 the NHS cost £72.1 bn.
○ By 2004–05 the NHS cost £79.3 bn.
○ By 2005–06 the NHS cost £87.2 bn, although a parliamentary answer quoted in Hansard is £76.4 bn and a business article says £77.6 bn.
○ By 2006–07 the NHS cost £95.9 bn, although another source says £96.2 bn.
○ By 2007–08 the NHS cost £105.6 bn or £104 bn or £105 less a surplus of £1.8 (=£103.2 bn).
○ For 2008–09 various figures have been quoted from £90 bn to £94 bn; much depends on the fate of the surplus from the previous financial year. The NHS Information Centre quotes a figure of £92.5 bn and the Darzi Report £96 bn.
○ In 2009–10 the NHS will cost £102.6 bn according to a parliamentary answer quoted in Hansard.
○ The 2010–11 figures are estimated by DoH to be £110.0 bn, although the financial

state of the country could alter that. At time of writing savings of £4.35 bn are planned.

The huge rise in funding equates to an average rise in spending over the full 60-year period of about 3% a year once inflation has been taken into account. However, in recent years investment levels have been double that to fund the modernisation pro-gramme. It also means that the NHS now costs about £2 billion a week.

o The DoH estimates that treatment and care of long-term conditions accounts for 69% of the total health and social care spend in England or almost £7 in every £10 spent.
o Some 60% of the NHS budget is used to pay staff.
o Some 20% pays for drugs and other supplies.
o The remaining 20% is split between buildings, equipment and training costs on the one hand and medical equipment, catering and cleaning on the other.
o Nearly 80% of the total budget is distributed by local trusts in line with the par-ticular health priorities in their areas.
o The NHS (England) spends over £1 million about every 5 minutes, equivalent to a little over £2000 per head in 2007.
o Just under half of NHS spending goes on acute services, over £800 per person per annum.
o The NHS accounts for 18% of all government spending.
o Some 77% of funding comes from general taxation, 12% from the NHS share of national insurance contributions and 2% from patient charges.
o Over 40% of total hospital and community health services expenditure is for people over 64 years of age, although they represent just 16% of the population.
o A one-week stay in hospital costs over £1100 and a night in intensive care costs over £500.
o The budget roughly equates to a contribution of more than £1500 for every man, woman and child in the UK.
o The NHS Scotland spent £11.2 bn in 2008/09, and The Scottish Parliament has budgeted £11.7 bn for 2009/10 and £12.2 bn for 2010/11.
o The NHS Wales spent £5.8 bn in 2008/09, and The National Assembly for Wales has budgeted £6.0 bn for 2009/10 and £6.2 bn for 2010/11.

Given that 60% of the budget goes on staff, it is worth considering the size of the NHS. Nationwide, the NHS employs more than 1.5 million people. Of those, just short of half are clinically qualified, including some 90 000 hospital doctors, 35 000 general practitioners (GPs), 400 000 nurses and 16 000 ambulance staff.

The NHS in England is far and away the biggest part of the system, catering to a population of 50 million and employing more than 1.43 million people. The NHS in Scotland, Wales and Northern Ireland employ 158 000, 71 000 and 67 000 people respectively.

Distribution of NHS funds

The NHS is the second largest government spending programme. The following paragraphs provide information about the allocation of NHS funding.

The DoH allocates resources to:

o **revenue allocations** (about 95%), i.e. staff salaries and wages, purchase of goods and services such as drugs and fuel, a small proportion for DoH administrative costs, for central miscellaneous services and agencies, research and development funds, medical costs of UK nationals treated in EU member states

o **capital allocations**, i.e. purchasing and maintaining assets such as land, buildings and medical equipment.

Revenue allocations

In England the funding supports hospital, community and family health services, and other centrally purchased services such as those outlined in Chapter 1. The basis for distributing the total NHS funds varies between England, Wales, Scotland and Northern Ireland.

Revenue allocations (i.e. for goods and services being purchased) to primary care trusts cover hospital and community health services (HCHS), prescribing, primary medical services, etc. PCT revenue allocations are made after each Spending Review. For example, following the 2007 Government Comprehensive Spending Review, the DoH announced in December 2007 £74 billion allocations for 2008–09, and then in December 2008 £164 billion allocations for 2009–10 and 2010–11.

To take England as the main example, the DoH allocates over 80% of the NHS budget to PCTs. The remaining 20% is allocated to strategic health authorities and NHS trusts directly as operational or strategic capital, or to fund specific developments, programmes or projects. By far the largest component of this budget is the funding provided to SHAs for workforce development and training.

The funding is allocated to PCTs on a per capita basis but is weighted depending on the nature of the population served. According to the DoH, it uses 'a complex mathematical formula developed by independent academic researchers and adapted by its resource allocation team to determine the level of funding'. The current formula was introduced in 2003 but was changed slightly for the 2006/07 and 2007/08 allocations.

PCTs then commission activity from acute trusts, foundation trusts, care trusts, mental health trusts and other healthcare providers. Thus these trusts receive most of their income from carrying out work for PCTs.

Budgets for individual practices or departments within NHS bodies are determined by the local practices of each health body. Each will have an annual budget-setting process, often led by their Finance Directors and management team. They are expected to set a budget that will not over-commit their incoming resources.

The funding formula aims to provide resources that reflect local needs for healthcare. Additional funds are then allocated to an area with high levels of deprivation, for example. Funding is weighted according to a number of factors, including age, socio-economic variables and indices of morbidity and mortality. Other elements include rates of HIV/AIDS, Personal Medical Services, prescribing and emergency ambulance cost adjustments. In 2004/05, for example, the per capita weighted allocations varied between £860 for individuals in the least deprived areas to £1166 in the most deprived.

A so-called Market Forces Factor (MFF) is added to the formula. This allows for the differences between areas of the unavoidable costs of providing healthcare, such as expenditure on the workforce. The funding formula generates a target allocation for each PCT. This indicates what is considered the PCT's 'fair share' of the national allocation, based upon the total impact of all of the weighted factors. The PCT's current allocation is then compared to this target and the gap, known as the Distance from Target, determines the level of increased allocation given in any one year. No PCT has a reduced allocation, and all receive a minimum level to cover the cost of inflation. Additional funding, or growth, is allocated in proportion to the PCT's Distance from Target, with those furthest away (i.e. the most under-funded) receiving a higher rate of growth than those at or near to Target.

The formula does not directly measure health needs. Instead it uses proxies of socio-economic status and assumptions associated with these variables, based on a series of statistical analyses from Resource Allocation Research Papers (RARPs), research commissioned by the Department's Advisory Committee on Resource Allocation (ACRA).

For example RARP 26 states:

> The allocation of resources for healthcare across geographical areas in the NHS is based on the principle that individuals in equal need should have equal access to care, irrespective of where they live. To implement the principle it is necessary to measure need for healthcare in different areas. But those allocating resources do not have sufficient information to measure need directly. Recent research on the funding formula is limited. However, some researchers have criticised the funding formula and argued that there is a connection between it and PCTs' levels of past deficits.

Deficit definitions

Deficits are spoken of in several different ways as part of government accounting procedure, depending on the period of time in question and whether the organisation is an NHS trust, PCT or SHA. The most common terms are:

o   the in-year deficit, which is used to describe an NHS trust's deficit (if the trust has a surplus, it is described as an 'in-year' surplus)
o   the overall net deficit, which is the total of in-year deficits and overspends, plus any surpluses, of all NHS organisations
o   the cumulative deficit, which is a trust's previous years' deficits added together.

Capital vs. revenue

You might think it easy to differentiate capital from revenue but according to the HMRC website at www.hmrc.gov.uk/manuals/bimmanual/bim35010.htm, it is not possible to draw up a list of items, the cost of which is capital, nor is it possible to draw up a list of items, the cost of which is revenue. The classification, capital or revenue, is not uniquely determined by the nature of the item involved, rather it is determined by the circumstances of the transaction. What is capital in one person's hands may well be revenue in another's. Although there is no universal recipe to decide in any given circumstance if an expenditure is on capital or revenue account, there are a number of broad criteria. Some may be more useful than others in particular cases.

However, as you are very unlikely to be involved in NHS finances, for our purposes let us assume the following as being acceptable.

Capital budgets

In contrast to revenue expenditure (that is, expenditure on goods and services and including wages and salaries, to be used in the financial current year), capital expenditure, typically buildings and very large items of equipment, will continue to provide benefits over a number of future years. Capital funding can be spent on anything over £5000 which fits the definition of 'capital' spend, so it could include items such as new buildings, extensions to existing buildings, new diagnostic equipment such as MRI scanners, and it can be used to replace or refurbish existing buildings. In the NHS this is generally taken to mean items that cost £5000 or more and are thus recorded on the balance sheet as fixed assets. For the first time, in 2005/06, capital budgets were made available to local health services for three years rather than one year. It was also the first time day-to-day operational capital was allocated directly to NHS trusts and primary care trusts.

The NHS 2008–09 capital budget was said to have an underspend but that could have been clawed back by the Treasury to fund its plans to lend money to stalled PFI schemes, as the Treasury announced plans to raise between £1 billion and £2 billion to lend to schemes over the following year, but NHS projects were not expected to be a priority. There were suggestions that many of the 110 PFI schemes that had been approved across all sectors were still searching for lenders from whom to borrow a total of around £13 billion. Thus the Treasury needed to borrow money itself to lend to the schemes and made it clear that its first port of call would be underspend by government departments.

The DoH has run up this substantial capital underspend over recent years partly due to slow progress on the national IT programme. One-fifth of the NHS capital is unspent; in 2007–08 the capital underspend was equivalent to 22% of the NHS budget. If the NHS continues to underspend at the same rate over the next three years, the Treasury could claim some £3.3 billion out of its total £15.1 billion capital budget to recycle but perhaps to other departments. The Treasury has not yet decided how it will prioritise which schemes it lends to. NHS projects could be vulnerable because they might not be seen as directly crucial to economic development. In a parliamentary answer the NHS capital budget for 2009–10 was said to be £5.4 billion (www. parliament.co.uk 2010).

Spending Reviews (SR) and Comprehensive Spending Reviews (CSR)

Spending Reviews and Comprehensive Spending Reviews both represent the process by which the government decides:
○ how much money it can allocate for public spending
○ how this money should be allocated
○ what its future priorities are ('Public Service Agreements') and how the money will be used to achieve them.

Spending Reviews normally take place every two years and cover a three-year period. Since 1998 there have been biennial spending reviews (in 1998, 2000, 2002 and 2004) to set out its public spending plans. The next in 2007 was in the form of a Comprehensive Spending Review announcing spending plans for the three fiscal years 2008 to 2011. At the time of writing because of the state of the economy and national debt the next spending review may be kicked into the post-election, long grass of autumn 2010, leaving it to a new administration. The Treasury's current projections require public spending to fall (and tax receipts to rise) as a share of national income over this three-year period if they are to meet their borrowing forecasts. This is in contrast to the previous four spending reviews which had all planned and delivered increases in public spending as a share of national income.

Comprehensive Spending Reviews are less frequent and on average take place about every 10 years. The last two CSRs have taken place in 1998 and 2007.

Public service agreement (PSA)

A major feature of spending reviews since 1998 has been the public service agreement (PSA). Each government department's PSA is a statement setting out the following.
○ *Aim:* a high-level statement of the role of the department.
○ *Objectives:* in broad terms, what the department is looking to achieve.
○ *Performance targets:* under most objectives, outcome focused performance targets.
○ *Value for money:* each department is required to have a target for improving the efficiency or value for money of a key element of its work.
○ A statement of who is responsible for the *delivery* of these targets.

The PSA system tries to accommodate the fact that problems do not fit neatly into the boundaries of government departments and agencies, the so-called crosscutting problem. So targets may be shared between two or more departments. Where targets are jointly held this is identified and accountability arrangements clearly specified.

The objectives of PSAs are stated to improve:
○ service standards
○ health and social care outcomes
○ value for money.

Examples for some of these objectives can be seen in the following more detailed list, some of which you may recognise.

Service standards

o Reduce the maximum wait for an outpatient appointment to three months and the maximum wait for inpatient treatment to six months by the end of 2005, and achieve progressive further cuts with the aim of reducing the maximum inpatient and day case waiting time to three months by 2008.

o Reduce to four hours the maximum wait in A&E from arrival to admission, transfer or discharge, by the end of 2004; and reduce the proportion waiting over one hour.

o Guarantee access to a primary care professional within 24 hours and to a primary care doctor within 48 hours from 2004.

o Ensure that by the end of 2005 every hospital appointment will be booked for the convenience of the patient, making it easier for patients and their GPs to choose the hospital and consultant that best meets their needs.

o Enhance accountability to patients and the public and secure sustained national improvements in patient experience as measured by independently validated surveys.

o By 2010 reduce inequalities in health outcomes by 10% as measured by infant mortality and life expectancy at birth.

Health and social care outcomes

o Reduce the under-18 conception rate by 50% by 2010.

o Improve life chances for children, including by DoH.

o Reduce mortality rates from major diseases by 2010: from heart disease by at least 40% in people under 75; from cancer by at least 20% in people under 75.

o Improve life outcomes of adults and children with mental health problems.

o Reduce the mortality rate from suicide and undetermined injury by at least 20% by 2010.

o Improve the quality of life and independence of older people so they can live at home wherever possible, by increasing by March 2006 the number of those supported intensively to live at home to 30% of the total being supported by social services at home or in residential care.

Value for money

o Value for money in the NHS and personal social services will improve by at least 2% per annum, with annual improvements of 1% in both cost efficiency and service effectiveness.

For more information of PSAs there is a pdf file from the NHS Health Development Agency at www.erpho.org.uk/Download/Public/6125/1/HDA%20PSA%20briefing. pdf.

Payment by results (PbR)

Historically, hospitals had been paid according to 'block contracts' – a fixed sum of money for a broadly specified service – or 'cost and volume' contracts, which attempted to specify in more detail the activity and payment. But there were no incentives for providers to increase throughput, since they got no additional funding. In the document *Delivering the NHS Plan: next steps on investment, next steps on reform* (DoH 2002), the idea of incentives for performance or payment by results was introduced. In October 2002 the DoH issued *Reforming NHS Financial Flows: introducing payment by results*, setting out plans for changes in the way that healthcare providers are paid in the NHS.

The plans indicated the government's intention to link the allocation of funds to hospitals to the activity they undertake. It stated that in order to get the best from extra resources there would be major changes to the way money flowed around the NHS and differentiation between incentives for routine surgery and those for emergency admissions. Hospitals would be paid for the elective activity they undertake and this is a system of payment by results. This reformed financial system attempted to offer incentives to reward good performance, to support sustainable reductions in waiting times for patients and to make the best use of available capacity.

In 2002–03 a start was made by testing different ways of moving resources with patients to establish the key principle that providers which fail to deliver lose money to those that can deliver. Experience of the internal market showed that price competition did not work, particularly for emergency cases that were admitted to the nearest hospital, and merely led to excessive transaction costs. In June 2004 the Audit Commission published a useful booklet, *Payment by Results: key risks and questions to consider for trust and PCT managers and non-executives*, which can still be viewed at www.audit-commission.gov.uk/SiteCollectionDocuments/AuditCommissionReports/National Studies/PaymentByResults_booklet.pdf.

A consultation paper, *Payment by Results: preparing for 2005*, identified the key decisions needed for implementing the payment by results scheme and outlined how it would apply to NHS foundation trusts from April 2004 and to all NHS trusts from April 2005. The information received in response to this exercise and feedback received from the NHS revealed two issues. First, non-elective and outpatient activity is not stable, incurring big increases in short-stay, emergency admissions. This meant that a tariff based on a previous year's practice was not reliable for pricing work the next year. Second, there were concerns about the consistency of approach by the NHS to the base-lining exercise. As a result it was decided to amend the phasing in of payment of results (PbR) to include elective care only in 2005–06, although by then NHS foundation trusts were already operating PbR.

The latest DoH publications on the subject, *Guidance and Supporting Information: confirmation of Payment by Results (PbR) arrangements for 2009–10*, can be viewed at www.dh.gov.uk/en/Publicationsandstatistics/Publications/PublicationsPolicy AndGuidance/DH_094183.

Reference costs

The White Paper, *The New NHS* (NHSE 1997), and later consultation document *A National Framework for Assessing Performance* (NHSE 1998), stressed the need to develop new methods to tackle inefficiency in the NHS rather than using the long criticised Purchaser Efficiency Index.

Among these instruments it was proposed to use Healthcare Resource Group (HRG) (see below) costs. Plans were published for a system of 'reference costs' itemising the cost of every treatment in every NHS trust. These reference costs were to be derived from HRGs with the aim of benchmarking cost improvement, measuring relative efficiency, identifying best practice, funding transfers and costing health-improvement programmes that created perverse incentives.

Without going into the various options and changes that occurred in this debate, by 2009 the NHS, with encouragement from DoH, was implementing patient-level information and costing systems (PLICS). The implementation of PLICS is still not mandatory but the DoH strongly supports it. It was claimed that the benefits of patient-level information costing systems were:

○ service-level economics reporting
○ understanding of the variations and their causes within services
○ a major improvement in clinical ownership of resource decisions
○ information to enable improved HRG classification
○ improved funding policy and evidence-based analysis in discussions with commissioners.

Patient-level information and costing systems

Patient-level information and costing systems can be defined as the ability to measure the resources consumed by individual patients. They represent a change in the method of costing in the NHS from a predominantly 'top-down' allocation approach, based on averages and apportionments, to a more direct and sophisticated approach based on the actual actions and events related to individual patients and the associated costs. The following are taken from the published guidance notes at www.dh.gov.uk/PolicyAndGuidance/OrganisationPolicy/FinanceAndPlanning/NHSReferenceCosts.

Patient-level costs are calculated by tracing resources used by a patient and the associated costs by using costs incurred by the organisation in providing the service. In other words, it can be defined as a measure of the resources used by a patient. Resources for inpatients are measured each day or part day from the time of entry and admission until discharge. For outpatients and non-admitted A&E patients, the consumption of resources is on a service basis.

It is said that, for example, a minimum set of costs driven by an activity should include emergency departments, operating theatres, critical care, wards, pathology, imaging, other diagnostics, special procedure suites, pharmacy services and drugs, prostheses, therapies and outpatients.

It is not sufficient to allocate ward costs by overall length of stay. Adjustments must be made for both the patients' admission and discharge days and for their acuity (i.e. severity, co-morbidities).

High-cost treatments and procedures in specialty hospitals should also be allocated to individual patients on an activity basis.

As far as is possible overheads should be allocated to these areas prior to allocation to patients, on the closest proxy to activity. It is not acceptable, however, to allocate any of the above resources as 'overheads'.

In the event that data is missing proxy allocations must be created. These might include standard costs (e.g. prosthesis by procedure) or service weights (i.e. data from other sources as substitutes).

Patient-level costing is the resourcing consequences of clinical activity and is primarily informed by the measurement of that clinical activity. Clinical validity is therefore underpinned by the accuracy and legitimacy of that core activity data. This necessitates the involvement of clinical staff in the definition, documentation and authentication of raw data inputs into a patient-level information and costing system.

You can find all this and more details at www.dh.gov.uk/PolicyAndGuidance/ OrganisationPolicy/FinanceAndPlanning/NHSReferenceCosts.

National Tariff

The National Tariff was used for commissioning services in 2005–06 when the system covered around half of the hospital and community health services spend and for large hospitals, typically some 70% of income was covered by the National Tariff. Later, as a result of consultations and contacts with other countries, modifications were made to the tariff to try to make it more sensitive and reflect the true cost of service delivery. However, during 2006–07 the National Tariff was deferred because of concerns that the process would lead to over-commitment of funds.

By 2009 there was Tariff reform and further attempts at efficiency for 2009/10 and 2010/11 when the government announced three-yearly allocations to its departments through the Comprehensive Spending Reviews. The national allocations policy by then, at least for PCTs, included the following.

o   Baseline allocation – the previous year's recurrent allocation adjusted for allocations issued during the year.
o   Fair share target – calculated by use of a fair share formula, applying age and need weights to PCT populations to determine a fair share to each PCT of the total resource available nationally.
o   Distance from target – the distance between baseline allocation and fair share target. Those PCTs having baseline allocations lower than fair share target are deemed to be 'under target' while those having baseline allocations higher than fair share target are deemed to be 'over target'.
o   Pace of change policy – a policy that governs the means by which PCTs' baseline allocations are moved towards fair share targets over time. In essence, those below target get an above average share of new (growth) funding, while those above target get a lower than average share.

Casemix Service

The Casemix Service develops clinical groupings and software that enables the NHS to record clinical activity that in turn enables the NHS to determine activity costs, inform national tariff setting processes, collect patient activity information (thus ensuring providers are paid for the services they deliver) and provide information to support epidemiological studies and service planning. The main method uses Healthcare Resource Groups.

Healthcare Resource Groups

HRGs are the main grouping method used by Casemix Service, the prime purpose of which is to assist the DoH to implement payment by results. HRGs are used as a means of determining fair and equitable reimbursement for care services rendered. They have been called 'units of currency' to support standardised healthcare commissioning across the service. HRGs represent groups of clinically similar treatments and diagnoses, which consume similar levels of healthcare resource. HRGs for inpatient surgical care have been in use since 1992.

HRGs was developed in the UK by the NHS Information Authority but was transferred to the Information Centre. With input from UK clinicians, to ensure UK clinical practice and UK patterns of service delivery were used, the current version is 3.5 although work on version 4 is taking place at time of writing.

Other countries (the US, Australia, the Nordic countries, Austria) have developed similar tools, often called Diagnostic Related Groups (DRGs). Most OECD and EU countries are now using, or planning to use, casemix tools in their provider payment systems. When DRGs were first introduced in the US there was a significant shift in the pattern of healthcare delivery. Purchasers could see the total cost of a treatment. They became very aware of the proportion of that cost that was due to hospitalisation. Therefore, in order to save money, they began to opt for the same care package but with a home-based patient. The result was a massive swing to homecare and the creation of a multi-billion dollar homecare industry to deliver a range of high-tech treatments, mainly focused on intravenous therapies such as chemotherapy together with the necessary nursing support.

The development of HRGs is an ongoing process that adapts to changes in clinical practice and the way services are configured. Reflecting modern clinical practice and aligned across all specialties, HRGs now include the following clinical specialties:
o   adult critical care
o   emergency medicine
o   pathology
o   radiology
o   chemotherapy
o   radiotherapy
o   specialist palliative care.

Other countries, such as the US, Canada and Germany, and have developed HRGs for acute patient care. The Casemix Service monitors developments of HRGs internationally, to adapt its work to best practice and share developments. For more information go to www.ic.nhs.uk/casemix.

Programme budgeting (and marginal analysis)

Tensions between doctors and managers and the differences between medical and managerial cultures have existed since the earliest provision of organised healthcare. In a resource allocation context, doctors are caricatured as taking the role of patient advocate while managers take the corporate, strategic view.

Delivery of efficient and equitable healthcare increasingly requires doctors to take responsibility for resources and to consider the needs of populations while managers need to become more outcome and patient centred. Programme budgeting and marginal analysis were felt to have the potential to align the goals of doctors and managers and create common ground between them.

In 2002 the DoH introduced programme budgeting, a retrospective review of resource allocation, broken down into programmes, with a view to tracking future resource allocation in those same programmes. It had its origins in the Rand Corporation in the USA in the 1950s. Its first major application was not in healthcare, but for the US Department of Defence in the 1960s where it was used as part of a cost accounting tool that could display, over time, the deployment of resources towards specific military objectives. Such objectives were looked at in terms of wars overseas, the support of NATO or the defence of the homeland, instead of the conventional 'inputs based' budgetary headings of tanks, missiles or diesel fuel. Allocation of new resources, or shifts between budgets, could be judged on their relative contribution to these specific objectives. Extensive research has been undertaken in the area of programme budgeting since its early application, in particular, when used in conjunction with marginal analysis (see below).

It was thought that such an approach could equally be applied to healthcare. So instead of seeing investment on the level of a hospital or drug budget, the focus switches to specific health objectives or medical conditions, the aim being to maximise health gain through deploying available resources to best effect, an aim relevant to the commissioning role of PCTs.

So, for example, primary care services are allocated to programmes of care based on the following 23 areas:

1 infectious diseases
2 cancers and tumours
3 blood disorders
4 endocrine, nutritional and metabolic problems
5 mental health problems
6 learning disability problems
7 neurological system problems
8 eye/vision problems
9 hearing problems
10 circulation problems (coronary heart disease)
11 respiratory system problems
12 dental problems
13 gastrointestinal system problems
14 skin problems
15 musculoskeletal system problems (excludes trauma)
16 trauma and injuries (includes burns)
17 genito-urinary system disorders (except infertility)
18 maternity and reproductive health
19 neonates

20 poisoning
21 healthy individuals
22 social care needs
23 other conditions.

2008/09 will be the sixth year of use in the NHS. A programme budgeting guide issued in June 2009 and contained in the guidance manual available at the website below has been developed by the national Programme Budget Project Board and agreed with its many stakeholders (including NHS, DoH, NAO, Audit Commission and HMT representatives): www.dh.gov.uk/en/Managingyourorganisation/Financeandplanning/Programmebudgeting/DH_4117326.

The terms programme budgeting, performance budgeting, and performance-based budgeting are often used interchangeably. The National Programme Budget Project aims to map some £50 billion of NHS expenditure into, currently, 23 programmes of care, as detailed above. You can obtain more information on the operating framework 2009–10 for NHS in England at www.dh.gov.uk/en/Managingyourorganisation/Financeandplanning/index.htm.

Expenditure data at PCT and SHA level are published annually on the DoH website, in the form of an Excel spreadsheet. Data is currently available for financial years 2003–04 to 2006–07. Comparative data shows how PCTs (and SHAs) distribute their allocations over the 23 programme budgeting categories and also allow for inter-PCT comparisons, with PCTs locally, nationally or which according to the Office for National Statistics (ONS) exhibit similar characteristics. The programme budgeting spreadsheet is designed to show PCTs how they distribute their allocations across programmes as well as allowing NHS trusts and foundation trusts to investigate commissioner expenditure. Finally, as the spreadsheet is published on the DoH's website, it can also be analysed by patients, academics and other interested parties.

Marginal analysis

Most often used in conjunction with programmed budgeting, programme budgeting and marginal analysis (PBMA) is defined as a technique used in microeconomics by which very small changes in specific variables are studied in terms of the effect on related variables and the system as a whole. It examines the incremental costs and benefits of shifting resources from one area to another, to provide insight into whether changes should be made.

One of the principal researchers in this field of PBMA, responsible for bridging the gap between military and healthcare applications in the USA, was Alain Enthoven, later an important influence on NHS reforms in the UK.

Funding for NHS in devolved parts of the UK

The funding of the various parts of the NHS in the UK is slightly different and can be reviewed on the relevant NHS websites.

NHS Scotland

The NHS Scotland has also undergone a radical reorganisation, but the NHSS remains the single largest budget item for which the Scottish Parliament is responsible, with around a third of the budget being spent by NHS Scotland.

For the year 2009/10 NHS Scotland's total budget is £11 billion. The NHS Scotland boards will share 78% (i.e. £8.6 bn), which includes £385 million for capital investment. General practices are funded separately as is some medical equipment and IT.

There are 14 geographically based boards and eight special boards, which include the ambulance service and national waiting times centre. The biggest board in funding terms is Greater Glasgow and Clyde, which will receive £1.8 billion in revenue funding. The smallest is Orkney, which will get £31 million.

The NHS Scotland has about 4.5 million outpatients attendances, 1.4 million new A&E attendances, over half a million attendances at nurse-led clinics, 77.3 million prescriptions and carried out 775 000 inpatient and day case principal operations.

The Accounts Commission for Scotland

The Accounts Commission is a statutorily independent body that ensures that NHS Scotland (and local government) achieve high standards of financial stewardship and value for money. Audit Scotland helps the Accounts Commission by investigating, on its behalf, various aspects of how public bodies work. It was set up in 1975, is independent of local councils and of government and can make recommendations and reports to Scottish ministers. It examines how Scotland's 32 councils and 41 joint boards manage their finances, helps these bodies manage their resources efficiently and effectively, promotes 'best value' and publishes information every year about how the bodies perform. The Accounts Commission has powers to report and make recommendations to the organisations it scrutinises and holds hearings and reports and makes recommendations to Scottish Government ministers. The Commission also has powers to take action against councillors and council officials if their negligence or misconduct leads to money being lost or breaks the law. Copies of reports and more information can be obtained from their website at www.audit-scotland.gov.uk/about/ac.

NHS Wales

The NHS Wales is Wales' biggest organisation, with 80 000 staff, and a total budget of £4.4 billion. The Welsh Assembly decides the size of the NHS budget, from within the total allocation it receives from the Chancellor. About 80% of this is allocated to the 22 local health boards according to a formula, which gives most money to those parts of Wales with the poorest health. This supports most hospital services. About 12% goes on GPs, dentists and others in the community, 5% is kept back to fund education and training for existing and future staff. The rest goes on various national public health initiatives and to fund research.

At the local level the 22 local health boards use their allocation to decide what the NHS trusts should provide, make decisions about the future of local hospitals, and hold the trusts to account. (The 14 NHS trusts are responsible for the day-to-day running of hospital services, for ambulances, and for staff such as district nurses and midwives.) In practice, the boards' freedom to manoeuvre is circumscribed by national policy as the Assembly's waiting times targets have to be met, by national contracts such as the national GP contract which states what GPs can be expected to do and by a historical factor as many budgets are simply rolled over from year to year.

Wales Audit Office

The Auditor-General for Wales, as head of the Wales Audit Office, either directly audits bodies, such as the Welsh Assembly Government and the NHS or, as in the case of local government, appoints auditors to do so. The Wales Audit Office covers all sections of government, except those reserved to the UK government. For more information go to www.wao.gov.uk/home.asp.

Capital in the NHS

This was formerly a government-funded capital grant, but is now a mixture of two elements: government funding and the private finance initiative, part of the PPP agenda. There have been growing concerns about the availability of capital funding for NHS schemes as some PCTs reported difficulties in confirming whether they have access to capital funding in 2009–10. This followed a £1 billion cut to the NHS's planned capital allocations between 2009 and 2011. Capital allocations were further hit by new international financial reporting standards, which meant most private finance initiative-style schemes will need to be reported as NHS capital, rather than revenue spending.

Public Private Partnership and Private Finance Initiative

These initiatives were intended to give the NHS (and other public sector organisations) access to private sector skills and expertise, as well as being a source of finance for capital investment. The PFI and PPP initiatives have spawned an industry and a collection of websites and literature that is not useful to cover in a book such as this.

Briefly, Public Private Partnership is the umbrella name given to a range of initiatives that involve the private sector in the operation of public services. The Private Finance Initiative is the most frequently used initiative. The key difference between PFI and conventional ways of providing public services is that the public does not own the asset. The public authority makes an annual payment to the private company who provides the building and associated services, rather like a mortgage. A company set up specially to run the scheme would own a typical PFI project. These companies are usually consortia including a building firm, a bank and a facilities management company. While PFI projects can be structured in different ways, there are usually four key elements: design, finance, build and operate.

The PFI scheme encourages private investment in public construction projects such as hospitals. This means that the private companies raise the capital and keep the borrowing off the nation's balance sheet. Having built it, the company then undertakes to run it for at least 25 years (sometimes up to 42 years), providing maintenance and upkeep, although not medical staff, and in return the NHS pays the company an annual rent to cover the interest on the money spent, the cost of maintenance and a profit margin for the company.

It is difficult to obtain a figure for total PFI and PPP contract debt that has been entered into by government, particularly as it is 'off book'. This is one reason why they are so attractive to government; they take debt off the government's balance sheets and assist the Treasury in not exceeding the EU rules on debt being no more than 40% of GDP. However, they are also beneficial in fees and profits for merchant banks, accountants, lawyers and construction companies who are pleased to encourage them. But they do commit large amounts of future governments' expenditure. From information that we have been able to ascertain it seems likely that as of October 2007 the total capital value of PFI contracts signed throughout the UK was £68 billion (Timmins 2009). However, this figure pales into insignificance compared with the commitment of central and local government to pay a further £215 billion (Timmins 2009) over the lifetime of these contracts. To break this down by region, the £5.2 billion of PFI investment in Scotland up to 2007 has created a public sector cash liability of £22.3 billion (Hellowell 2007) and the investment of £618 million via PFI in Wales up to 2007 has created a public sector cash liability of £3.3 billion (Hellowell and Pollock 2007).

The problem, however, may be that the commitment to the future 'mortgage payments' may prove a significant burden as this alone could represent 20% of a trust's future income. Another more recent problem has been that, unfortunately, in 2009 because of the credit crisis the government had to lend £2 billion of public money to the private firms building projects under PFI to maintain the system. At the time of writing there appears to be 69 schemes already, of which three are currently under construction. Another 18 schemes are planned to go ahead in the next two years (2010–12) (They Work For You 2009), bringing the total to 87 with a target of 100.

For a detailed discussion on the subject go to www.parliament.uk and under advanced search type in 'The Private Finance Initiative' you will then see a selection of reports and Hansard Written Answers (but some of them are fairly old now).

So as a result of PFI and PPP, NHS estate management has undergone major changes in recent years and even more challenges may yet occur. Once estate management was an accepted part of the NHS, but since the emergence of the private finance initiative in the 1990s NHS bodies have been encouraged to concentrate on providing clinical services rather than constructing and managing buildings. In 20 to 30 years' time, there may be few buildings managed by NHS organisations, with many owned by the private sector.

Under some early PFI schemes, long leases were granted after the concession period had ended. This practice was quickly dispensed with in favour of a PFI structure, with a lease and lease back just through the concession period. Finally, this was replaced with a 'contract debtor structure', providing a more tax-efficient arrangement and making the public sector the owner throughout. These arrangements reflected a core message – that NHS bodies should not sell the 'family silver'. However, increasing numbers of NHS organisations are still considering ways of converting outdated property stock into cash and in some cases replacing traditional facilities with more versatile ones owned by the private sector.

All trusts, whether foundation, acute or primary care, face challenges in relation to their estate ownership and provision of facilities as a result of new commissioning models and increased private sector competition.

Primary care trusts have to demonstrate evidence of competition and contestability in the commissioning of services. This may be difficult to show if their provider arms or bodies are the owners of the only appropriate facilities for a particular service. It may not be cost-effective to create new facilities, and unless commissioners have the power to require estate to be transferred, or at the very least to grant leases to a competitively selected service provider, there could be challenges and claims of bias.

Commissioning arms of PCTs may hold on to their estate when they release their provider arms or seek new providers – otherwise they may need to include break provisions in leases or call options in freehold transfers. This may be particularly important when they are setting up interim hosting arrangements with other NHS bodies or managing their provider arms out of the PCT and into new provider entities in the form of community interest companies or community foundation trusts. Conversely, providers need sufficient control over premises to ensure services are not disrupted because of maintenance or access problems. Furthermore, if services are put fully out to tender, ownership and control of the relevant premises could be a trump card in retaining the provider role. So we are left with a potential conflict at the time of commissioner–provider separation. The commissioner arm and the provider arm will each wish to have control and be able to retain or divest itself of the property at the appropriate time. The solution would appear to be for commissioners to retain the freehold, with provider bodies receiving a lease that is coterminous with the length of the services contract they are operating under.

Facilities in the future may need to be more sustainable and flexible than ever to ensure that they provide value for money. Facilities that were once used for a couple of daytime clinics may need to be used for much longer periods. The traditional 25-year lease to general practitioners may become outmoded and in some cases may need to be replaced with a more flexible so-called 'hot surgery' or 'hot clinic' option.

The flow of procedures from traditional secondary care to primary care environments and the streamlining of care pathways may require buildings and facilities that are fit for that purpose. Foundation trusts in particular are likely to be eager to bid for services from PCTs. Having appropriate facilities (or the ability to acquire such facilities) will be a prerequisite for this.

There are fewer large PFI schemes developing, but it is a structure that might be considered where several facilities are needed in one area. However, where there is a significant amount of retained estate or existing structures, a different solution may be preferable.

Many health sector private developers are now locating sites and funding and developing facilities on a more speculative basis. This is a challenge to banks and funders, which require long-term payment commitments upfront to justify the level of borrowing required. However, there is a shift in that some of the established private medical companies do not need funding investment as they can afford the initial construction themselves. They are then freer to anticipate the facilities needed by the NHS market for future services. In some situations, this may erode the provider arm's advantage, as ownership/control of existing estate may not be quite the passport to provide services that it once was.

As an aside and in relation to the costs and debts of PFI and PPP, it is interesting to note that for NHS bodies that are involved in private finance initiative or public private partnership projects, the application of international accounting standards that were to be applied at the time of writing have been delayed by 12 months. Many in the NHS were concerned that the changes would shift PFI and PPP debt (including existing debt) onto their balance sheets. Now they have another year to prepare for these changes.

Local Improvement Finance Trust (NHS LIFT)

NHS LIFT is an attempt at improving and developing primary and community care facilities. Commencing in 2001, it allowed PCTs to invest in new premises in new locations and not merely reproduce existing services. Only 40% of primary care premises were purpose built, almost half being either adapted residential buildings or converted shops. Fewer than 5% of GP surgeries were co-located with a pharmacy and around the same proportion were co-located with social services. Around 80% of surgeries were considered to be below the recommended size. NHS LIFT's aim, therefore, was to provide modernised integrated services in purpose-built primary care premises. It has provided a range of GP premises, one-stop primary care centres, integrated health and local authority service centres and community hospitals.

The National Audit Office (NAO)

Established under the National Audit Act 1983, the NAO's role is to ensure account-ability to Parliament and the taxpayer for all monies voted by Parliament. The Comptroller and Auditor-General (C&AG) also has statutory powers to certify a wide range of public sector accounts, and statutory powers to report to Parliament on the economic efficiency and effectiveness with which departments and other bodies have used their resources.

The National Audit Office audits the accounts of all central government depart-ments and agencies, as well as a wide range of other public bodies, and reports to Parliament on the economy, efficiency and effectiveness with which they have used public money.

The audit and inspection rights are vested in the head of the National Audit Office, the C&AG. The staff of the National Audit Office carry out these tasks on behalf of the C&AG.

The NAO holds the government to account for the way it uses public money by:
o supporting and helping public service managers improve performance

o safeguarding the interests of citizens who as taxpayers are responsible for paying for public services

o championing the interests of citizens as users of public services.

They are an independent organisation in that the C&AG is an Officer of the House of Commons, appointed by the Queen in an address proposed by the Prime Minister with the agreement of the Chairman of the Committee of Public Accounts and approved by the House of Commons. The C&AG then appoints the professional staff of NAO, currently numbering around 850, who are not civil servants and therefore independent of government.

The C&AG and the NAO have comprehensive statutory rights of access to the bodies they audit.

Their budget is set by Parliament, not the government of the day. About a fifth of the budget comes from income generated, including audit fees paid by international clients.

Oversight of the NAO is carried out by the Parliamentary Public Accounts Commission who appoint external auditors and scrutinise performance. For further information go to www.nao.org.uk.

The NAO does not audit the spending of the devolved governments in the rest of the UK or publish statistical information.

Audit Commission

In respect of health, the Commission audits NHS trusts, PCTs and SHAs, to review the quality of their financial systems. They also provide services to foundation trusts and those aspiring to become foundation trusts through their Trust Practice. For more information go to www.audit-commission.gov.uk/Pages/default.aspx and click on Health.

The Audit Commission also publishes independent reports highlighting risks and good practice to improve the quality of financial management in the health service and encourage continual improvement in public services, including public health and health inequalities.

Office for National Statistics

The Office for National Statistics produces independent information to improve understanding of the UK's economy and society because reliable and impartial statistics are vital for planning the proper allocation of resources, policy-making and decision making to ensure a fair society. For more details go to www.statistics.gov.uk/default.asp.

As the Office covers only England, for other devolved regions and for government spending in the rest of the UK go to:

o Audit Scotland at www.audit-scotland.gov.uk

o Wales Audit Office at www.wao.gov.uk

o Northern Ireland Audit Office at www.niauditoffice.gov.uk.

Finances at local level

Trusts obtain most of their income from provision of patient care services from NHS bodies (principally primary care trusts) and from other agencies. This includes income not directly related to patient care, such as education, training, research, payroll services for other bodies, car parking, meals to staff, etc.

Agreements with PCTs set out the treatment or services the trust agrees to provide in return for funding. Agreements can include quality clauses and requirements to meet targets for equal opportunities, respond to complaints and provide information to the public. Trusts have the power to make their own investment decisions and, with their financial freedom, can develop services for patients. The single financial obligation of the trust is to break even.

Financial control within NHS trusts

Members of trust boards have to ensure that the trust:
○ publishes a strategic direction document every third year covering the next five-year period
○ publishes a summary business plan by 31 March each year
○ ensures that the annual income and expenditure budget is realistic
○ makes adequate provision for inflation
○ receives a monthly report showing financial position with a forecast of year-end position
○ organises its management in an effective manner within limits set by the NHS.

Trusts must comply with certain requirements in pricing their services:
○ prices must equal costs for NHS agreements
○ costs must include depreciation and a 6% return on the value of assets employed
○ there must be no cross-subsidising between services
○ marginal costs can only be charged where unplanned spare capacity exists
○ for private contracts, charges should be what the market will bear.

The SHA is responsible to the DoH for the accumulated financial position of its constituent PCTs, NHS trusts and its own financial position each year. The DoH sets each SHA a 'control total' level of accumulated underspending each year, which it expects the local health economy to achieve, as part of a national NHS financial position.

NHS Employers

NHS Employers is an organisation that represents trusts in England on workforce issues. It is part of the NHS Confederation, an independent body for the full range of organisations that make up the NHS. It represents 99% of NHS organisations as well as a growing number of independent healthcare providers. It aims to influence policy, support leaders through networking, and share information and learning.

There is a policy board with members drawn from a range of organisations and professions. Over the last year they have signed off evidence to the pay review bodies, responded to the Tooke Report and the future direction of NHS Careers.

The board also has two national forums – the Medical Workforce Forum and the Healthcare Professions Advisory Board that facilitates debate and has its own work programme to support employers. In addition, the policy board is setting up a Primary Care subgroup, which will advise the board on the strategic direction of travel that General Medical Services contract negotiations might take over the longer term.

The policy board meets around five times a year and is made up of 27 members who are elected to bring the perspective of a particular work area or profession.

The policy board members comprise a chair and two vice-chairs supported by:

- immediate past chair
- two acute trust chief executives
- two acute trust HR directors
- two PCT chief executives
- two PCT HR directors
- two senior mental health trust/learning disability representatives
- one senior care trust representative
- one senior ambulance trust representative
- two chair/non-executive directors
- two nurse directors from any NHS organisation
- one acute trust medical director
- one PCT medical director
- one senior allied health professional/senior healthcare scientist representative from any NHS organisation
- one SHA workforce lead representative
- one SHA chief executive
- one senior SHA representative
- one finance director from any NHS organisation.

Elections are conducted by the independent organisation the Electoral Reform Services using a fair and transparent process that is in accordance with the NHS Confederation's policy and with best practice.

NHS Employers provides a range of services to meet the needs of members, made up of mental health trusts, primary care trusts, acute trusts, foundation trusts, ambulance trusts, and independent sector providers that deliver services on behalf of the NHS and SHAs, and works to address their needs through networks, forums and special interest groups.

It also runs an NHS European Office to inform NHS organisations about key EU developments and to promote the priorities and interests of the NHS in Europe. The Welsh NHS Confederation and the Northern Ireland Confederation support members in their countries and NHS Employers also provides a subscription service for NHS organisations in Scotland.

NHS Employers manages the negotiation infrastructure that supports discussions between NHS employers and unions on pay and terms and conditions. It negotiates specific contracts on behalf of employers, leads on pensions and ill health retirement reviews, provides evidence to pay review bodies and oversees the development of *Agenda for Change* (AfC; see below).

In their last Written Evidence to the Doctors' and Dentists' Review Body (DDRB) in October 2008, the DoH stated that it would commission NHS Employers to conduct work to look at the 'effectiveness and value for money of the current contractual arrangements for doctors in training'.

NHS Employers, with DoH and employers, was also asked to consider:
○ the current contractual arrangements for doctors and dentists in hospital training (the New Deal Contract introduced in 2000), identifying issues, strengths and weaknesses with clear evidence of all findings
○ evidence on the financial and other consequences of keeping the current contractual arrangements in place, and amending them
○ an appraisal of possible changes to the contractual arrangements, including a full assessment of all related costs, including pension costs for both employer and employee, and the cost of reform itself (which should begin from the assumption that any changes should be achieved with overall cost neutrality)
○ a full assessment of the value-for-money gain of any potential reform in both cost and productivity terms
○ the interface with contractual arrangements for doctors and dentists in the practice/ community settings of GP or dental vocational training.

The government's evidence to the Doctors' and Dentists' Review Body said this work should take account of:
○ the direction of travel resulting from the government's response to the Tooke Enquiry into Modernising Medical Careers
○ the NHS Next Stage Review (England)
○ Reshaping the Clinical Workforce (Scotland)
○ the current reform programme in Wales.

Findings were to be presented to the DoH by November 2009. For more information on this go to www.nhsemployers.org/Pages/home.aspx and follow the links to the various subjects.

Agenda for Change

Agenda for Change is described as the most radical shake up of the NHS pay system since the NHS began in 1948. It applies to the over one million NHS staff across the UK. NHS Employers is responsible for representing the views of employers in national negotiations on *Agenda for Change*, and provides support and assistance for trusts introducing the new systems through the *Agenda for Change* Implementation Team. NHS Employers' Pay and Negotiations team offers support and advice to employers in the NHS. Individual members of staff are advised to seek advice from their employer, professional representatives or trade union.

AfC is basically the single pay system in operation in the NHS. It applies to all directly employed NHS staff with the exception of doctors, dentists and some very senior managers so most readers of this book will not be affected. If you need further details go to www.nhscareers.nhs.uk/details/Default.aspx?Id=766.

In passing interest, there is a page at the above website briefly introducing the career of a doctor. It will tell you that doctors are responsible for the diagnosis, care and treatment of illnesses, infections, diseases and the well-being of people. They may work in a variety of settings such as in hospital or as a family doctor. It will further inform you that contemporary medicine is both challenging and exciting, with new discoveries making their impact on medical practice, doctors now qualifying will see even more dramatic changes in the future, with the developments of many new techniques, involving not only drugs, but methods arising from research in genetics, electronics, nuclear physics and molecular biology. There are links in a menu giving further information on issues such as starting, training and returning to a career in medicine.

The information on this website primarily relates to working and training to work in England. For information about opportunities elsewhere in the UK there is a site for Scotland at www.paymodernisation.scot.nhs.uk/AfC/docs/afc_staffbooklet.pdf.

Healthcare worldwide

The costs of delivering a high-quality healthcare system continue to rise inexorably in all countries due to a combination of factors. Central among these factors are an ageing population, increasing life expectancy, development of ever more effective drugs and technological interventions, which not only help prolong and sustain good-quality life, but may also lead to a need for resources for the management of other chronic yet treatable conditions.

At the same time, public expectations and demands about the standards of care and responsiveness within healthcare services continue to rise. There are also demands for patients to be able to exercise greater choice over the type of treatment they receive, the time they wait before being treated, and the location where treatment is delivered.

The nature of healthcare financing systems varies widely across developed countries. With the exception of the US and South Africa, all of the developed countries have implemented some kind of national health insurance system. Some countries (such as Germany and France) require employers to offer and employees to purchase a health insurance plan with payroll taxes as the major source of funding for this. In other countries, such as Canada, general tax revenues supply the major source of funding for their health insurance systems. Healthcare financing in the US is fundamentally different from that in most other developed countries because there is no national health insurance plan. There is a variety of third-party payers such as government programmes (Medicare and Medicaid), insurance companies (which can be either for-profit or not-for-profit), self-insured plans operated by employers and provider sponsor organisations (providers that contract directly to provide healthcare services). Each of these types of third-party payers offers different health plans that have different financing rules.

Healthcare systems models

o Purely private enterprise healthcare systems are comparatively rare. Where they exist, it is usually for a comparatively well-off subpopulation of a poorer country with a poorer standard of healthcare.
o Countries with a majority private healthcare system with residual public service (e.g. the US with Medicare, Medicaid).
o The other major models are all some form of public insurance systems.

In almost every country with a government healthcare system a parallel private system is allowed to operate. This is sometimes referred to as two-tier healthcare. The scale, extent, and funding of these private systems is very variable. The following give a greatly simplified view of healthcare systems in different countries. It is important to realise that systems change in other countries too, so if you are interested in one it would be best to visit the country's government health organisations websites, which often give extensive details for current information.

Australia
Medicare was instituted in 1984. It coexists with a private health system. Medicare is funded partly by an income tax but mostly out of general revenue. An additional levy is imposed on high earners without private health insurance. As well as Medicare, there is a separate Pharmaceutical Benefits Scheme that subsidises prescription medications.

Canada
Canada has a federal-sponsored, publicly funded Medicare system, with most services provided by the private sector. It is known as a single-payer system, where basic services are provided by private doctors, with the entire fee paid for by the government at the same rate. All GPs receive a fee per visit. Rates are negotiated between the provincial governments and the province's medical associations, on an annual basis. A doctor cannot charge a fee for a service that is higher than the negotiated rate – even to patients who are not covered by the publicly funded system – unless he or she opts out of billing the publicly funded system altogether. Pharmaceutical costs are set at a global median by government price controls. Other areas of healthcare, such as dentistry and optometry, are wholly private.

Cuba
Cuba has a government system that guarantees universal coverage but does charge fees for elective conditions in patients from abroad, although tourists who fall ill are treated freely in Cuban hospitals. Cuba attracts patients from Latin America and Europe by offering care of comparable quality to a developed nation but at much lower prices.

Finland
Public medical services at clinics and hospitals are run by local government and funded mostly by taxation but partly by patients. Taxation funding is partly local and partly

national. Patients can claim reimbursement of part of their prescription costs. There is a small private medical sector in which about 8% of doctors work and some choose also to work in the public sector. Private patients can claim a contribution towards their private medical costs (including dentistry) if they choose to be treated in the more expensive private sector, or they can join private insurance funds.

France

Most doctors work in private practice but there are both private and public hospitals. Social Security consists of several public organisations, distinct from the state government, with separate budgets that refunds patients for care in both private and public facilities. It generally refunds patients most of their healthcare costs, and all costs in costly or long-term conditions. Supplemental coverage may be bought from private insurers, most of them not-for-profit, mutual insurers.

Germany

Germany has a universal multi-payer system with two main types of health insurance: compulsory health insurance (Gesetzlich) and private insurance (Privat). Compulsory insurance applies to those below a set income level and is provided through private non-profit sickness funds at common rates for all members, paid for with joint employer/employee contributions. Private supplementary insurance to sickness funds of various sorts is available.

Ghana

Most healthcare is provided by the government, but hospitals and clinics run by religious groups also play an important role. Some for-profit clinics exist, but they provide less than 2% of health services. Healthcare is very variable through the country. The major urban centres are well served, but rural areas often have no modern healthcare. Patients in these areas either rely on traditional medicine or travel great distances for care.

Hong Kong

Both private and public clinics are common, while public hospitals account for the majority of the market.

India

Hospitals are run by government, charitable trusts and by private organisations. The government hospitals in rural areas are called the primary health centre (PHC). Major hospitals are located in district headquarters or major cities. Apart from the modern system of medicine, traditional and indigenous medicinal systems like Ayurvedic and Unani systems are in practice throughout the country.

Ireland

The public healthcare system of the Republic of Ireland was introduced by the Health Act 2004, which established a new body responsible for providing health and personal social services to everyone living in Ireland. The new National Health Service came into being officially on 1 January 2005. In addition to the public sector, there is also a large private healthcare market.

Israel
Israel has a publicly funded medical system that is universal and compulsory. Payment for the services is shared by labour unions and government.

Italy
A public system has the unique feature of paying its doctors a fee per capita per year, a salary system that does not reward repeat visits, testing and referrals. Italy has one of the highest doctor per capita ratios.

Japan
Services are provided either through regional/national public hospitals or through private hospitals/clinics, and patients have universal access to any facility, though hospitals tend to charge higher for those without referral. Public health insurance covers most citizens/residents and pays most of the cost for care and prescribed drugs. Patients are responsible for part of the cost with an upper limit. The insurance system is funded by tax from each household and employer. Supplementary private health insurance is available but only to cover the co-payments or non-covered costs, and usually makes fixed payment per days in hospital or per surgery performed, rather than per actual expenditure.

Netherlands
Since January 2006 healthcare has been provided by a system of compulsory insurance backed by a risk equalisation programme so that insured are not penalised for age or health status. This is meant to encourage competition between healthcare providers and insurers. Children under 18 are insured by the government and special assistance is available to those with limited incomes.

New Zealand
The health system is made up of public, private and voluntary sectors, with over 75% of healthcare funded publicly. Hospitals run by district health boards are public and treat citizens or permanent residents free. District health boards plan, fund and provide government-funded healthcare services for their local populations, within capped budgets. A national accident compensation insurance scheme provides accident insurance for all citizens, residents and temporary visitors. Healthcare in rural areas is limited since most specialists work in large towns and cities. There are part charges for visits to GPS and most prescriptions, and charges for dental care.

South Africa
Parallel private and public systems exist. The public system serves the vast majority of the population but is chronically underfunded and understaffed. The wealthiest

20% of the population uses the private system and are far better served. This division perpetuates racial inequalities created in the pre-apartheid segregation era.

Sweden
A publicly funded medical system is comprehensive and compulsory. Doctors and hospital services take a small patient fee, but their services are funded through the taxation scheme of the County Councils of Sweden.

United States
The US is alone among developed nations for its absence of a universal healthcare system, although this may change soon. However, there are significant publicly funded components. Medicare covers the elderly and disabled with a historical work record, Medicaid is available for some but not all of the poor and the State Children's Health Insurance Program covers children of low-income families. The Veterans Health Administration directly provides healthcare to US military veterans through a nationwide network of government hospitals; active duty service members, retired service members and their dependants are eligible for benefits through TRICARE. Together, these tax-financed programmes cover about 27% of the population and make the government the largest health insurer in the nation.

Privately owned hospitals or doctors in private practice generally provide care, but public hospitals are common in older cities. About 60% of Americans receive health insurance through an employer, although this number is declining and the employee's expected contribution to these plans varies widely and is increasing as costs escalate.

A significant and growing number of people cannot obtain health insurance through their employer or are unable to afford individual coverage so that about 16% of the US population, or 47 million people, are uninsured. A few states have taken serious steps towards universal healthcare coverage, most notably Minnesota and Massachusetts. The Indian Health Service provides publicly funded care for indigenous peoples.

Funding in the future
As NHS costs increase many doctors call for more debate about the future funding of the NHS. The members of Royal College of Physicians of Edinburgh were reported recently as saying a debate was needed about how long the country could afford to pay for free healthcare, as the NHS finds itself under increasing financial pressure. Issues faced include new and expensive drug treatments, an ageing population with increasing life expectancy, significant challenges in the form of rising obesity and alcohol-related disease and a reduction in public spending in the future.

In view of the country's financial problems in 2009, even without cuts from 2011 onwards the NHS faces a significant financial challenge. Analysis by researchers at The King's Fund and the Institute for Fiscal Studies (2009) outlined three plausible funding futures for the NHS in England over the next two comprehensive spending review periods from 2011/12 to 2016/17. If the NHS budget were frozen in the next two spending reviews, this would be the tightest six-year settlement in its history.

The report suggested that the gap in funding could, in principle, be filled by increasing NHS productivity. However, to do this over the period from 2011/12 to 2016/17 it would need to make gains of between £23.5 billion (£3.9 bn pa) and £48.9 billion (£8.2 bn pa). This is equivalent to improvements of 3.7 to 7.7% per year. Private sector productivity growth is about 2% a year, while the ONS estimates average NHS productivity between 1997 and 2007 has fallen each year by 0.4%.

The King's Fund (2009) added:

The scale of what is about to hit the healthcare system is unprecedented. If as seems likely the NHS will have at least three or four years of low or zero growth that will be the first time in its history that it has had to go for such a long period with rising demand and little or no new money. It would be a grave mistake to underestimate the challenge ahead.

Clearly, there are very tough choices in the future.

Related reading

The websites listed throughout Chapter 1 will provide the latest information, but please check the date on the articles you find on them, as there is much that is outdated. However, you might want to read The King's Fund and Institute for Fiscal Studies' (2009) *How Cold Will it Be? Prospects for NHS funding: 2011–17*, referred to above, by Appleby, Crawford and Emmerson. It is available as a pdf file at www.kingsfund.org.uk/research/publications/how_cold_will_it_be.html.

Hellowell M. *Written Evidence to the Finance Committee of the Scottish Parliament with Regards to its Inquiry into the Funding of Capital Investment.* Edinburgh: University of Edinburgh; 2007.

Hellowell M, Pollock AM. *Written Evidence to the National Assembly for Wales Finance Committee with Regards to its Inquiry on Public Private Partnerships.* Edinburgh: University of Edinburgh; 2007.

NHSE. *The New NHS.* Leeds: NHS Executive; 1997.

NHSE. *A National Framework for Assessing Performance.* Leeds: NHS Executive; 1998.

Timmins N. Projects seek partners. *Financial Times.* 24 February 2009.

They Work For You. Written parliamentary answers 2009. NHS Private Finance Initiative. Available online at www.theyworkforyou.com/wrans/?id=2009-02-23f.255300.htm

Parliament UK. Departmental public expenditure. 2010. Available online at http://services.parliament.uk/hansard/Commons/ByDate/20090513/writtenanswers/part010.html

Acts, circulars, reports and inquiries

The aim of this chapter is to provide you with information about health-related Acts of Parliament including Statutory Instruments (SIs), Health Service Circulars (HSC), Executive Letters (EL), Reports, Inquiries, Green Papers, White Papers, Codes of Practice and other Guidance Notes and publications issued by various bodies such as the GMC, medical royal colleges etc., that you may find useful, instructive or that you may need to know. I have divided it into three sections:

- health-related and other useful Acts of Parliament including Statutory Instruments
- health circulars, and guidance notes on codes and best practice
- government-inspired reports and inquiries.

Health-related Acts of Parliament and legislation including Statutory Instruments

The following list covers Acts of Parliament, Health Service Circulars, and Executive Letters (ELs). There has been an enormous output of these documents since the last edition of this book and although I have tried to be as comprehensive as possible, not everything can be included. Some publications have been omitted as I felt the size of the list had to be reduced. Clearly, for any individual doctor some will be totally irrelevant; for example, all the mental health papers, while they may be of interest to psychiatrists, may be of no interest to general surgeons or physicians and papers referring to abortion are only likely to interest those pursuing a career in obstetrics and gynaecology.

I have included Statutory Instruments known as secondary or subordinate legislation. They normally consist of an order, regulations, rules or a scheme and are made under powers conferred by primary legislation (an enabling Act). They are normally signed by a Minister and then laid before Parliament. On a given date they come into force and become law. In general, subordinate legislation makes detailed provisions, which supplement the enabling Act. Subordinate legislation is also used when frequent or speedy changes in the law are required.

Births and Deaths Registration Act 1953

Parents have a legal duty to register the details (child's name, sex, date and place of birth, parents' name, places of birth, address and father's occupation) of a birth with the local registrar within 42 days. The doctor or midwife normally has a duty to inform the district medical officer of the birth within six hours. Stillbirths (a baby born dead after the twenty-fourth week of pregnancy) must also be registered. Doctors attending patients during their last illness must sign a death certificate, giving cause of death (to their best knowledge). The certificate must be sent to the registrar. The registrar must inform the coroner of any death that occurs without attendance of a doctor at the last illness, or during an operation, or while the effects of an anaesthetic persist.

Abortion Act 1967

Under the terms of the Abortion Act of 1967, termination is legal up to the twenty-fourth week of pregnancy, subject to approval from two doctors. To 'qualify' for an abortion, a woman must prove that having a baby would cause her or her family greater physical or mental damage than not having one. The Act was amended and updated by the Abortion Regulations 1991.

The Family Law Reform Act 1969

This was passed in order to: amend the law relating to the age of majority, to persons who have not attained that age and to the time when a particular age is attained; to amend the law relating to the property rights of illegitimate children and of other persons whose relationship is traced through an illegitimate link; to make provision for the use of blood tests for the purpose of determining the paternity of any person in civil proceedings; to make provision with respect to the evidence required to rebut a presumption of legitimacy and illegitimacy; to make further provision, in connection with the registration of the birth of an illegitimate child, for entering the name of the father; and for connected purposes.

Misuse of Drugs Act 1971

Covers dangerous or otherwise harmful drugs and related matters.

NHS (Venereal Diseases) Regulations 1974

These require health authorities to take all necessary steps to ensure that information capable of identifying patients with sexually transmitted diseases does so not only for the purpose of treating people with the disease but also in preventing its spread. Such disclosure, furthermore, can only be made to a doctor, or to someone working on a doctor's instruction in connection with treatment or prevention. This allows contact tracing. However, it does not allow those working in a genito-urinary clinic to inform an insurance company of a patient's sexually transmitted disease – even with the patient's consent. Case notes from genito-urinary clinics are kept separate from other hospital records. GPs are not routinely informed of the patient's attendance at such clinics, although the patient may request that the GP is informed.

Health and Safety at Work etc. Act 1974

Sets out the relevant responsibilities of employers and people at work. The legal obligations ensure, as far as is reasonably possible, that employees and members of the public are not exposed to unacceptable risk as a result of the organisation's activities.

Sex Discrimination Act 1975

Makes it illegal for employers, professional bodies and trade unions to discriminate either directly or indirectly on the grounds of sex or marital status, except where marital status or a particular sex can be clearly shown to be a genuine requirement.

Medicines Labelling Regulations 1976

Rules about how medicines should be labelled.

Race Relations Act 1976

Aims to eliminate racial discrimination and to remedy individual grievances. It makes unlawful direct or indirect discrimination on the grounds of race, ethnicity or nationality in the fields of, for example, employment, education or housing.

Medical Act etc. 1983

As amended by the Professional Performance Act 1995, the European Primary Medical Qualifications Regulations 1996, the NHS (Primary Care) Act 1997, the Medical Act (Amendment) Order 2000, the Medical Act 1983 (Provisional Registration) Regulations 2000, the Medical Act 1983 (Amendment) Order 2002, and the National Health Service Reform and Health Care Professionals Act 2002, The European Qualifications (Health Care professions) Regulations 2003, the European Qualifications (Health & Social Care Professions and Accession of new Member States) Regulations 2004, the Medical Act 1983 (Amendment) and Miscellaneous Amendments Order 2006, and The European Qualifications (Health and Social Care Professions Regulations 2007).

Sets up and specifies the role of the GMC and its role in the registration and maintenance of a register of doctors.

For details go to www.gmc-uk.org/about/legislation/medical_act.asp.

Mental Health Act 1983 (MHA)

Provides the statutory framework under which mentally ill patients are detained and cared for in hospital. Includes patient admission (under strict guidelines) for assessment, treatment and emergency detention, and outlines the power of the courts, placing of safety orders and consent to treatment. A patient should be made aware of his or her admission to hospital and has a statutory right of appeal. Amended by Mental Health Act 2007.

Data Protection Act 1984

Brings the UK into line with other Western countries in terms of the rights, duties and obligations of all persons and organisations concerned with computers and computerised data. The Act recognises the specific importance of personal data and an individual citizen's rights. It allows individuals right of access to information about themselves that is held on computer.

The Registered Homes Act 1984

Sets standards for the independent healthcare sector. Sets out basic standards for facilities, staffing and procedures of a registered home.

Public Health (Control of Diseases) Act 1984 (Notifiable Diseases)

A doctor must notify the relevant local authority officer (usually a public health consultant) if he or she suspects a person of having a notifiable disease or food poisoning. The following information must be provided (by completing a specific certificate): patient's name, age, sex, address, suspected disease, approximate date of outset, date of admission to hospital (if appropriate).

Police and Criminal Evidence Act 1984

Gives the police power to apply to a court for access to records to assist in an investigation.

Access to Medical Reports Act 1988, Access to Health Records Act 1990 or Access to Health Records (Northern Ireland) Order 1993

Gives people right of access to their own health records and provides for the correction of inaccurate information in manually held records. Repealed by Data Protection Act 1998.

Road Traffic Act 1988

Gives powers to police to require doctors, on request, that might identify a driver alleged to have committed a traffic offence. This would not normally justify providing clinical information without the patient's consent, or a court order.

The Children's Act 1989

Provides the foundation for law on children in Britain. Principles laid down include that, wherever possible, children should be cared for by their own family in a safe and protected environment, that parents still have responsibility for their children not living with them, and that both the parents and the child should be kept informed and involved in decisions about the child's future. The Act requires collaboration between agencies in the provision of services to, and the protection of, children deemed to be in need. It also places responsibilities on local authority Social Services Departments (SSD) in relation to children in need. The Act emphasises the rights of a child to make informed decisions in relation to her or his own medical care. This has major implications about consent to treatment in children.

Prevention of Terrorism Act (Temporary Provision) Act 1989

All citizens, including doctors, must inform police, as soon as possible, of any information that may help to prevent an act of terrorism, or help in apprehending or prosecuting a terrorist.

National Health Service and Community Care Act 1990 (NHSCCA)

Covers the establishment of NHS trusts, the financing of the practices of medical practitioners, the provision of accommodation and other welfare services by local authorities, and the establishment of the Clinical Standards Advisory Group. Also defined membership of health authorities, established the family health services authorities (FHSA), and created the internal market, NHS trusts, GP fundholders and a significant change in community-based care arrangements.

Food Safety Act 1990

Specifies appropriate qualifications for food examiners and analysts.

Human Fertilisation and Embryology Act 1990

To make provision in connection with human embryos to prohibit certain practices; to establish a Human Fertilisation and Embryology Authority; to make provision about the persons who in certain circumstances are to be treated in law as the parents of a child; and to amend the Surrogacy Arrangements Act 1985.

Human Fertilisation and Embryology (Disclosure of Information) Act 1992

To relax restrictions on disclosure of information imposed by section 33(5) of the Human Fertilisation and Embryology Act 1990 and require licensing and monitoring of performance of fertility treatment clinics, and any research using human embryos. It covers three main activities: any fertility treatment which involves the use of donated eggs or sperm (for example, donor insemination) or embryos created outside the body (IVF – in vitro fertilisation); the storage of eggs, sperm and embryos; and research on early human embryos. The Act was amended in 2000 and 2001, to allow the use of a dead person's sperm in IVF and to allow the creation of embryos for therapeutic cloning research. The Human Fertilisation and Embryology Act 2008 now amends the Act further. (*see* p. 172)

Working Together under the Children Act (1989): a guide to arrangements for the protection of children from abuse, 1991, DoH

Covers arrangements for cross-agency working on child protection policies and procedures.

Welsh Language Act 1993

Sets out provisions for the use of the Welsh language in healthcare. This requires health authorities and trusts to translate all documents, information leaflets and signs into Welsh

Mental Health (Patients in the Community) Act 1995

Sets out the requirements for supervised discharge for severely mentally ill people. This Act supplements Section (1) 18 of the Mental Health Act 1983.

Children's (Northern Ireland) Order 1995

Replaces the provisions of the Children and Young Persons Act (Northern Ireland) 1968 and amends the law relating to illegitimacy and guardianship.

Carers (Recognition and Services) Act 1995 (DDA)

Covers carers who are either providing, or plan to provide, a substantial amount of care on a regular basis. Under the Act, the carer is entitled to request an assessment, the results of which should be taken into account along with the needs of the patient.

Disability Discrimination Act 1995 (DDA)

Aimed to end the discrimination which many disabled people face. It gave disabled people rights in the areas of employment, access to goods, facilities and services, and buying or renting land or property. The employment rights and first rights of access came into force in 1996 with further rights in 1999, and the remainder in 2004. In addition the Act allowed the government to set minimum standards so that disabled people could use public transport easily. For more information go to www.disability. gov.uk/law.html.

Employment Rights Act 1996

About the employment right of employees. Requires that certain terms and conditions must be set out in a single document – this can be a written 'contract of employment' or a 'statement of the main terms and conditions of employment'. The written terms and conditions will contain both contractual and statutory rights, that is, both those protected by law and those negotiated directly between the employer and the employee or representative. The Act has been amended, the last occasion being in 2004.

Mental Health Act 1983 – memorandum on Parts I to VI, VIII and X 1998

Designed to assist those who work with the Mental Health Act 1983, it offers guidance on the main provisions of the Act. The publication advises on appropriate application of the Act, and clarifies its interpretation with regard to the following areas: admission procedures; consent to treatment; court powers; mental health review tribunals; supervised discharge and aftercare; and supplementary provisions of the Act.

Data Protection Act 1998

About access for patients to their medical records. Updates previous Acts and replaces Access to Medical Records Act 1990.

Audit Commission Act 1998

Set up the Audit Commission and passed legislation enabling it to access information to carry out its functions.

Human Rights Act 1998

Makes it unlawful for any public body to act in a way that is incompatible with the European Convention on Human Rights unless the wording of an Act of Parliament means they have no other choice.

Health Act 1999

Under the Health Act 1999, money can be pooled between health bodies and health-related local authority services, and resources and management structures can be integrated. The arrangements, which have been in use since April 2000, allow the joining up of existing services and the development of new, co-ordinated services.

Employment Relations Act 1999

An Act based on the measures proposed in the White Paper *Fairness at Work*.

The Race Relations (Amendment) Act 2000

Is concerned with outlawing discrimination on the grounds of race in public life. For more information go to www.swap.ac.uk/widen/raceact.asp.

Adults with Incapacity (Scotland) Act 2000

To help people (aged 16 and over) who lack capacity to make some or all decisions for themselves. It enables carers or others to have legal powers to make welfare, healthcare and financial decisions on their behalf.

Care Standards Act 2000

Established a major regulatory framework for social care to ensure high standards of care and improve protection of vulnerable people. Implementation led to the establishment of the independent National Care Standards Commission (NCSC).

Health and Social Care Act 2001

To provide regulations for functions of Care Trusts under partnership arrangements. For more information go to www.legislation.hmso.gov.uk/acts/acts2001.

Employment Act 2002

Providing statutory rights to paternity and adoption leave and amending law on statutory maternity leave and pay. For more information go to www.legislation.hmso.gov. uk/acts/acts2002.

NHS Reform and Health Care Professions Act 2002

Establishing Commission for Patient and Public Involvement in Health. This Act reformed the distribution of functions between strategic health authorities and primary care trusts, extended the role of the Commission for Health Improvement, reformed the structures for patient and public involvement in the NHS, provided for joint working between NHS bodies and the prison service and reformed the regulation of the healthcare professions, including the establishment and functions of the Council for the Regulation of Health Care Professionals. For more information go to www. legislation.hmso.gov.uk/acts/acts2002.

Health and Social Care Act 2003

The Health and Social Care Act 2003 introduced a raft of new dental legislation.

Sex Discrimination Act 1975 (Amendment) Regulations 2003

Made some amendments to the original 1975 Sex Discrimination Act and more information go to www.lg-employers.gov.uk/relations/law/discrimination/sex.html.

Health (Community Health and Standards) Act 2003

Gives Commission for Healthcare Audit and Inspection access to fulfil its statutory obligations.

Mental Health (Care and Treatment) Scotland Act 2003

Replaces the 1984 Act and establishes new arrangements for the detention, care and treatment of persons who have a mental disorder. It also refines the role and functions of the Commission and establishes the Tribunal as the principal forum for approving and reviewing compulsory measures for the detention, care and treatment of mentally disordered persons.

Gender Recognition Act 2004

Previously transsexuals were defined by the gender they were born into. This Act allows them to apply for a Gender Recognition Certificate for which doctors may be asked to provide supporting medical evidence.

Freedom of Information Act 2004

Gives the public new rights on information held by approximately 100 000 public authorities. It gives them rights to ask how services are organised and managed, how much they cost and how they can make complaints. The organisation must reply to people's requests within 20 working days. There are exceptions, some absolute such as court records and some non-absolute such as commercial interests. For more information go to www.informationcommissioner.gov.uk.

Health Protection Agency Act 2004

To establish the Health Protection Agency and make provision as to its functions.

Human Tissue Bill 2004

To provide a consistent legislative framework for issues relating to whole body donation and the taking, storage and use of human organs and tissue and to make provision about the transfer of human remains from certain museum collections, and for connected purposes. For more information go to www.publications.parliament.uk.

Children Bill 2004

The Children Bill represents the biggest ever change in the organisation of Children's Services. New management models must be developed to support integrated services and all the key agencies must commit to the service model. Its aim is to prevent the abuse and killing of children. It creates an obligation for healthcare providers to safeguard and promote the health and well-being of children to be achieved by undertaking new guidance on doctors' roles and responsibilities in promoting children's rights and contributing to improving their access to good-quality healthcare services. Key aspects are ensuring respect for the privacy and confidentiality of the child, protecting children from harm and providing children and young people with accessible information. Details can be seen at a number of websites including www.publications. parliament.uk, www.gmc-uk.co.uk or www.nspcc.org.uk.

Mental Capacity Bill 2004

People with limited mental capacity will be encouraged to take as many decisions for themselves as possible under this legislation. The Mental Capacity Bill aims to protect more than two million adults who may be unable to take decisions for themselves. For more information go to www.direct.gov.uk. Amended by Mental Health Act 2007.

Mental Health Bill 2004

The Mental Health Bill is part of the government's strategy to improve the provision of mental health services and make them more focused on the needs of the individual. For more information go to www.dh.gov.uk.

Assisted Dying for Terminally Ill Bill 2004

This Bill, which sought to legalise physician-assisted suicide (PAS) and euthanasia, was considered by a special select committee of the House of Lords, which reported in April 2005. The committee did not reach a conclusion on the principle of whether PAS or euthanasia should become legal, but identified a number of issues which would need to be overcome before any further attempt to introduce legislation on this issue is made. The Select Committee report was debated in the House of Lords in October 2005. However, the Bill fell when the General Election was called earlier in 2005 and did not progress further. For more information go to www.publications.parliament.uk.

Domestic Violence, Crime and Victims Act 2004

An Act to amend Part 4 of the Family Law Act 1996, the Protection from Harassment Act 1997 and the Protection from Harassment (Northern Ireland) Order 1997; to make provision about homicide; to make common assault an arrestable offence; to make provision for the payment of surcharges by offenders; to make provision about alternative verdicts; to provide for a procedure under which a jury tries only sample counts on an indictment; to make provision about findings of unfitness to plead and about persons found unfit to plead or not guilty by reason of insanity; to make provision about the execution of warrants; to make provision about the enforcement of orders imposed on conviction; to amend section 58 of the Criminal Justice Act 2003 and to amend Part 12 of that Act in relation to intermittent custody; to make provision in relation to victims of offences, witnesses of offences and others affected by offences; and to make provision about the recovery of compensation from offenders. Amended by the Mental Health Act 2007. For more information go to www.opsi.gov.uk/acts/acts2004/ukpga_20040028_en_1.

The Disability Discrimination Act 2005
Amends the Disability Discrimination Act (DDA 1995); for more information go to www.disability.gov.uk/legislation/dda/ddaintro.

Mental Capacity Act 2005
To clarify and reform the common law provisions that had governed the ways in which society dealt with people lacking decision-making capacity. It is supplemented by new statutory schemes for advanced decision making and court-based resolution of disputes or difficulties. The Act covers decisions relating to an individual's property and financial affairs, together with decisions regarding healthcare treatment and more everyday decisions, such as personal care.

Mental Capacity Act 2005
Provides a statutory framework to protect vulnerable people, carers and professionals. It makes it clear who can take decisions in which situations and how they should go about this. It starts from the fundamental point that a person has capacity and that all practical steps must be taken to help the person make a decision.

Consolidation of NHS law in England and Wales 2006
Most health legislation made since 1977 has been summarised within three Acts of Parliament that received Royal Assent in 2006 and came into effect in 2007 (subject to a few exceptions). All those who refer to the law governing the NHS need to make sure that, where necessary, they replace their earlier copies of statutes with the three new Acts: NHS Redress Act 2006, Health Act 2006 and Mental Capacity Act 2005.

Human Tissue (Scotland) Act 2006
To modernise the legal framework for organ and tissue donation by strengthening the existing system, based on giving effect to people's wishes.

NHS Redress Act 2006
The government's objective was to reform the way lower value clinical negligence cases are handled in the NHS to provide appropriate redress, including investigations, explanations, apologies and financial redress where appropriate, without the need to go to court, thereby improving the experience of patients using the NHS.

Health Act 2006
Makes provision:
o for the prohibition of smoking in certain premises, places and vehicles

○ for amending the minimum age of persons to whom tobacco may be sold
○ in relation to the prevention and control of healthcare infections
○ in relation to the management and use of controlled drugs
○ in relation to the supervision of certain dealings with medicinal products and the running of pharmacy premises, and about orders under the Medicines Act 1968 and orders amending that Act under the Health Act 1999
○ about the NHS in England and Wales and about the recovery of NHS costs
○ for the establishment and functions of the Appointments Commission
○ about the exercise of social care training functions.

The Health and Social Care (Community Health and Standards) Act 2003, Order 2006

About the NHS recovering the costs of hospital treatment and ambulance services where people receive compensation for injuries.

The Personal Injuries (NHS Charges) Regulations 2006

Provides for the recovery of charges in cases where an injured person who receives a compensation payment in respect of his or her injury has received NHS hospital treatment or ambulance services. The charges are payable by persons who pay compensation to the injured person.

The National Health Service (Pharmaceutical Services) (Amendment) Regulations 2006

Makes amendments to Regulations relating to community pharmaceutical services.

The Smoke-free (Premises and Enforcement) Regulations 2006

Specifies the meanings of 'enclosed' and 'substantially enclosed' premises. Premises are enclosed if 'they have a ceiling or roof and, except for doors, windows and passageways, they are wholly enclosed either permanently or temporarily'. Premises are substantially enclosed 'if they have a ceiling or roof and less than half of their perimeter consists of openings in the walls, other than windows, doors or openings which can be shut'. And also defines 'roof' for the purposes of the regulation to include 'any fixed or moveable structure that is capable of covering all or part of the premises'.

The National Health Service (Charges to Overseas Visitors) (Amendment) Regulations 2006

For the making and recovery of charges in respect of certain services provided under the NHS Act 1977 to persons not ordinarily resident in the UK, i.e. overseas visitors.

The National Health Service (Charges to Overseas Visitors) (Amendment) Regulations 2006

Extend exemption from charges to an overseas visitor who is a missionary and the spouse, civil partner or child of some overseas visitors who are exempt.

The Controlled Drugs (Supervision of Management and Use) Regulations 2006

Contain measures relating to arrangements about the safe management and use of controlled drugs in England and Scotland.

The Medicines for Human Use (Clinical Trials) Amendment (No.2) Regulations 2006

Amended the Medicines for Human Use (Clinical Trials) Regulations 2004 that implement Directive 2001/20/EC on the laws, regulations and administrative provisions of the EC Member States relating to the implementation of good clinical practice in the conduct of clinical trials on medicinal products for human use.

The Mental Capacity Act 2005 (Independent Mental Capacity Advocates) Regulations 2006

Adjust the obligation to make arrangements as to the availability of independent mental capacity advocates (IMCAs).

The Mental Capacity Act 2005 (Appropriate Body) (England) Regulations 2006

Defines 'appropriate body' and for the purposes of Act provides that certain research carried out on or in relation to a person without capacity is unlawful unless it is carried out as part of a project which is approved by an appropriate body and satisfies further requirements specified in the Act.

The National Health Service (Complaints) Amendment Regulations 2006

Amend the NHS (Complaints) Regulations 2004 that detail the procedure for the handling of complaints made relating to NHS bodies and prescribe the Healthcare Commission's role in respect of NHS complaints.

The Blood Safety and Quality (Amendment) Regulations 2006

Further amend the Blood Safety and Quality Regulations 2005. They implement Directive 2002/98/EC of the European Parliament and Council, setting out the standards of quality and safety for the collection, testing, processing, storage and distribution of human blood and blood components. They also implement Commission Directive 2004/33/EC, which contains certain technical requirements relating to blood and blood components.

The Medicines for Human Use (National Rules for Homoeopathic Products) Regulations 2006

Implement the provisions of Directive 2001/83/EC on the Community Code relating to medicinal products for human use relating to marketing authorisations, to introduce a new scheme for applications for such authorisations for certain homoeopathic medicinal products. Article 16(2) of the 2001 Directive permits Member States to introduce in their territory specific rules for pre-clinical tests and clinical trials of such products.

The Medicines for Human Use (Clinical Trials) Amendment Regulations 2006

Implement Directive 2001/20/EC on the approximation of the laws, regulations and administrative provisions of the Member States relating to the implementation of good clinical practice in the conduct of clinical trials on medicinal products in human use.

The Mental Capacity Act 2005 (Independent Mental Capacity Advocates) (General) Regulations 2006

Define 'NHS body' and 'serious medical treatment' for the purposes of certain provisions of the Mental Capacity Act 2005 that deals with independent mental capacity advocates. The Regulations also contain provision as to who can be appointed to act as an IMCA and as to an IMCA's functions when he or she has been instructed to represent a person in a particular case.

The Strategic Health Authorities (Establishment and Abolition) (England) Amendment Order 2006

This Order amends the Strategic Health Authorities (Establishment and Abolition) (England) Order 2006 by correcting the name of the County of North Somerset.

The Strategic Health Authorities (Establishment and Abolition) (England) Order 2006

Abolishes the listed strategic health authorities and establishes in their place new strategic health authorities again listed identifying each successor strategic health authority for each of the old authorities. It also provides for the transfer of property, rights, liabilities and staff from the old authorities to the new authorities, for the accounts and the winding up of the affairs of the old authorities and for the continuity of the exercise of functions between the old authorities and the new authorities.

The Health Authorities (Membership and Procedure) Amendment (England) Regulations 2006

Remove the requirement for one of the non-officer members of an Authority to be a person who holds a post in an institution within the higher education sector that provides education leading to registration in certain health professions. Also remove the provision as to termination of such a person's appointment as a member of the Authority where the person ceases to hold such a post.

The National Health Service (Performers Lists) Amendment Regulations 2006

To 'permit a doctor, who is undertaking the post-registration part of the foundation programme for newly qualified doctors, to perform primary medical services without being a general medical practitioner or on a list, but only in so far as the performance of primary medical services constitutes part of that programme'.

The Medical Act 1983 (Amendment) and Miscellaneous Amendments Order 2006

Miscellaneous amendments to the Medical Act 1983. The register of medical practitioners with limited registration, kept by the GMC, is abolished, and as a consequence the GMC will now only keep one register ('the GMC register'). Medical practitioners will no longer be able to apply for limited registration, but those on the register of medical practitioners with limited registration prior to the abolition of that register will transfer to the GMC register, with certain exceptions, but will initially have to work in an approved practice setting.

The training requirements for newly qualified medical practitioners with provisional registration are revised. Under the new arrangements, medical practitioners with provisional registration who are in training in the UK are required to complete a programme for provisionally registered doctors (PPRD), recognised by the Education Committee, of the GMC, before they can become fully registered medical practitioners. The requirements of PPRDs will be determined by the Education Committee who will also be responsible for determining which bodies may be involved in PPRDs – and for the arrangements for monitoring those bodies. PPRDs will be open to all provisionally registered doctors, including those who have qualified overseas.

In addition, the GMC is given powers to limit, by regulations, the length of time for which medical practitioners may be provisionally registered. Also, it will become possible for bodies other than universities to hold qualifying examinations, where the Education Committee recommends this and the Privy Council makes the necessary Order.

The arrangements for the registration of medical practitioners who have qualified outside the European Economic Area or Switzerland have been revised. Previously, except in the case of certain specialists and qualified general practitioners, and in the case of practitioners who were registering under the arrangements for temporary registration, such practitioners were given limited registration, but now they are to be given full registration, provided that they have an acceptable overseas qualification and have demonstrated that they have the requisite knowledge, skills and experience.

If the Registrar determines that the medical practitioner does not yet have the requisite knowledge, skills and experience, but has sufficient knowledge and skills to embark upon a PPRD (or, transitionally, to be employed as a house doctor), the Registrar may provisionally register the medical practitioner to enable him or her to participate in a PPRD (or, transitionally, to be employed as a house doctor). There are separate arrangements for those only needing temporary registration, which again have been fully revised.

A new category of temporary registration is also created for overseas practitioners who will be employed or engaged within the UK to provide particular medical services for persons who are not nationals of the UK. The registration of these practitioners is conditional upon them only providing particular medical services at particular establishments, and only providing those services to patients who are not nationals of the UK, except in an emergency. Visiting eminent specialists will also have their own separate registration arrangements.

Entitlement to registration under any provision of the Act is now conditional upon the applicant's fitness to practise not being impaired. The Registrar is given new, extended powers to obtain information about whether a medical practitioner's fitness to practise is, or was, impaired at the time of registration – and he may remove medical practitioners from the GMC register (subject to rights of appeal) either if new information comes to light showing that their fitness to practise was impaired at the time of registration but this was not disclosed at the time or if a practitioner refuses to co-operate with the new information-gathering arrangements. Decisions to refuse to restore a person to the register for a fitness to practise reason, if they left it voluntarily or for non-payment of fees, are now appealable through the courts.

There are also changes to the fitness to practise procedures for medical practitioners post registration. The GMC is given powers to apply to a court to require production of documents from third parties relating to fitness to practise investigations, where these have not been supplied within 14 days. It is also made clear that the GMC has the power to disclose information relating to a medical practitioner's fitness to practise, whenever or wherever the matter to which it relates arose, where it sees it as being in the public interest to do so, and to take decisions to disclose particular classes of information.

A list is also provided of the decisions of panels and committees that have to be published, although the GMC is given powers to withhold, in the course of publication of these decisions, information concerning a person's physical or mental health, where it considers the information to be confidential. Allowance is made for the possibility that a medical practitioner will concede, during an investigation into his or her fitness to practise, that his or her fitness to practise is impaired – and in these circumstances, the GMC may make rules in respect of the agreement of undertakings to be observed by the practitioner, and in respect of the procedure to be followed where such undertakings are breached. Fitness to practise hearings are to be in public, except to the extent that rules made by the GMC provide otherwise. There is also a change to the arrangements for the making of legal assessors' rules.

If a person's registration has been suspended, the provisions of the Act relating to voluntary erasure from the GMC register, and those relating to fraudulent or incorrect entry, will now apply to him. Furthermore, the provisions of the Act relating to fraudulent or incorrect entry are amended so that the Registrar rather than the GMC deals with cases covered by these provisions, with rights of appeal to Registration Appeals Panels.

There are also changes to ensure that revalidation of a medical practitioner's licence to practise can take place at any time, and to allow the GMC to make regulations about requiring medical practitioners to supply information to assist licensing authorities in determining when and how to revalidate them. There are also transitory arrangements enabling the GMC, a licensing authority or a future licensing authority to obtain information to assist them in preparing for the introduction of revalidation. Additionally, licence to practise appeals will have to be held in public, except to the extent that rules provide otherwise.

There is a new requirement on all medical practitioners who hold a licence to practise that they are covered by an adequate and appropriate indemnity arrangement, such as a policy of insurance. There are new information-gathering powers relating to this requirement, and applicants for licences to practise who cannot demonstrate that they will have adequate cover may be refused a licence to practise. Medical practitioners may face disciplinary proceedings or withdrawal of their licence to practise if they breach either the notification requirements relating to the new requirement or the requirement itself. Provision is made for appeals and in respect of restoration of those who are subject to erasure. There are transitional arrangements if the new requirement is brought into force before the introduction of licences to practise, so that the requirement will instead temporarily apply to all registered doctors.

All medical practitioners who are newly fully registered, newly restored to the register or transferred from the register of medical practitioners with limited registration (except those with rights of establishment under European Community Law or where the GMC directs otherwise) will have to work in an approved practice setting until the first revalidation of their fitness to practise by the GMC. There are transitional arrangements to cover what will happen if the revalidation arrangements are brought into force after the provisions relating to approved practice settings come into force. Medical practitioners who are newly fully registered or newly restored and who are exempt from this requirement may be given guidance by the GMC on suitable practice settings for them.

There are miscellaneous amendments in connection with fees. If medical practitioners wish to remain registered, they are required to pay a retention fee, and the regulation-making power in respect of setting the fee is amended so that it need not necessarily fall due on the anniversary of first registration. In addition, the Privy Council is no longer required to approve fees regulations. Also, the limitations under the Act on persons other than registered medical practitioners being entitled to recover charges through the courts for certain medical services are amended so as not to prohibit recovery of charges by other specified providers of such services.

In view of the importance of this you can see all the details at www.opsi.gov.uk/si/si2006/20061065.htm.

The National Health Service (Travel Expenses and Remission of Charges) Amendment Regulations 2006

Amend the National Health Service (Travel Expenses and Remission of Charges) Regulations 2003 to increase the amounts used as the basis for calculating entitlement to the payment of travel expenses and the remission of charges under those Regulations.

The Medicines for Human Use (Prescribing) (Miscellaneous Amendments) Order 2006

Makes provision for nurses and pharmacists who meet certain conditions ('nurse independent prescribers' and 'pharmacist independent prescribers') to prescribe and administer prescription-only medicines, and remove provisions which applied to 'extended formulary nurse prescribers'.

The Medicines (Sale or Supply) (Miscellaneous Amendments) Regulations 2006

Make amendments to Regulations relating to the sale or supply of medicines. Mainly an amendment so that a 'health prescription' includes a prescription issued by a community practitioner nurse prescriber, a nurse independent prescriber or a pharmacist independent prescriber, under legislation relating to the NHS.

The NHS (Miscellaneous Amendments Relating to Independent Prescribing) Regulations 2006

These regulations make changes to three sets of NHS Regulations that apply in England that arise out of new arrangements for the independent prescribing of drugs and appliances by nurses and pharmacists. Independent nurse prescribers, unless they are community practitioner nurse prescribers, will no longer be limited to prescribing from a particular formulary, and nor will a new category of independent prescriber known as pharmacist independent prescribers.

The Private and Voluntary Health Care (England) (Amendment) Regulations 2006

Affect the frequency of inspections.

The Medicines for Human Use and Medical Devices (Fees Amendments) Regulations 2006

Specifies amendments to the Medicines (Homoeopathic Medicinal Products for Human Use) Regulations 1994 and other fees payable relating to marketing authorisations, licences and certificates in respect of medicinal products for human use.

The Functions of Primary Care Trusts (Dental Public Health) (England) Regulations 2006

Set out the functions of PCTs in England in relation to oral health. Those functions relate to oral health promotion programmes, dental inspection of pupils in schools maintained by local education authorities and oral health surveys.

Mental Health Act 2007

Amends the Mental Health Act 1983, the Domestic Violence, Crime and Victims Act 2004 and the Mental Capacity Act 2005 in relation to mentally disordered persons; to amend section 40 of the Mental Capacity Act 2005; and for connected purposes. Introduces a number of changes to the 1983 Act and the MCA. The following are the main changes to the 1983 Act.

○ *Definition of mental disorder:* it changes the way the 1983 Act defines mental disorder, so that a single definition applies throughout the 1983 Act, and abolishes references to categories of disorder.
○ *Criteria for detention:* it introduces a new test of whether a person's ability to make decisions about medical treatment is significantly impaired because of mental disorder.

○ *Professional roles:* it is broadening the group of practitioners who can take on the role of the approved social worker (ASW) and responsible medical officer (RMO).
○ *Nearest relative (NR):* it gives to patients the right to make an application to displace their NR and enables county courts to displace a NR where there are reasonable grounds for doing so.
○ *Supervised community treatment (SCT):* it introduces SCT for patients following a period of detention in hospital.
○ *Mental Health Review Tribunal (MHRT):* it introduces an order-making power to reduce the time before a case has to be referred to the MHRT by the hospital managers. It also introduces a single Tribunal for England and one in Wales.
○ *Abolition of finite restriction orders:* it removes the possibility of restriction orders being made for a limited period, so that they may remain in force for as long as the offender's mental health problem poses a risk of harm to others.

Access to all the documents is at www.dh.gov.uk/en/Healthcare/Mentalhealth/DH_063423.

The Local Government and Public Involvement in Health Act 2007
First introduced to Parliament in 2006, it introduces a number of measures relating to local government as well as involvement of local communities. One of the measures it introduces is the establishment of Local Involvement Networks (LINks), which replace Patients' Forums, and the Commission for Patient and Public Involvement in Health in 2008. Also clarifies and strengthens the existing duty on NHS bodies to involve and consult patients and the public in the planning and provision of services. For more information go to www.dh.gov.uk/en/Publicationsandstatistics/Publications/PublicationsLegislation/DH_076445.

The European Qualifications (Health and Social Care Professions) Regulations 2007
Relate to the removal of barriers to the freedom of movement of professionals across the EU by standardising the principles applicable across all professions.

The Smoke-free (Signs) Regulations 2007
These regulations relate to the display of no-smoking signs in smoke-free premises and vehicles in England.

The Smoke-free (Exemptions and Vehicles) Regulations 2007
Regulations that apply only to England provide exemptions from the smoke-free requirements of the Health Act 2006 and provide for most public and work vehicles to be smoke-free.

The Children and Young Persons (Sale of Tobacco etc.) Order
Order substituting the age of 18 for the age of 16 in that related to the prohibition on the sale of tobacco products and cigarette papers to young persons in England and Wales.

The Blood Safety and Quality (Amendment) Regulations 2007

These regulations further amend the Blood Safety and Quality Regulations 2005, which implement Directive of the European Parliament and of the Council setting out the standards of quality and safety for the collection, testing, processing, storage and distribution of human blood and blood components. It also corrects an error in earlier regulation that imposes requirements on blood establishments, hospital blood banks and facilities where blood transfusion takes place to report serious adverse reactions and events, ensuring that such establishments, blood banks and facilities must make an annual report to the Secretary of State on serious adverse events.

Human Fertilisation and Embryology Act 2008

The Act mainly amends the Human Fertilisation and Embryology Act 1990. Key provisions are as follows.

o Ensure that all human embryos outside the body – whatever the process used in their creation – are subject to regulation.

o Ensure regulation of 'human-admixed' embryos created from a combination of human and animal genetic material for research.

o Ban sex selection of offspring for non-medical reasons. This puts into statute a ban on non-medical sex selection currently in place as a matter of Human Fertilisation and Embryology Authority policy. Sex selection is allowed for medical reasons; for example, to avoid a serious disease that affects only boys.

o Recognise same-sex couples as legal parents of children conceived through the use of donated sperm, eggs or embryos. These provisions enable, for example, the civil partner of a woman who carries a child via IVF to be recognised as the child's legal parent.

o Retain a duty to take account of the welfare of the child in providing fertility treatment, but replace the reference to 'the need for a father' with 'the need for supportive parenting' – hence valuing the role of all parents.

o Alter the restrictions on the use of HFEA-collected data to help enable follow-up research of infertility treatment.

For more information go to www.dh.gov.uk/en/Publicationsandstatistics/Legislation/Actsandbills/DH_080211 and for explanatory notes go to www.opsi.gov.uk/acts/acts2008/en/ukpgaen_20080022_en_1.htm.

Health and Social Care Act 2008

Contains four main policy areas as follows.

o Care Quality Commission is the new integrated regulator for health and adult social care, bringing together existing health and social care regulators into one regulatory body, with powers to ensure safe and high-quality services.

o Professional regulation to enhance public and professional confidence in the system of professional regulation and strengthen clinical governance as part of the government's response to the Shipman Inquiry.

o Public health protection measures providing a comprehensive set of public health measures to help prevent and control the spread of serious diseases caused by infection and contamination.

o Health in Pregnancy Grant, a one-off payment to expectant mothers ordinarily resident in the UK, to help with the costs of a healthy lifestyle, including diet, in the later stages of pregnancy.

And a number of smaller measures that can all be seen at www.dh.gov.uk/en/Publications andstatistics/Legislation/Actsandbills/HealthandSocialCareBill/index.htm.

The National Health Service (Charges to Overseas Visitors) (Wales) Regulations 2009

State that an asylum seeker whose application for asylum has failed will not be charged for services forming part of the health service.

The NHS Trusts (Transfer of Staff, Property, Rights and Liabilities) (Wales) Order 2009

Provides for the transfer of staff, property, rights and liabilities from the NHS trusts dissolved by the NHS Trusts (Dissolution) (Wales) to the new local health boards established by the Local Health Boards (Establishment and Dissolution) (Wales) Order 2009.

The Local Health Boards (Transfer of Staff, Property, Rights and Liabilities) (Wales) Order 2009

This Order provides for the transfer of staff, property, rights and liabilities from the local health boards dissolved by the Local Health Boards (Establishment and Dissolution) (Wales) Order 2009 to the new local health boards established by that Order.

The Working Time (Amendment) Regulations 2009

These regulations implement the third subparagraph of Article 17(5) of Directive of the European Parliament and of the Council 2003 concerning certain aspects of the organisation of working time. These amendments provide for the 48-hour working time limit for doctors in training to be increased to 52 hours for certain doctors in training until 2011. Regulation 3 inserts a new Schedule into the Working Time Regulations 1998, which lists those categories of doctors in training to whom this 52-hour working time limit applies. You can read the full text at www.opsi.gov.uk/si/si2009/uksi_20091567_en_1.

The Mid Yorkshire Hospitals National Health Service Trust (Establishment) Amendment Order 2009

This Order amends the Mid Yorkshire Hospitals NHS Trust and the Pinderfields and Pontefract Hospitals NHS Trust and the Dewsbury Health Care NHS Trust (Dissolution) Order 2002 that established the Mid Yorkshire Hospitals NHS Trust.

The Human Fertilisation and Embryology (Statutory Storage Period for Embryos and Gametes) Regulations 2009

These regulations provide for embryos and gametes to be stored in certain circumstances for longer than the period of 10 years laid down by the Human Fertilisation and Embryology Act 1990 as amended by the Human Fertilisation and Embryology Act 2008.

The National Health Service (Travel Expenses and Remission of Charges) Amendment Regulations 2009

These regulations, which apply to England, amend the NHS (Travel Expenses and Remission of Charges) Regulations 2003. Also Regulation 2 updates the reference to the publication which describes additional loans paid under the Education (Student Loans) (Scotland) Regulations 2007. These loans are disregarded in the calculation of a student's loan income when a person's entitlement to the payment of NHS travel expenses and the remission of NHS charges is being established under the Travel Expenses and Remission of Charges Regulations.

Health Bill 2009

Proposes measures to improve the quality of NHS care, the performance of NHS services and to improve public health. It contains a number of features including establishing a framework for the NHS Constitution, and the creation of new Quality Accounts, enabling direct payment of healthcare with initial pilots as a first step to personal health budgets. This latter by provision of powers to allow the Secretary of State (in practice devolved to primary care trusts) to make direct payments to people, enabling them to arrange and pay for their own healthcare. Initially, the payments would be made by specific primary care trusts as part of a pilot programme. The Bill allows for the detail of the pilot schemes, e.g. the types of services for which direct payments can be used, to be set out in regulations. If the pilots are successful, direct payments for healthcare may be rolled out nationally through secondary legislation, subject to the approval of Parliament.

Various health-related Regulations, Guidance Notes and Codes of Conduct and Good Practice

Health and Safety (First Aid) Regulations 1981

Identify the necessary requirements to ensure first aid can be provided in the workplace.

Ionising Radiations Regulations 1985

The Ionising Radiations Regulations 1985, which came fully into operation on 1 January 1986, provided a coherent set of requirements for all forms of work with ionising radiation. Since replaced by The Ionising Radiations Regulations 1999 (IRR99), which came into force in 2000.

Guidelines for the Safe and Secure Handling of Medicines, 1988
Also known as the Duthie (RB) Report.

Control of Substances Hazardous to Health Regulations 1988 (COSHH)
Often referred to as the 'COSHH requirements'. Now replaced by new regulations.

Ionising Radiation (Protection of Persons Undergoing Medical Examination or Treatment) Regulations 1988 (SI.1988 No.778)
State that in the interest of persons (or patients) undergoing medical examinations, employers must ensure that their employees (carrying out such examinations with ionising radiation) are qualified and can produce a certificate to that effect. Employers must also keep a record of their employees' training.

Guidelines for Change in Postgraduate and Continuing Medical Education, 1990
A set of guidelines for a model of change in post-basic medical education. Ask for Gale and Grant, *Guidelines for Change in Postgraduate and Continuing Medical Education*. British Postgraduate Medical Federation and Open University; March 1990.

Heads of Agreement: ministerial group on Junior Doctors' Hours, 1990, NHS Executive
Usually known as *Junior Doctors: the new deal*.

Care Programme Approach for People with a Mental Illness Referred to the Specialist Psychiatric Services, HC(90)23
Sets out the general principles of the care programme approach.

Welfare of Children and Young People in Hospital, 1991, DoH
Covers all aspects of caring for children and young people in hospital.

Changing Childbirth, 1992, HMSO
Guidelines for the development of maternity services.

Strategy for Information Management and Technology (IM&T) in the NHS, 1992, NHS Executive
Describes a common way forward for information management and technology for all sectors of the health service in England. Information management includes both computer- and paper-based systems.

Health of the Nation: a strategy for health in England, 1992, HMSO
The first attempt of a government to produce a strategy document aimed at improving the nation's health. Produced as a White Paper it set national targets for disease prevention and health promotion in five areas to be achieved by 2000. These were coronary heart disease, cancers, mental illness, HIV/AIDS and sexual health, and

accidents. It identified approaches to include public policies such as food labelling, healthy surroundings, healthy lifestyles and high-quality health services. For this to be achieved, links were necessary with schools, local authorities and voluntary agencies. Ask for DHSS/NHS, *Health of the Nation*. HMSO; 1992.

Health and Safety (Display Screen Equipment) Regulations 1992
State the minimum requirements for workstations with display screen equipment activities (in line with EC directive 901770 EEC).

Post-Registration Education and Practice for Nurses (PREP), 1992, UKCC
Introduces new legislation for the renewal of registration for nurses, midwives and health visitors and restructures all specialist post-registration education. Sets out the United Kingdom Central Council for Nursing's requirements for education and practice following registration.

Management of Food Services and Food Hygiene in the NHS (England and Wales only), HSG(92)34
All about food-handling services in the NHS.

Management of Health and Safety at Work Regulations 1992
These set out broad general duties which apply to almost all work activities. Replaced by new Act 1999.

An Introduction to the NHS in Scotland, 1993
A simple explanation of the health services in Scotland, which are slightly different to England and Wales. Ask for Ham C, Haywood S, *An Introduction to the NHS in Scotland*. MDG Library, Scottish Health Service Centre, Crewe Road South, Edinburgh EH4 2LF. Now somewhat dated in the light of subsequent legislation.

Tomorrow's Doctors, 1993
Superseded by versions published in 2003 and then 2009. GMC recommendations on undergraduate medical education. Recommended a revision of the curriculum framework, a core curriculum, special study modules and the regulation of the undergraduate course.

Mental Health Act (1983) Code of Practice, 1993, HMSO
Provides guidance on the application of the Mental Health Act, section 118.

Guidance and Ethics for Occupational Physicians, 1993, Faculty of Occupational Medicine

Introduction of Supervision Registers for Mentally Ill People, HSG(94)5
Covers the requirements of the supervision register. Set up to ensure continuity of care

for mentally ill people, to identify those people with a severe mental illness who may be a significant risk to themselves or others and to ensure that follow-up is effective.

Guidance on the Discharge of Mentally Disordered People and their Continuing Care in the Community, HSG(94)27

Covers the discharge of people with a serious mental illness. Risk assessment illness is given extensive coverage.

Maternity Allowance and Statutory Maternity Pay Regulations 1994

Social Security Maternity Benefits and Statutory Sick Pay (Amendment) Regulations 1994

The Pre-Registration House Officer Experience, 1994

A consensus statement from the UK Postgraduate Deans on the PRHO year. Covers standards and responsibilities, working conditions, appropriateness of clinical work, workload, education and training, educational supervision, approval of posts and living conditions. Ask for *The Pre-Registration House Officer Experience: implementing change.* COPMED UK Conference of Postgraduate Deans; 1994.

Education of Sick Children, HSG(94)24

Covers aspects of providing education to children in hospital.

Ethnic Monitoring of Staff in the NHS: a programme of action, EL(94)12

A programme aimed at achieving the equitable representation of minority ethnic groups at all levels in the NHS, reflecting the ethnic composition of the local population.

Codes of Conduct and Accountability Guidance, 1994, EL(94)40, NHS Executive

Codes concerned with the conduct and account of NHS boards and their members. Standing orders should reflect the guidance that deals mainly with exchequer funds. Areas covered include annual reports, remuneration, terms of service committees, declaration of interests and register of interests.

The Patient's Charter, 1991 (updated 1995)

An attempt to make public services more responsive to consumers. These were stated as basic rights and expectations as applied to the NHS. They include the following:

The Patient's Charter, (96)43

Updated in April 1995, this expanded charter sets out new rights and standards and aims to reduce waiting times. It also aims to promote the respect of dignity, privacy and patient choice.

The Patient's Charter: a charter for patients in Wales
As above but for Wales.

The Patient's Charter: services for children and young people
Sets out new rights for children and young people.

The Patient's Charter: services for children and young people in Wales
As above, again for Wales.

The Patient's Charter: mental health services
This sets out new rights for users of mental health services.

Code of Practice on Openness in the NHS, 1995
Aimed at increasing access to information in the NHS. Required trusts and health authorities to make available or publish information about services, targets, standards, results, cost-effectiveness, important changes in service delivery, local health service management and who is responsible, details of public meetings, etc., and access to personal health records.

Collection of Ethnic Group Data for Admitted Patients, EL(94)77
The introduction of ethnic monitoring systems in hospitals became mandatory from April 1995.

New Deal: Plan for Action, EL(94)17
A planned approach for reducing junior doctors' hours.

Advance Statements about Medical Treatment, 1995, BMA
Gives guidance on dealing with advance directives.

Assessment of Mental Capacity: guidance for doctors and lawyers, 1995, BMA/The Law Society
Gives guidance on assessing a person's capacity to give valid consent.

Building Bridges: a guide to requirements for interagency working for the care and protection of severely mentally ill people, 1995, DoH
Describes best practice on caring for the severely mentally ill and the importance of interagency working.

Towards Evidence-Based Practice: a clinical effectiveness initiative for Wales, 1995, Welsh Office
Plans to develop evidence-based practice in Wales.

Code of Practice on Openness in the NHS, EL(95)42

Sets out the basic principles underlying public access to information about the NHS. It complements the code of access to information which applies to the DoH/NHS Executive and builds on the progress made by The Patient's Charter in this area. Requests for information should be responded to positively, except in certain circumstances, such as patients' records which must be kept safe and confidential.

Reporting of Injuries, Diseases and Dangerous Occurrences Regulations (RIDDOR), 1995, HMSO

Identifies the injuries, diseases and dangerous substances that must be reported, and the relevant authorities to which they should be reported.

Hospital Infection Control: guidance on the control of infection in hospitals, HSG(95)10

Contains a number of recommendations for health authorities regarding the surveillance, prevention and control of hospital infection.

Developing the Care Programme Approach: building on strengths, 1995, NHS Training Division

A resource pack, developed by the NHS Training Division, enabling organisations to develop good practice around the care programme approach.

Baseline IT Security Policy in the NHS in Wales, DGM(96)100, and IT Security Policy in the NHS in Wales, DGM(95)199

Cover issues of security in relation to patient information.

European Specialist Medical Qualifications Order, 1995

Requires the GMC to be responsible for publishing a register of specialists that states the individual's speciality.

The Patient's Charter Monitoring Guide: key standards, April 1996

The guide covers key Patient's Charter standards which need to be monitored nationally, and guidance on monitoring local Patient's Charter rights and standards.

Promoting Clinical Effectiveness, 1996, NHS Executive

Describes sources of information on clinical effectiveness, suggests ways in which changes to services can be encouraged (based on well-founded information about effectiveness) and describes how changes can be assessed to see whether improvements have resulted.

Protection and Use of Patient Information, HSG(96)18

Guidance on the protection and use of patient information, builds on existing legislation and guidance such as the Data Protection Act and Code of Practice on Openness in the NHS.

NHS Information Management and Technology Security Manual, HSG(96)15

Sets out guidance on the best information-systems security practice to be adopted by the NHS.

Protection and Use of Patient Information in the NHS in Wales, DGM(96)43

Covers issues of confidentiality and security.

Clinical Negligence and Personal Injury Litigation, EL(96)11

First of a linked series of guidance notes which set out the action required by trusts and health authorities in claims handling.

NHS Complaints Procedure, EL(96)19

Arose out of the recommendations of the Wilson Report, *Being Heard*, and came into force on 1 April 1996.

Health and Safety (Consultation with Employees) Regulations 1996

Set out the requirements for consultation with employees on health and safety issues.

Guidance on Supervised Discharge (After-Care under Supervision) and Related Provisions, WHC(96)11 and WOC 6196

Cover the discharge of seriously mentally ill people in Wales.

NHS Waiting Times: guidelines for good administrative practice, 1996

This document updates guidance issued in 1990 to waiting list managers. It gives guidance on when patients should be added to the list and the systems required to maintain it effectively. Regular reviews of the lists are necessary and the guide sets out review criteria. Procedures for the admission of patients or transfer to alternative providers are also included. It considers the role of accurate information on waiting lists in hospital management, detailing the information required by clinicians, managers and GPs.

Communication Skills: learning from patients – a training tool to help doctors reflect on their communication with patients, 1996

This report presents the findings of the second stage of a College of Health project to develop a tool that will encourage doctors to think about how well they communicate with patients. Reservations were expressed about the validity of the results, but there was general agreement that the tool could be useful in training junior staff.

The New NHS Number: the key to sharing patient information, 1996

The new NHS number attempts to ensure unique and unambiguous identification of each patient. The old NHS number, in 22 different formats, is prone to transcription errors and is unsuitable for computer applications. In order to overcome these shortcomings, the NHS Executive as part of its Information Management and Technology Strategy has devised the new numbering system. This booklet describes how the new

NHS number is being introduced with the support of a National Implementation Team, over a two-year period.

NHS Waiting Times: good practice guide, 1996
Setting out the Patient's Charter guarantees and standards for waiting times as of April 1995, this guide considers the goal of delivering shorter waiting times with a booked admission date, and maintenance of local clinical priorities.

Code of Practice in the Appointment and Employment of HCHS Locum Doctors, 1997
Originates from the recommendations of the Working Group on Locum Doctors, set up in December 1993. All locum appointments should comply with the Code. The main action points for trusts and others using locum agencies are listed. Details are given for the employment of locums: standards and conditions of appointment; references; health declarations; and criminal convictions.

Primary Health Care Teams Involving Patients: examples of good practice, 1997
This document aims to promote awareness and stimulate thinking about appropriate ways for primary healthcare teams to involve patients.

The NHS Number: putting the NHS number to work, 1997
Part of the NHSE Information Management and Technology Strategy has led to the introduction of a new NHS number that will uniquely identify each patient and allow patient information to be readily accessible but with suitable security safeguards. This booklet is intended for NHS staff and explains the benefits of the new NHS number.

National Lottery White Paper healthy living centres, EL (97)44
The Department of Health and Department of Culture Media and Sport published this paper on the use of Lottery Funds.

A Guide to Specialist Registrar Training ('The Orange Book'), 1998, DoH
This is the official and full guide to the appointment, training and assessment of specialist registrars.

National Specialist Commissioning Advisory Group Annual Report, 1997–98
NSCAG is responsible for managing and developing highly specialised services selected for central purchasing.

Partnership in Action (new opportunities for joint working between health and social services): a discussion document, 1998
As part of the White Paper *The New NHS: modern, dependable*, the government made a commitment to encourage more joint working between health and social services.

This document sets out plans to make partnerships a reality so that people whose needs span both health and social services have those needs met in the most efficient and cost-effective way.

Shared Contributions, Shared Benefits: the report of the Working Group on Public Health and Primary Care, 1998

This working group was set up by the DoH in 1995 with the aim of making practical proposals that would promote better co-operation between public health and primary care. The Primary Care Act 1997 enables health authorities, primary care and public health practitioners to become involved in joint enterprises. The recent White Paper *The New NHS* supports this with the development of primary care groups and health action zones.

An Enquiry into Mentoring, 1998

Supporting doctors and dentists at work – an enquiry into mentoring. A report from The Standing Committee on Postgraduate Medical and Dental Education (SCOPME).

Seeking Patients' Consent: the ethical considerations, 1998, GMC

Sets out the principles of good practice which doctors are expected to follow when seeking patients' informed consent to investigations, treatment, screening or research.

Public Appointments Annual Report, 1998

A second annual report covering public appointments made by and on behalf of the Secretary of State for Health. The report details those people in posts at 1 March 1998 and relates to chairpersons and non-executives in the following bodies: executive non-departmental public bodies (ENDPBs); advisory non-departmental public bodies (ANDPBs); health authorities; NHS trusts; special health authorities; and the Dental Practice Board. Appointments to the boards of health authorities and NHS trusts are listed by body and the NHS region in which they are located.

The New NHS Finance Function: modern, dependable. A medium-term development programme, 1998

This is a response from the Finance Staff Strategy Group to the government White Paper of the same title. The identified key changes are structural, organisational, functional and external, and the support offered to help individuals manage change will be training, personal development programmes and guidance on good practice.

Composite Directory of NHS Ethnic Health Unit Projects, 1998

The NHS Ethnic Health Unit (NHS EHU) was set up in 1994 to work with ethnic minority community organisations to foster confidence in the NHS among black and minority ethnic people. This publication provides details of the 123 projects funded by the EHU between 1994 and 1997.

General Practice Vacancies: revised selection procedures – a quick reference guide for health authorities on the revised arrangements for dealing with GP practice vacancies, 1998

The NHS (Primary Care) Act 1997 set out new procedures for the selection of candidates for general practice vacancies. This document provides health authorities with a reference guide on handling vacancies.

Research and Development: towards an evidence base for health services, public health and social care – information pack, 1998

Describes elements of the NHS R&D programme, the DoH's policy research programme and related research matters.

A Review of Continuing Professional Development in General Practice: a report by the Chief Medical Officer, 1998

The report of a multidisciplinary group chaired by the CMO, which set out to review the current state of continuing professional development in general practice, and suggest directions for improvement. The group's main recommendation is that the educational process should be integrated through the creation of a practice professional development plan (PPDP).

The Early Years, 1998, GMC

GMC recommendations on Senior House Officer (SHO) training.

The Doctor as Teacher, 1999, GMC

Sets out the expectations required of those who provide a role model to junior colleagues as well as medical students.

Prescription Cost Analysis, England, 1999

Prescription items dispensed in the community in England, listed alphabetically within chemical entity by therapeutic class with cost analysis and statistical data.

Getting Patients Treated: the Waiting List Action Team Handbook, 1999

A handbook about reducing waiting lists and good practices relating to this in the NHS.

Quality and Performance in the NHS: clinical indicators, 1999

Data was collected on six clinical quality indicators in the NHS: deaths in hospital within 30 days of surgery by method of admission; emergency admission with a hip fracture; or heart attack; emergency readmission to hospital within 28 days of discharge; returning home after treatment for a stroke within 56 days (aged 50 plus); and hip fracture within 28 days (aged 65 plus). Data is given for each area in England, classified using the 11 Office of National Statistics groups, and also by type of hospital (nine types listed). The source data was over 11 million patient episode records (1995–98).

Modernising the NHS in London, 1999

A progress report on implementing the recommendations of the Turnberg Report on London's health services, one year on. These include the building programme, health action zones, NHS Direct, reduced waiting lists and improved co-ordination and integration with other services.

Ionising Radiations Regulations 1999

Statutory requirements to specify radiological protection measures in medical, hospital and dental work, including researchers. Replaces Ionising Radiations Regulations 1985. It sets dose limits on workers but these dose limits do not apply to those undergoing medical treatment or examination (involving ionising radiation), or to 'comforters & carers'. A 'comforter/carer' is someone who 'knowingly and willingly incurs an exposure resulting from the support given to another person undergoing (or has undergone) medical exposure'. For more information go to www.ionactive.co.uk/regguidancelist.html?part=15&section=34.

Control of Substances Hazardous to Health Regulations 1999

Replace the Control of Substances Hazardous to Health Regulations 1988.

Management of Health and Safety at Work Regulations 1999

Broad guidelines of regulations that apply to almost all work activities. Replace Management of Health and Safety at Work Regulations 1992.

Guidance on Providing Online Public Information about Local Healthcare Services, 2000

In August 2000, the NHS Executive issued 10 targets associated with an additional £60 million for investment in information and IT. One relates to the online provision of accurate, standard and timely information on local healthcare services and their performance. Guidance is available on the definitive list of core information to be provided and the way in which it will be collected and published. The website nhs.uk will host and provide the main portal to the core information which will also be featured and accessed through NHS Direct Online.

The Vital Connection: an equalities framework for the NHS – working together for quality and equality, 2000

A framework for equal opportunities in the NHS is described and a strategy is set out for putting equality aims into action. Actions to be taken by the NHS and other organisations to implement the framework are specified. Priorities for 2000–04 are listed.

Millennium Executive Team Report on Winter 1999/2000

Explains preparations taken for winter throughout the health authorities, covering resources and planning, social care, public information and immunisation programmes. The Report describes the impact of winter 1999/2000 and the consequent demand for services. A list of conclusions and recommendations is given.

UK Antimicrobial Resistance Strategy and Action Plan, 2000

This document identifies surveillance, prudent antimicrobial use and infection control as the key elements to controlling antimicrobial resistance. The strategy and plan specifies eight areas for action. The aims are to minimise morbidity and mortality due to antimicrobial resistant infection and maintain the effectiveness of antimicrobial agents used in the treatment of humans and animals.

The Declaration of Helsinki, 2000

The Declaration of Helsinki is the most important international guideline on biomedical research involving humans. Published by the World Medical Association, it is the WMA's best-known policy statement. It was first adopted in 1964 and has been amended five times since, most recently in 2000. Notes of clarification were added to para. 29 in 2002 and to para. 30 in 2004. The current (2004) version is the only official one; all previous versions have been replaced and are only cited for historical purposes. You can access it at www.wma.net/e/ethicsunit/helsinki.htm.

The NHS Plan: a plan for investment, a plan for reform, 2000

Sets out how increased funding and reform are aimed to redress geographical inequalities, improve service standards and extend patient choice.

Good Medical Practice, 2001, GMC

Describes the principles of good medical practice and standards of competence, care and conduct expected of doctors in all aspects of their professional work.

Working Together, Learning Together: a framework for lifelong learning for the NHS, 2001

Outlines the lifelong learning strategy for the NHS, a strategic framework setting out a co-ordinated approach to lifelong learning in healthcare. It sets the direction for delivering systematic development for all NHS staff.

Health Service Circular: *Good Practice in Consent*, 2001

About good practice in obtaining consent and the NHS Plan commitment to the practice of patient-centred consent.

Health Service Circular: *Violent and Abusive Patients*, 2001

About withholding treatment from violent and abusive patients in NHS trusts and the NHS zero-tolerance zone.

Health Service Circular: *Reintroduction of Matrons*, 2001

Implementing the NHS Plan for modern matrons and strengthening the role of ward sisters and introducing senior sisters.

First Report of Select Committee on Health: IV The Private Finance Initiative, 2002

A useful and informative discussion on 'What is the Private Finance Initiative?' Can be accessed at www.parliament.uk and under advanced search type in 'IV The Private Finance Initiative' or 'Select Committee Reports'.

Withholding and Withdrawing Life-prolonging Treatments: good practice in decision-making, 2002, GMC

Develops the advice given in the GMC booklets *Good Medical Practice* and *Seeking Patients' Consent*. It sets out the standards of practice expected of doctors when they consider whether to withhold or withdraw life-prolonging treatments. It was the subject of a Judicial Review focusing on whether the guidance complied with the European Convention on Human Rights that handed down a ruling in July 2004. The GMC appealed and in July 2005 Court of Appeal upheld and endorsed the GMC guidelines.

NHS Reform and Health Care Professions Act 2002

Amending the law about the NHS to establish a Commission for Patient and Public Involvement in Health, thus creating Patient and Public Involvement Forums (PPI Forums) and to make provision in relation to arrangements for joint working between NHS bodies and the prison service, and between NHS bodies and local authorities in Wales and to make provision in connection with the regulation of healthcare professions.

Shifting the Balance of Power, 2002

The name for the programme of changes to reform the way the NHS works. The aim was to design a service centred on patients and put them first. It also aimed to be faster, more convenient and offer patients more choice. The main feature of the change was to give local PCTs the role of running the NHS and improving health in their areas. This also meant creating new strategic health authorities that cover larger areas and have a more strategic role.

Tomorrow's Doctors, 2003

Superseded by version published in 2009. GMC recommendations on undergraduate medical education. Recommended a revision of the curriculum framework, a core curriculum, special study modules and the regulation of the undergraduate course.

Health Service Circular: Child Abuse, 2003

Advice on what to do if you are worried a child is being abused.

Health Service Circular: Protecting Staff and Delivering Services, 2003

About implementing the European Working Time Directive for doctors in training.

Making Amends: clinical negligence reform, 2003

A consultation paper by CMO sets out proposals for reforming the approach to clinical negligence in the NHS. The aims of these proposals are to ensure that the emphasis of the NHS is directed at preventing harm, reducing risks and ensuring safety.

Building on the Best: choice, responsiveness and equity in the NHS, December 2003, DoH

This strategy paper draws out and develops the main themes that emerged from the 'Choice, Responsiveness and Equity' consultation, which closed in November 2003. This document broadly sets out how the government will make NHS services more responsive to patients, by offering more choice across the spectrum of healthcare. Its main aim is to improve patient and user experience and build new partnerships between those who use health and social care and those who work in them.

Delivering the NHS Plan: next steps on investment, next steps on reform, April 2004, DoH

In this document the Secretary of State for Health presented a progress report on the NHS Plan. He detailed what had been achieved to date and the programme of changes yet to come. This document presented a progress report on the NHS Plan up to 2002. Achievements to this point and planned changes to the programme were detailed.

Confidentiality: protecting and providing information, 2004, GMC

Doctors hold information about patients that must not be disclosed without the patient's consent. This booklet gives guidance on the principles of confidentiality, disclosures required by law, the public interest and what to do when the patient cannot give consent, such as with children and disclosures after a patient's death. When it can be released you should act promptly.

Standards for Better Health, 2004

The document establishes the core and developmental standards covering NHS healthcare provided for NHS patients in England.

The NHS Improvement Plan, 2004

The NHS Improvement Plan was published in June 2004 and set out the way in which the NHS needed to change in order to become patient-led, moving away from a centrally directed system. Claiming that the previous five years had been about building capacity and capability, it stated that the next would be about improving quality, giving best value for money and using the new capacity and capability to build a truly patient-led service. It introduced the concept of Community Matrons (*see* Chapter 1).

Review of Arm's Length Bodies, 2004

The Secretary of State announced his intention to carry out the review in 2003. It was prompted because many frontline staff reported that ALB activities generated considerable levels of bureaucracy, because of the amount of overlap and duplication in their functions. In 2004, the objectives of the ALB review were announced. By 2007/08, the ALB Review would deliver a 50% reduction in the number of ALBs, savings of approximately £0.5 billion and a 25% reduction in the number of posts. In 2004 the report *Reconfiguring the Department of Health's Arm's Length Bodies* was published, which set out the government's conclusions based on the analysis of the review and the input of the ALBs.

The New Doctor: recommendations on general clinical training, 2005, GMC

This edition is transitional. It is effective from January 2005 until July 2007, when the legal requirements for Pre-Registration House Officer (PRHO) training will change. The current legal requirements for obtaining full registration will remain in place until then. The main purpose of this document is to ensure that by July 2007 both trainers and PRHOs are aware of the list of competencies that will become necessary to be eligible for full registration.

Withholding and Withdrawing Life-prolonging Treatments: good practice in decision-making (judicial review of), 2005, GMC

There had been a lot of coverage in the media of a court case involving the GMC booklet on *Withholding and Withdrawing Life-Prolonging Treatments: good practice in decision-making*. In February 2004 Mr Leslie Burke, who has a progressively disabling brain disease, sought a judicial review of the guidance. Based on his understanding of how it might be applied in managing his care, he believed some aspects of the guidance would be seen as unlawful. The guidance was subject to intense scrutiny by the courts. In July 2005 the appeal court was able to reassure Leslie Burke that his fears about the actions of doctors following the guidance were unfounded. They would not be able to deny him (or patients in a similar position) artificial nutrition and hydration when it was necessary to prolong his life and in the face of his clear wish to receive it. Not only would such denial be against the guidance, it would be unlawful. The court also provided reassurance for patients more generally that the contents of the guidance not only reflects current law, but represents good standards of practice which can protect the interests of patients, whether they are able to make decisions about treatment for themselves or have become incapacitated. The GMC promised to consider what steps it could take to raise public and professional awareness of the contents of the guidance, and to help ensure that good practice is followed across the NHS and other healthcare settings. Copies of the guidance and details about the court ruling can be read online at www.gmc-uk.org.

Creating a Patient-led NHS: delivering the NHS Improvement Plan, March 2005, DoH

Explains how the NHS Improvement Plan will be delivered and describes the major changes under way and how some of the biggest changes will be carried forward for a patient-led health service.

New Developments in Sexual Health and HIV/AIDS Policy White Paper, DoH July 2005

Sets out the government's response to the Health Select Committee's *New Developments in Sexual Health and HIV/AIDS Policy: third report of the session 2004/05*. Includes discussion of service improvement; charges for overseas visitors for HIV treatment; chlamydia screening; workforce and training; primary care and sex and relationships education.

Now I Feel Tall: what a patient-led NHS feels like, December 2005, DoH

Provides examples of good practice, showing how the NHS is improving the patient's emotional experience. Outlines the policy context and explains why improving the emotional experience of patients matters. It claims to make the NHS more aware of the importance of improving patients' emotional experience and the relevance of this to creating a patient-led NHS.

NHS Redress, November 2005, DoH

Plans for establishing an NHS Redress Scheme as an alternative to clinical negligence legal action.

Walport Report, 2006

Called *Medically- and Dentally-qualified Academic Staff: Recommendations for training the researchers and educators of the future*. UKCRC and MMC; 2005. It is the report of the Academic Careers Sub-Committee of Modernising Medical Careers and the UK Clinical Research Collaboration. Can be downloaded in full as a pdf file from www.nccrcd.nhs.uk/intetacatrain/index_html/copy_of_Medically_and_Dentally-qualified_Academic_Staff_Report.pdf.

Good Doctors, Safer Patients, 2006, DoH

A Department of Health report (sometimes known as the Donaldson Report) aimed at creating a new approach to promoting and assuring good medical practice and protecting patients from bad practice. The CMO was asked to undertake this broad review of medical regulation, following Dame Janet Smith's inquiry into the circumstances surrounding the murders committed by Hyde GP, Dr Harold Shipman. The report advises Ministers on measures to strengthen the arrangements in place for the protection of patients. It contains 44 detailed recommendations. Proposed changes include devolving some of the powers of the GMC to a local level, changing its structure and function, and creating a new framework for revalidation. The Secretary of State for Health welcomed the publication and launched a period of consultation. You can download all the documents as pdf files from www.dh.gov.uk/en/Publicationsandstatistics/Publications/PublicationsPolicyAndGuidance/DH_4.

Good Medical Practice, 2006, GMC

The definitive guide to the principles and values on which good practice is founded; these principles together describe medical professionalism in action. The guidance is addressed to doctors, but it is also intended to let the public know what they can expect from doctors. It is available from the GMC website at www.gmc-uk.org/guidance/good_medical_practice/index.asp as a pdf file in both English and Welsh.

Competence and Curriculum Framework for the Medical Care Practitioner: a consultation, 2006, DoH

Provides the proposed national educational and practice standards and proposed regulatory framework that future healthcare workers will need to meet before being able to treat patients as a medical care practitioner.

Cooksey Report, 2006

A report into UK health research funding. It can be downloaded at www.hm-treasury.gov.uk/d/pbr06_cooksey_final_report_636.pdf.

Local Government and Public Involvement in Health Act 2007

Among other provisions to abolish Patients' Forums and the Commission for Patient and Public Involvement in Health.

UK Revalidation Programme Board, 2007

Terms of Reference, Membership and related documents can be downloaded from links on the GMC website at www.gmc-uk.org/doctors/licensing/revalidation_board/index.asp.

The Operating Framework for the NHS in England 2008/09, 2007, DoH

The business and financial arrangement for 2008/09, the first of a three-year planning cycle, sets out in greater detail the ambitions for the next three years. Superseded by one for 2009/10 and then 2010/11 (*see* p. 192).

NHS Next Stage Review: leading local change, 2008, DoH

This document sets out how, where necessary, the NHS can change through the leadership of clinicians and the support of patients and the communities in which they live. It makes five pledges, which PCTs should have regard to, demonstrating commitment to delivering the most effective change possible: needs of everyone; universal is not the same as uniform; different places have different and changing needs; local needs are best met by local solutions.

On Your Best Behaviour: new guidance for medical students, 2009, GMC

GMC guidance outlining the professional behaviour and values expected of UK medical students and outlining professional values and fitness to practise. It is available at www.gmc-uk.org/education/undergraduate/undergraduate_policy/professional_behaviour.asp.

As well as advising students on professional conduct it also advises medical schools on how to develop consistent procedures for dealing with students when their fitness to practise is called into question.

The National Health Service Constitution, 2009, DoH

A document published first in 2008 as a result of the Darzi Reports, consultation on a draft and the final text of the NHS Constitution was published on 21 January 2009. Discussed in Chapter 1, documents can be downloaded from www.dh.gov.uk/en/ Publicationsandstatistics/Publications/PublicationsPolicyAndGuidance/DH_085814 or www.dh.gov.uk/en/Healthcare/NHSConstitution/DH_093184. The NHS Constitution aims to bring together in one place what staff, patients and public can expect from the NHS. As well as describing the purpose, principles and values of the NHS, the Constitution brings together a number of rights, pledges and responsibilities for both staff and patients. These rights and responsibilities are the result of extensive discussions and consultations with staff, patients and public and reflect what matters to them. Subject to parliamentary approval, all NHS bodies, and private and third-sector providers supplying NHS services in England will be required by law to take account of the Constitution in their decisions and actions. The government will have a legal duty to renew the Constitution every 10 years. No government will be able to change the Constitution, without the full involvement of staff, patients and the public. The full text can be seen at www.dh.gov.uk/en/Publicationsandstatistics/Publications/ PublicationsPolicyAndGuidance/DH_093419.

Tomorrow's Doctors, 2009

Tomorrow's Doctors: outcomes and standards for undergraduate medical education supersedes earlier versions published in 1993 and 2003. It is a statement on the duties of a doctor registered with the GMC and sets out the responsibilities of the GMC, the medical schools, all NHS organisations, doctors and students. Can be downloaded from www.gmc-uk.org/education/documents/GMC_TD_2009.pdf.

Being Open, 2009

The NPSA guidelines, *Being Open*, urge 'effective communication' with patients, their families and carers. It states that the NHS should be open with patients when things go wrong – including being ready to say sorry. Further information is at the NPSA website www.nrls.npsa.nhs.uk/resources/?entryid45=65077, where you can download the three documents: *Being Open – communicating patient safety incidents with patients, their families and carers*; *Being Open – supporting information*; and *Being Open – framework*.

The NHS in England: the operating framework for 2009/10, 2008, DoH

Superseded by the operating framework for the NHS in England for 2010/11, see next item.

The Operating Framework for the NHS for 2010/11, Dec 2009, DoH

Sets out the same five priorities for the NHS for the year ahead.
1 improving cleanliness and reducing healthcare associated infections
2 improving access through achievement of the 18-week referral to treatment pledge and improving access (including at evenings and weekends) to GP services

3 keeping adults and children well, improving their health and reducing health inequalities
4 improving patient experience, staff satisfaction, and engagement
5 preparing to respond in a state of emergency such as an outbreak of pandemic flu, learning from our experience of swine flu.

During 2010/11, the NHS must also continue its work to reduce local variation and eliminate poor performance.

For full details go to www.dh.gov.uk/en/Publicationsandstatistics/Publications/PublicationsPolicyAndGuidance/DH_110107.

NHS 2010–2015: from good to great, DoH

Five-year plan to reshape the NHS to meet the demands of an aging population and increased prevalence of lifestyle diseases. See www.dh.gov.uk/en/Publicationsand statistics/Publications/PublicationsPolicyAndGuidance/DH_109876.

Toolkit for High Quality Neonatal Services, 2009, DoH

A Neonatal Taskforce was established to identify ways of improving services. Bliss (the baby charity) has helped to develop the toolkit, which provides evidence-based guidance for all neonatal services. Details can be accessed and downloaded from www.dh.gov.uk/en/Publicationsandstatistics/Publications/PublicationsPolicyAnd Guidance/DH_107845.

Key health-related reports

This alphabetical list includes Green Papers and White Papers with both their short and official titles where appropriate, and official government-initiated health-related reports and inquiries.

Note: White Papers are issued by the government as statements of policy, and often set out proposals for legislative changes, which may be debated before a Bill is introduced. Green Papers set out for discussion proposals that are still at a formative stage. This section lists White and Green Papers issued by the DoH, and certain other preliminary legislative proposals.

The short titles of reports are often derived from the name of the person who chaired the group or committee that produced the report. Each entry often provides the item's full title and some brief details. Reports are available via the government, NHS or DoH websites.

Agenda for Change, 1999–2004

Negotiations began in 1999 when the four Health Departments of England, Scotland, Wales and Northern Ireland published a document called *Agenda for Change* (AfC). The document highlighted the need for changes to pay, career structures and conditions of employment of all directly employed staff within the NHS except very senior managers and those covered by the Doctors' and Dentists' Pay Review Body. Talks came to an end in November 2002, and the proposals were published in January 2003. It is said by some authorities to have resulted in huge cost increases for minimal return. The full text of the proposals can be found on the DoH website (www.dh.gov.uk).

An Organisation with a Memory, 2000

An Organisation with a Memory: report of an expert group on learning from adverse events in the NHS, chaired by the Chief Medical Officer.

Acheson Report, 1988

The Report of the Committee of Inquiry into the Future Development of the Public Health Function.

Acheson Report, 1998

Report of the Independent Inquiry into Inequalities in Health, carried out under the chairmanship of Sir Donald Acheson.

Allitt Inquiry, 1994 (also known as the Clothier Report)

Independent Inquiry Relating to Deaths and Injuries on the Children's Ward at Grantham and Kesteven General Hospital.

Ashton Report, 2000

Review of the Cardiac Unit at the Royal Liverpool Children's Hospital NHS Trust Alder Hey.

Ayling Enquiry, 2004

Independent Investigation into How the NHS Handled Allegations about the Conduct of Clifford Ayling report. For more information go to www.dh.gov.uk and search for Ayling Enquiry.

Banks Report, 1994

Review of the Department of Health.

Barlow Report, 1994

Report by the Advisory Group on Osteoporosis.

Bevan Report, 1989

Staffing and Utilisation of Operating Theatres: a study conducted under the guidance of a steering group.

Beveridge Report, 1942

Social Insurance and Allied Services report.

Black Report, 1980

Inequalities in Health: report of a research working group. Revised editions have since been published by Penguin.

Blom Cooper Report, 1992

Two volumes of the *Report of the Committee of Enquiry into Complaints about Ashworth Hospital.*

Bonham-Carter Report, 1969

Report on the Committee on the Functions of the District General Hospital.

Boyd Report, 1994

Confidential Inquiry into Homicides and Suicides by Mentally Ill People.

Bradbeer Report, 1954

Report by a Committee of the Central Health Services Council on the Internal Administration of Hospitals

Briggs Report, 1972

Report of the Committee on Nursing.

Building a Safer NHS for Patients: improving medication safety, 2004

This report explores the causes and frequency of medication errors, highlights drugs and clinical settings that carry particular risks, and identifies models of good practice to reduce risk.

Butler Report, 1975

Report of the Committee on Mentally Abnormal Offenders.

Butterworth Report, 1994

Mental Health Nursing Review: Team Working in partnership: a collaborative approach to care.

Cadbury Report, 1992 (and *Standards of Business Conduct*, 1993)

Outlines a code of practice that members of boards have a responsibility to the public to manage services efficiently and effectively with proper regard to corporate govern-ance, i.e. a duty to act honestly and diligently. Concern at the time of its publication over certain managerial conduct in the NHS led to the NHSE issuing guidance entitled *Standards of Business Conduct*, as it was felt that the Cadbury Report was not directly transferable to the NHS.

Caldicott Committee Report, 1997

Report on the Review of Patient–Identifiable Information.

Calman Report, 1991

Report on junior doctors. Sometimes referred to as *Junior Doctors: the New Deal*.

Calman Report, 1993

The report of the Working Group on Specialist Medical Training for hospital doctors' training in the future. It reviewed current specialist training and changes necessary for consistency with EC law. Also identified areas for further review and development. The report reviewed progress with the development of structured and planned training programmes, and noted the potential for the duration of specialist training to be reduced, a single training grade and introduction of Certificate of Completion of Specialist Training (CCST). Ask for *Hospital Doctors: training for the future. The Report of the Working Group on Specialist Medical Training*. DoH; 1993.

Calman-Hine Report, 1995

A Policy Framework for Commissioning Cancer Services: a report by the Expert Advisory Group on Cancer to the Chief Medical Officers of England and Wales.

Canterbury Report, 1984

Report based on an interdisciplinary workshop conference held at Canterbury in 1983 on coronary heart disease prevention and suggested plans for action.

Carter Review, 2006

DoH independent review set up in 2005 into commissioning arrangements for specialised services headed by Scotland's former CMO, Professor Sir David Carter. The *Report of the Review into Commissioning Arrangements for Specialised Services* (the Carter Review) and its recommendations for improvement were published in May 2006. For more information go to www.ncg.nhs.uk/index.php/key-documents/the-carter-review.

Cave Report, 1921

Two reports an interim and final report on voluntary hospitals and their services.

Ceri Davies Report, 1983

Underused & surplus property in the National Health Service: report of the enquiry. Report of an inquiry into ways of identifying surplus and under-used land and property in the NHS.

CHI Reports, 2003

CHI, the independent regulator of NHS performance, produces ratings for NHS trusts in England. The first year in which primary care trusts and mental health trusts received star ratings was 2003. The government is responsible for setting the priorities, which in turn determine the indicators relating to key targets. Other indicators designed by CHI and the DoH cover a wide range of performance issues, following consultation with the service and other stakeholders.

Children's Green Paper, 2003

The report *Every Child Matters* can be downloaded as a pdf file at www.rcu.gov.uk/articles/news/everychildmatters.

Clinical Monitors and Alarms, 1995

Report of the Working Party on Alarms on Clinical Monitors. Medical Devices Agency; 1995.

Clothier Report, 1972

Report of the Committee appointed to inquire into the circumstances, and production, which led to the use of contaminated infusion fluids in the Devonport section of Plymouth General Hospital.

Clothier Report, 1994

Independent Inquiry Relating to Deaths and Injuries on the Children's Ward at Grantham and Kesteven General Hospital. This is the report of the Allitt Inquiry (see above).

Clyde Report, 1992

Also known as The Orkney Enquiry, a *Report of the Enquiry into the Removal of Children from Orkney in February 1991.*

Cogwheel Reports, 1967–74

First report of the Joint Working Party on the Organisation of Medical Work in Hospitals. It was followed by a second report and a third report published in 1974.

Collins Report, 1992

Also known as *When the Eagles Fly*, a report on resettlement of people with learning difficulties from long-stay institutions.

Commission on the Provision of Surgical Services, 1988

A report of the working party on the composition of a surgical team. Covers general surgery, orthopaedics and otolaryngology. Ask for *Commission on the Provision of Surgical Services.* Royal College of Surgeons of England; 1988.

Commissioning a Patient-led NHS, 2005

Follow on from *Creating a Patient-led NHS* in March 2005 and focuses on how the Department of Health will develop commissioning throughout the whole NHS system, with some changes in function for primary care trusts and strategic health authorities. In future both will concentrate on three main areas:
o promoting health improvement and reducing inequalities
o securing safe and high quality services for their population
o emergency planning.

The document asks SHAs to work with their local health communities to consider roles and responsibilities of organisations in their areas, and sets out criteria for assessing any local proposals for change. It also commits to a development process for PCTs and SHAs similar to that for NHS trusts to prepare them fully for their new roles.

Court Report, 1976
Also called *Fit for the Future*, a report of the Committee on Child Health Services.

Cranbrook Report, 1959
Report of the Maternity Services Committee.

Crown Report, 1989
Report of the Advisory Group on Nurse Prescribing. Followed by a *Final Report of the Review of Prescribing, Supply and Administration of Medicines.*

Cullen Report, 1991
Chief Nursing Officers of the UK reporting on *Caring for People: mental handicap nursing.*

Culyer Report, 1994
A report to the Minister of Health on supporting research and development in the NHS. Makes a variety of recommendations about the research and development funding systems and related topics in the NHS. An implementation plan was issued by the NHS Executive in April 1995. Ask for *Implementing Research and Development in the NHS*, EL(96)47.

Cumberlege Report, 1986
Report on Neighbourhood Nursing: a focus for care.

Cumberlege Report, 1993 (2 vols.)
Changing Childbirth.

Curtis Report, 1946
Report of the Care of Children Committee.

The Darzi Report, 2008
High Quality Care for All: NHS Next Stage Review and final report 2008. The final report of Lord Darzi's NHS review. It responds to the 10 SHA strategic visions and sets out a vision for an NHS with quality at its heart. It is described in more detail in Chapter 1. Or to see the full report go to www.dh.gov.uk/en/Publicationsandstatistics/Publications/PublicationsPolicyAndGuidance/DH_085825.

Data Protection Act 1998
All businesses that keep any information on living and identifiable people must comply with the Data Protection Act. The Act applies to computerised personal information

and to some structured manual records about people. Some businesses must register under the Act and ensure their information is properly managed. But others only need to observe data-protection principles – enforceable rules of good practice for handling personal information. See www.opsi.gov.uk/ACTS/acts1998/19980029.htm or www.dh.gov.uk/PolicyAndGuidance/OrganisationPolicy/RecordsManagement/DataProtectionAct1998 concerning its application to the NHS.

Davies Report, 1973
Report of the Committee on Hospital Complaints Procedure.

Dawson Report, 1920
Interim report on the future provision of medical and allied services.

Developing NHS Direct, 1998
A study commissioned by the Operational Research Branch of the NHS Executive advocating the introduction of the nationwide 24-hour telephone advice line. *See* p. 34 for further details.

The Doctors' Tale, 1995
An Audit Commission report on the work of hospital doctors in England and Wales. Ask for The Audit Commission, *The Doctors' Tale*. London: HMSO; 1995.

Donaldson Report, 2001
Report of a census of organs and tissues retained by pathology services in England.

Donaldson Report, 2006
More usually known as *Good Doctors, Safer Patients* (*see* p. 189). A DoH report aimed at creating a new approach to promoting and assuring good medical practice and protecting patients from bad practice. The CMO was asked to undertake this broad review of medical regulation, following Dame Janet Smith's inquiry into the circumstances surrounding the murders committed by Hyde GP, Dr Harold Shipman. The report advises Ministers on measures to strengthen the arrangements in place for the protection of patients. The report contains 44 detailed recommendations. Proposed changes include devolving some of the powers of the GMC to a local level, changing its structure and function, and creating a new framework for revalidation. You can download all the documents as pdf files from www.dh.gov.uk/en/Publicationsandstatistics/Publications/PublicationsPolicyAndGuidance/DH_4.

Dowie Reports, 1991
On patterns of hospital medical staffing. It included a series of nine reports entitled: Overview; Anaesthetics; General Medicine; General Psychiatry; General Surgery; Obstetrics & Gynaecology; Ophthalmology; Paediatrics; Trauma and Orthopaedic Surgery.

Duthie Report, 1988
Guidelines for the Safe and Secure Handling of Medicines.

Ethics of Xenotransplantation, 1997
Animal Tissue into Humans: the report of the Advisory Group on the Ethics of Xenotransplantation outlines the government's proposed course of action following consideration of the Advisory Group's report by government departments.

Fallon Report, 1999
Report of the Committee of Enquiry into the Personality Disorder Unit, Ashworth Special Hospital. With Volume II entitled *Expert Evidence on Personality Disorder.*

Farquharson-Lang Report, 1966
Report on the Administrative Practice of Hospital Boards in Scotland.

Farwell Report, 1995
Aseptic Dispensing for NHS Patients.

First Green Paper, 1968
On administrative structure of the medical and related services in England and Wales.

Firth Report, 1987
Public Support for Residential Care: report of a joint central and local government working party.

Forrest Report, 1986
Breast Cancer Screening: report to the health ministers of England, Wales, Scotland and Northern Ireland.

Gillie Report, 1963
The Field of Work of the Family Doctor.

Glancy Report, 1974
Revised Report of the Working Party on Security in NHS Psychiatric Hospitals.

Goodenough Report, 1944
Report of the Interdepartmental Committee on Medical Schools.

Green Paper, 1970
National Health Service: the future structure of the National Health Service in England.

Green Paper, 1986
Primary Health Care: an agenda for discussion.

Green Paper, 1991

Health of the Nation: a consultative document for health in England.

Green Paper, 1998

Our Healthier Nation. The Green Paper stressed that health-promoting settings were key to a public health improvement strategy – and a commitment was made to develop health-promoting hospitals (HPHs).

Griffiths Report, 1983

Report on the effective use and management of resources in the NHS set up by Sir Norman Fowler, then Secretary of State for Social Services. Consists of a short report in the form of a letter comprising only 24 pages. Ask for DHSS, *NHS Management Enquiry. Griffiths Report.* DA(83)38. London: HMSO; 1983.

Griffiths Report, 1988

Community Care: agenda for action.

Guillebaud Report, 1956

Cost of the National Health Service: report of the Committee of Enquiry.

Hall Reports, 1989–

Report of the Joint Working Party on Child Health Surveillance: health for all children. Published in four editions commencing in 1989.

Halsbury Report, 1974

Report of the Committee of Enquiry into the Pay and Related Conditions of Service of Nurses and Midwives.

Halsbury Report, 1975

Report of the Committee of Enquiry into the Pay and Related Conditions of Service of the Professions Supplementary to Medicine and Speech Therapists.

Harding Report, 1981

The Primary Health Care Team: report of a joint working group of the Standing Medical Advisory Committee and the Standing Nursing and Midwifery Advisory Committee.

Harvard Davies Report, 1971

The Organisation of Group Practice: report of a sub-committee of the Standing Medical Advisory Committee.

Health Service Ombudsman Report for Wales, 2004/05

Can be accessed at www.wales.nhs.uk/documents/Ombudsmanannualreport04–05. pdf.

Health and Safety at Work Act 1974

Details how employers are responsible for employees being kept safe at work by emphasising the need for assessment of risks and adequate training. But also there is a responsibility on the employee to take reasonable steps to safeguard their own safety and health at work.

Health and Social Care (Community Health and Standards) Act 2003

Legislation that allows the government to take forward some of the reforms it outlined in the NHS Plan – a plan to 'modernise and rebuild' the health service and 'reshape' the health service from the patient's point of view.

Heathrow Debate, 1994

The Challenges for Nursing and Midwifery in the 21st Century: a report of the Heathrow debate between Chief Nursing Officers of England, Wales, Scotland and Northern Ireland.

Hill Report, 1968

Hospital Treatment of Acute Poisoning: report of the joint sub-committee of the standing medical advisory committees. Central and Scottish Health Councils.

Hinchliffe Report, 1959

Final Report of the Committee on the Cost of Prescribing.

Hunt Report

Report of the Committee on Hospital Supplies Organisation.

Hunter Report, 1972

Report of the Working Party on Medical Administrators.

Implementing the Tooke Report: an update, 2008

This was the response to the Tooke Report 2008 and published by the Parliamentary Health Select Committee (HSC) as the findings of their own inquiry into MMC. One of the HSC recommendations was that the Department of Health should publish an updated response to the 47 recommendations in Sir John's original report. For this go to www.dh.gov.uk/en/Publicationsandstatistics/Publications/Publications PolicyAndGuidance/DH_090286.

Ingall Report, 1958

Training of District Nurses: report of the Advisory Committee.

Jay Report, 1979 (2 vols.)

Report of the Committee of Enquiry into Mental Handicap Nursing and Care.

Judge Report, 1985

The Education of Nurses: a new dispensation.

Kennedy Report, 2001

Learning from Bristol: the report of the public enquiry into children's heart surgery at the Bristol Royal Infirmary, 1984–1995. The Final Report has two principal sections. Section One considers paediatric cardiac surgical services in Bristol during the years 1984–95. Section Two responds to the last element of the Enquiry's Terms of Reference: 'to make recommendations which could help to secure high quality care across the NHS'. The full report can be accessed at www.bristol-enquiry.org.uk.

Kerr Report, 2005 (2 vols.)

A report by The Scottish Executive entitled *The National Framework for NHS Scotland: building a health service fit for the future*. It comes in two volumes, the first is basically the report and the second the executive summary. Go to www.show.scot.nhs.uk.

Körner Report, 1982

First report of the Steering Group on Health Services Information.

Lewin Report, 1970

Organisation and staffing of operating departments.

Limerick Report, 1998

Expert Group to investigate cot death theories: toxic gas hypothesis final report.

Lung Report, 1996

British Lung Foundation on Lung disease: a shadow over the nation's health.

Lycett Green Report, 1963

Report of the Committee of Enquiry into the recruitment, training and promotion of administrative and clerical staff in the hospital service.

The Mackenzie Report, 1986

Report on general practice in UK medical schools suggesting increasing financial commitment by the NHS to support academic general practice.

Making Amends, 2003

Report by Sir Liam Donaldson CMO on proposals for reform of clinical negligence system. More information at www.dh.gov.uk/cmo.

Mansell Report, 1993

Services for People with Learning Disabilities and Challenging Behaviour or Mental Health Needs: report of a project group.

Mant Report, 1998

Research and Development in Primary Care: national working group report.

Mayston Report, 1969
Working Party on Management Structure in the Local Authority Nursing Services.

McCarthy Report, 1976
Making Whitley work.

McColl Report, 1986
Review of Artificial Limb and Appliance Centre Services.

Merrison Report, 1975
Report of the Committee of Enquiry into the Regulation of the Medical Profession.

Merrison Report, 1979
Royal Commission on the National Health Service.

Monks Report, 1988
Report of the Working Group to Examine Workloads in Genito-urinary Medicine Clinics.

Montgomery Report, 1959
Maternity Services in Scotland.

Neale Enquiry, 2004
Report of an Independent Investigation into how the NHS Handled Allegations about the Performance and Conduct of ex-Consultant Obstetrician and Gynaecologist Richard Neale. For more information go to www.dh.gov.uk and search for Neale Enquiry.

Nodder Report, 1980
Organisational and Management Problems of Mental Illness Hospitals: report of a working group.

Noel Hall Report, 1957
Grading Structure of the Administrative and Clerical Staff in the Hospital Service.

Noel Hall Report, 1978
Report of the Working Party on the Hospital Pharmaceutical Service.

Omega File, 1984
Published by the Adam Smith Institute on health and social services policy.

Orkney Report, 1992
Report of Enquiry into the Removal of Children from Orkney in February 1991.

Patient's Charter Monitoring Guide: key standards, 1996

The guide covers key Patient's Charter standards which need to be monitored nationally, and guidance on monitoring local Patient's Charter rights and standards.

Peach Report, 1999

Report of the UKCC Commission for Nursing and Midwifery and Education on Fitness for Practice. You can access details at www.nmc-uk.org/nmc/main/splash.html.

Peel Report, 1970

Report of the Standing Maternity and Midwifery Advisory Committee on Domiciliary Midwifery and Maternity Bed Needs.

Peel Report, 1972

The Use of Foetuses and Foetal Material for Research.

Pennington Report, 1997

Report on the Circumstances Leading to the 1996 Outbreak of Infection with E. coli 0157 in Central Scotland, the Implications for Food Safety and the Lessons to be Learned.

Pilkington Report, 1960

Royal Commission on Doctors' and Dentists' Remuneration.

Platt Report, 1959

Report of a Committee of the Central Health Services Council on the welfare of children in hospital.

Polkinghorne Report, 1989

Review of the Guidance on the Research Use of Foetuses and Foetal Material.

Powell Report, 1946

Report of the Sub-committee of Central Health Services Council. Ministry of Health appointed to study the pattern of the inpatients' day.

Professor Protti's 7th World View Report on PHRs, 2005

This is the seventh report in a series; it describes how the introduction of web-based Personal Health Records (PHR) demonstrates an emerging era in healthcare that will revolutionise communication between patients and clinicians. The important issue for Professor Protti is the key role of patients in taking responsibility for their healthcare.

RAWP Report, 1976

Resource Allocation Working Party: sharing resources for health in England.

Red Book, 1992
A statement of fees and allowances payable to general medical practitioners in England and Wales from April 1990.

Redfern Report, 2001
Report by Michael Redfern QC on the retention and use of children's organs at the Royal Liverpool Children's Hospital (Alder Hey). The full text of the *Report of the Royal Liverpool Children's Enquiry* can be seen at www.rlcenquiry.org.uk.

Reed Report, 1992/93
Review of mental health and social services for mentally disordered offenders and others requiring similar services: in five volumes including final summary report, service needs, finance, staffing and training, the academic and research base and special issues and differing needs.

Reed Report, 1994
High Security and Related Psychiatric Provision.

Reed Report, 1994
Services for People with Psychopathic Disorder.

Richards Report, 1997
Report of an independent task force chaired by Sir Rex Richards of Committee of Vice-Chancellors and Principals of the Universities of the UK on clinical academic careers.

Ritchie Report, 2000
Report of the Enquiry into Quality and Practice within the NHS Arising from the Actions of Rodney Ledward.

Rothschild Report, 1971
The Organisation and Management of Government Research and Development.

Rothschild Report, 1972
A Framework for Government Research and Development.

Rubery Report, 1993
Report of the Chief Medical Officer's Expert Group on the Sleeping Position of Infants and Cot Deaths.

Safeguarding Patients, 2007
A DoH publication of the government's response to the recommendations of the Shipman Inquiry's fifth report and to the recommendations of the Ayling, Neale and Kerr/Haslam Inquiries. You can download it as a pdf from www.dh.gov.

uk/en/Publicationsandstatistics/Publications/PublicationsPolicyAndGuidance/
DH_065953.

Sainsbury Report, 1967

*Report of the Committee of Enquiry into the Relationship of the Pharmaceutical Industry
with the National Health Service.*

Salmon Report, 1966

Report of the Committee on Senior Nursing Staff Structure.

Salmon letter

Although not a report, it is included here as the most convenient place for insertion.
A 'Salmon letter' is a letter which gives organisations under scrutiny by an inquiry
advance warning of potential criticisms. For example, in 2003 the GMC received a
'Salmon letter' that the Shipman Enquiry was required to write to all organisations
that had contributed to the Enquiry to outline areas of potential criticism. It advises
the recipient of their rights, including having a lawyer through the whole Enquiry who
would be able to ask questions and to assist in asking questions of other witnesses and
cross-examining other witnesses.

Schofield Report, 1996

The Future Healthcare Workforce. University of Manchester, Health Services Management
Unit, Project Steering Group on the future healthcare workforce.

Scottish Green Paper, 1968

Administrative Reorganisation of the Scottish Health Services.

Second Green Paper, 1970

National Health Service: the future structure of the National Health Service in England.

Seebohm Report, 1968

Report by the Committee on Local Authority and allied social service.

Seeing the Wood, Sparing the Trees, 1996

Efficiency Scrutiny Report by NHS Executive about bureaucracy in the NHS and the
'burdens' of paperwork in NHS trusts and health authorities.

Sheldon Report, 1971

Report of the Expert Group on Special Care Babies.

Shields Report, 1996

Scottish Office, Department of Health, Working Group on the Roles and
Responsibilities of Health Boards: *Commissioning Better Health: report of the short life
working group on the roles and responsibilities of health boards.*

Shipman Enquiry, 2002–2005

The Shipman Enquiry was chaired by Dame Janet Smith and published six reports. The first, *Death Disguised*, published in 2002, the second, *The Police Investigation of March 1998*, published in 2003 together with the third report *Death Certification and Investigation of Deaths by Coroners*. The fourth report, *The Regulation of Controlled Drugs* was published in 2004 followed later that year by the fifth report, *Safeguarding Patients: lessons from the past – proposals for the future*. This considered the handling of complaints against general practitioners, the raising of concerns about GPs, General Medical Council procedures and its proposal for revalidation of doctors. Dame Janet Smith made recommendations for change based upon her findings. The sixth report, *Shipman: the Final Report*, was published in 2005 and considered how many patients Shipman killed during his career as a junior doctor at Pontefract General Infirmary between 1970 and 1974. She also considered a small number of cases from Shipman's time in Hyde, which the Enquiry became aware of after the publication of the First Report. She also considered the claims by a former inmate at HMP Preston regarding alleged claims by Shipman about the number of patients he had killed. The Enquiry has its own website where all the data can be accessed at www.the-shipman-enquiry. org.uk or go to www.dh.gov.uk/cmo.

Short Guide to NHS Foundation Trusts, 2005

This DoH document provides information and 10 key points about NHS foundation trusts.

Short Report, 1980

Second Report from the Social Services Committee on perinatal and neonatal mortality.

Short Report, 1984

Third Report from the Social Services Committee on perinatal and neonatal mortality, follow up.

Spens Report, 1946

Report of the Inter-departmental Committee on the Remuneration of General Practitioners.

Spens Report, 1948

Report of the Inter-departmental Committee on the Remuneration of General Dental Practitioners.

Stewart Report, 2000

Report of the Independent Expert Group on Mobile Phones. It can be accessed at www. iegmp.org.uk.

Tilt Report, 2000

Report of the Review of Security at the High Security Hospitals.

Todd Report, 1968
Report of the Royal Commission on Medical Education.

Tomlinson Report, 1992
Report of the Enquiry into London's Health Service, Medical Education and Research. The latest of a series of reports on the future of London's health services. Ask for *The Tomlinson Report*. London: HMSO; 1992.

Tooke Report, 2008
This report, *Aspiring to Excellence: findings and final recommendations of the Independent Inquiry into Modernising Medical Careers*, looked at the recruitment process after thousands of junior doctors were left without training posts in 2007 and was also designed to cut the number of years it took for junior doctors to reach consultant level. It said a new independent body called NHS Medical Education England should be set up to manage postgraduate medical training, with cash ring-fenced to prevent trusts raiding budgets to help with debts. The DoH said it would assess the report, before setting out procedures. To download the report go to www.medschools.ac.uk/Publications/Pages/Aspiring-to-Excellence.aspx or the link at the MMC website www.mmc.nhs.uk or go to www.personneltoday.com/articles/2008/01/09/43841/tooke-report-on-modernising-medical-careers-calls-for-independent-body-to-manage-doctors-training.html. The Parliamentary Health Select Committee (HSC) then published the findings of their own inquiry into MMC. See *Implementing the Tooke Report: an update*. One of the HSC recommendations was that the DoH should publish an updated response to the 47 recommendations in Sir John's original report. For this go to www.dh.gov.uk/en/Publicationsandstatistics/Publications/PublicationsPolicyAndGuidance/DH_090286.

Tunbridge Report, 1968
Report of the Joint Committee of the Central and Scottish Health Services Councils on the Care of the Health of Hospital Staff.

Turnberg Report, 1998
A Strategic Review of Health Services in London.

Turner Report, 1991
Report of the Expert Working Group enquiring into the hypothesis that toxic gases evolved from chemicals in cot mattress covers and cot mattresses are a cause of SIDS.

Utting Report, 1991
Children in the Public Care: a review of residential care.

Wagner Report, 1988
Residential Care: a positive choice [Report of the independent review of residential care].

Wanless Report, 2002

Securing Our Future Health: taking a long-term view – an independent review by Derek Wanless – is the first ever evidence-based assessment of the long-term resource requirements for the NHS. It concluded that in order to meet people's expectations and to deliver the highest quality healthcare over the next 20 years, the UK would need to devote more resources to healthcare and that this must be matched by reform to ensure that these resources are used effectively. See www.hm-treasury.gov.uk/consult_wanless_final.htm.

Wanless Report, 2004

Securing Good Health for the Whole Population. An update of the challenges to be faced in implementing the 2002 report above. See www.hm-treasury.gov.uk/wanless.

Warnock Report, 1984

Report of the Committee of Enquiry into Human Fertilisation and Embryology.

Wells Report, 1997

Review of Cervical Screening Services at Kent and Canterbury Hospitals Trust.

Welsh Green Paper, 1970

Reorganisation of the Health Service in Wales.

White Paper, 1972

NHS Reorganisation England.

White Paper, 1977

Prevention and Health.

White Paper, 1981

Growing Older.

White Paper, 1987

Promoting Better Health: the government's programme for improving primary healthcare.

White Paper, 1989

Caring for People: community care in the next decade and beyond. Note: a separate white paper on this topic was published for Northern Ireland: *People First: community care in Northern Ireland for the 1990s.*

White Paper, 1989

Working for Patients, published in 1989, summarises the last Conservative Government's Strategy and Programmes for the Reforms of the NHS. The proposals in the paper were incorporated into the NHS and Community Care Act 1990 (NHSCCA). Ask for *Working for Patients.* London: HMSO, 1989.

White Paper, 1991

Primary Care: delivering the future. Sets out a series of measures to develop primary care.

White Paper, 1992

Health of the Nation: a strategy for health in England. Suggested a number of health-promoting settings should be developed, including in hospitals.

White Paper, 1996

A Service with Ambitions. Establishing mechanisms for assessing the extent to which existing policies for professional development and training support the objectives of the NHS, encourage team working and create effective partnerships to ensure that educational objectives reflect changing patterns of service. It also tries to determine whether better use could be made of budgets to meet the needs of employers, and the concerns of the main professional groups.

White Paper, 1996

Choice and Opportunity – Primary Care: delivering the future. Presenting a programme for action both nationally and locally, building on recent changes. It considers developing partnerships in primary care, and between primary and secondary care and local authorities. The education and training of primary care professionals, the role of research and development and the importance of clinical audit are then discussed. Proposals are made for the fairer distribution of resources and their effective use. There is also a review of workforce planning and employment opportunities, together with plans for improvements in primary care premises. The final section considers the better organisation of primary care by linking practices together, improved management support and increased use of information technology.

White Paper, 1996

Health Related Behaviour: an epidemiological overview. The Health of the Nation White Paper in 1992 emphasised the fact that an individual's health is dependent, at least in part, on their own chosen lifestyle. This paper underlines the key role of behaviour, and an understanding of health-related behaviours and the factors which influence them. Behavioural epidemiology is an important public health issue for the future. This provides an overview of the existing knowledge in this area.

White Paper, 1997

The New NHS: modern, dependable formed the basis of a 10-year programme for the NHS, which it hoped to improve through evolutionary change rather than organisational upheaval. The changes would build on what has worked, and discard what has failed. The needs of patients would be central to the new system. It set out how the internal market would be replaced by a system called 'integrated care', based on partnership and driven by performance. Key tasks for health authorities were defined, as an assessment of health needs, including reference to health improvement programmes

(HImPs), primary care groups (PCGs), National Institute for Health and Clinical Excellence (NICE) and Commission for Health Improvement (CHI).

White Paper NHS Scotland, 1997

The NHS in Scotland's *Designed to Care*. There have always been differences and variations in approach and this is reflected in this White Paper. The main differences relate to primary care. Primary care trusts came into force in Scotland in April 1999.

White Paper NHS Wales, 1998

The Welsh Office brought out this equivalent White Paper to *The New NHS: modern, dependable*, applicable to the NHS in Wales.

White Paper, 1998

Smoking Kills sets out the government's concerted plan of action to stop people smoking.

It notes action already taken by the government on tobacco advertising and taxation. It goes on to present a series of measures for reducing smoking among young people, new cessation services for adults, and action on smoking among pregnant women. It then outlines proposals for abolishing tobacco advertising and promotion, altering public attitudes, preventing tobacco smuggling and supporting research. It describes further proposals for working in partnership with businesses to restrict smoking in public places, places of work and government offices, and for working with other governments at European and global levels.

White Paper, 1998

Modernising Social Services: promoting independence, improving protection, raising standards. This White Paper presents the government's plans for modernising social services provision. It states the principles underlying the government's 'third way' in relation to social care.

White Paper, 1999

The White Paper *Saving Lives: our healthier nation* was published in 1999 together with *Reducing Health Inequalities: an Action Report*. All can be downloaded from the NHS website (www.nhs.uk).

White Paper, 1999

Modernising Government deals with public services and their administration, the civil service, management of change and government policy in these areas.

White Paper, 1999

Our Healthier Nation offered more direction on health-promoting settings.

White Paper, 2000

Adoption: a new approach sets out what the government will do, including the new legislation they will introduce, to make adoption work more clearly, more consistently, and more fairly.

White Paper, 2001

Valuing People: a new strategy for learning disability for the 21st century is the first White Paper on learning disability for 30 years and sets out an ambitious and challenging programme of action for improving services. The proposals are based on four key principles: civil rights, independence, choice and inclusion. *Valuing People* takes a lifelong approach, beginning with an integrated approach to services for disabled children and their families and then providing new opportunities for a full and purposeful adult life. It has cross-government backing and its proposals are intended to result in improvements in education, social services, health, employment, housing and support for people with learning disabilities and their families and carers.

White Paper, 2003

Our Inheritance, Our Future: realising the potential of genetics in the NHS. A Genetics White Paper published in June sets out a vision of how genetic techniques could benefit patients via a £50 million, three-year plan of implementation. New initiatives include substantial investment in upgrading genetics laboratories, a boost to the genetics workforce and more genetics counsellors, consultants and laboratory scientists. More than £7 million would be spent on new initiatives to introduce genetics-based healthcare into mainstream NHS services. A new Genetics Education and Development Centre would spearhead education and training in genetics for all healthcare staff. New research programmes in pharmacogenetics, gene therapy and health services research would help turn the science into real patient benefit.

This strategy aims to help put the NHS on a sound footing to cope with future developments in genetic knowledge and technology. The White Paper also sets out the safeguards and controls against inappropriate or unsafe use of developments in genetics. In addition to existing controls on gene therapy and use of genetic test results by insurance companies, the government will introduce new legislation to ban DNA theft: it will become an offence to test someone's DNA without their consent except for medical or police purposes. The government also recognises the importance of openness and public debate, and will continue to be responsive to new developments and shifts in public attitudes. See also the DoH Departmental Report of 2005, *see* p. 214.

White Paper (Summary), 2004

The previous Genetics White Paper in short summary form.

White Paper, 2004

Choosing Health: making healthier choices easier and 'to enable the public to set the health agenda for the future'. This White Paper sets out how the health service is being reformed to educate people about their health, help them make the right choices and focus on the promotion of good health. The key principles for supporting the public to make them healthier and more informed about choices in regards to their health. The government plans to provide information and practical support to get people motivated and improve emotional well-being and access to services so that healthy choices are easier to make. A further White Paper *Choosing Health FAQ* was published the same year, answering some of the questions the public might have about the White Paper.

White Paper, 2004

Published by The Council of Europe. A White Paper on the human rights of people with mental illness, especially those subject to compulsory detention. The White Paper contains a draft recommendation No.R (83) 2 concerning the legal protection of persons suffering from mental disorder placed as involuntary patients.

White Paper, 2005

Commissioning a Patient-led NHS: delivering the NHS improvement plan. A White Paper that follows on from earlier publication of the same name, and focuses on how commissioning will develop throughout the whole NHS, with some changes in function for PCTs and SHAs who in future will concentrate on three main areas, promoting health improvement and reducing inequalities, securing safe and high-quality services for their population and emergency planning. The document asks SHAs to work with their local health communities to consider roles and responsibilities of organisations in their areas, and sets out criteria for assessing any local proposals for change within a realistic timetable. It also commits to a development process for PCTs and SHAs similar to that for NHS trusts to prepare them fully for their new roles.

White Paper, 2005

Action on obesity, sexually transmitted diseases, alcohol abuse and smoking is at the top of the agenda in this White Paper on public health. Key points include an overhaul of sexual health services, so that patients can receive appointments at a genito-urinary (GUM) clinic within 48 hours, and a nationwide chlamydia screening programme to be set up by 2007. Each primary care trust will have a specialist obesity service, with access to a dietician and advice and support on changing behaviour. The National Institute for Clinical Excellence will prepare definitive guidance on prevention, identification and management of treatment of obesity by 2007. It also plans action to ensure that children have the healthiest possible start in life, with all advertising, promotion and sponsorship of unhealthy foods and drinks to be restricted voluntarily.

White Paper *Response to Health Select Committee Report on Continuing Care*, 2005

Sets out the government's response to the Health Select Committee's Sixth Report of Session 2004–05 on NHS continuing care. Sets out clearly the difference between fully funded NHS continuing care and the registered nursing care contributions.

White Paper, 2005

Departmental Report for 2005. As a result of the Genetics White Paper 2003 the capacity of specialist genetic services had been developed and modernised through increased training places for counsellors and laboratory scientists and an £18 million investment in new laboratory equipment to modernise and expand laboratory capacity and support reduced waiting times for test results.

It also stated that a NHS Genetics Education and Development Centre had been established to provide a focal point for genetics education and training in the NHS. The Department was also funding a number of pilot projects testing out ways of integrating genetics into other clinical areas; this included coronary heart disease prevention and a collaborative project with Macmillan Cancer Relief to develop services for patients with a family history that puts them at increased risk of developing cancer.

The DoH had also supported research to generate new knowledge, including £4 million funding for research into pharmacogenetics for existing common drugs and £6.5 million for gene therapy for single gene disorders such as cystic fibrosis, haemophilia and muscular dystrophy.

White Paper, 2006

Review of the Human Fertilisation and Embryology Act: proposals for revised legislation (including establishment of the Regulatory Authority for Tissue and Embryos) (Cm 6989). A paper detailing proposals for revision of the law on assisted reproduction and embryo research, including the proposed Regulatory Authority for Tissue and Embryos (RATE), which will replace existing regulatory bodies (the Human Fertilisation and Embryology Authority, and the Human Tissue Authority). These proposals formed the basis of the Human Fertilisation and Embryology Act 2008.

White Paper, 2006

Our Health, Our Care, Our Say: a new direction for community services (Cm6737). This White Paper claimed to set a new direction for the whole health- and social care system. It confirmed the vision set out in the Department of Health Green Paper, *Independence, Well-being and Choice*. There was to be a radical shift in the way services were delivered, ensuring that they were more personalised and fitted into 'people's busy lives'. It promised people a stronger voice so that they were the major drivers of service improvement. You can view contents at www.dh.gov.uk/en/Publicationsandstatistics/Publications/PublicationsPolicyAndGuidance/DH_4127453.

White Paper, 2007

Trust, Assurance and Safety: the regulation of health professionals. Sets out the programme of reform to the UK's system for the regulation of health professionals, based on consultation on the two reviews of professional regulation published in July 2006: *Good Doctors, Safer Patients* by the Chief Medical Officer for England and the DoH's *The Regulation of the Non-medical Healthcare Professions*. It is complemented by the government's response to the recommendations of the Fifth Report of the Shipman Enquiry and recommendations in the Ayling, Neale and Kerr/Haslam Inquiries, *Safeguarding Patients*, which sets out a range of measures to improve clinical governance in the NHS. It is particularly important because of its references to (re)licensing, and (re)validation, (re)certification of specialists and the appraisal process that will include a summative element. Go to www.dh.gov.uk/en/Publicationsandstatistics/Publications/PublicationsPolicyAndGuidance/DH_065946.

White Paper, 2008

Pharmacy in England: building on strengths – delivering the future (Cm7341). Sets out a vision for improvements in pharmaceutical services. It includes the government's response to the Review of NHS Pharmaceutical Contractual Arrangements conducted by Anne Galbraith, former chair of the Prescription Pricing Authority, which the government commissioned in 2007. It also considers views put forward by the All Party Pharmacy Group's report *The Future of Pharmacy* (published in 2007) and considers the complementary but important work of dispensing doctors and appliance contractors.

The Wilson Report, 1994

Entitled *Being Heard*, the report of a review committee on NHS complaints procedures.

Winterton Report, 1992

House of Commons Health Select Committee Second Report on the Maternity Services. Vol. 1: Report together with appendices and the proceedings of the Committee. Vol. 2: The Minutes of Evidence. Vol. 3: Appendices to the Minutes of Evidence.

Woolf Report, 1996

Lord Woolf's proposals for reform of the Clinical Negligence Scheme. *Interim Report. Access to Justice*, HMSO; 1995. *Final Report.* HMSO; 1996. Or you can access on the Internet.

Zuckerman Report, 1968

Hospital Scientific and Technical Services.

Glossary of NHS terminology

The aim of this chapter is to provide you with information on useful terms and a glossary of health service, management, non-clinical and medico-legal terms along with some definitions.

I'm afraid that further new terms continue to be introduced, many related to new information technology. Some are fairly obvious and have been included not just for the sake of completeness but just in case they need clarification. Beware – quite often they are terms that have only a loose connection with their real meaning. You may need to check this out when you hear the expressions, but do not be surprised if the speaker is not aware of the correct meaning. The meaning may also relate to a specific connection. A few terms are attempts that have been made to transfer manufacturing terminology to medical work.

Abduction   In clinical terms a form of logical inference, commonly applied in the process of medical diagnosis. Given an observation, abduction generates all known causes. (*See also* deduction, induction and inference.)

Absenteeism   Absence from work not authorised through appropriate channels.

Access rate   An estimate of the availability of facilities to people living in an identified locality, irrespective of where they are treated. The measure is stated as discharges and deaths per 1000 population.

Accident   Any unexpected or unforeseen occurrence, especially one that results in injury or damage.

Accident and Emergency (A&E)   The title given to the hospital department previously termed 'Casualty' and now frequently called 'Emergency'. The Accident and Emergency patient may be brought by ambulance or car, or may arrive on foot.

Accident report   A written report of an accident. The format of the report is laid down in health and safety legislation.

Accommodation (children)   Being provided with accommodation replaces the old voluntary care concept. It refers to a service that the local authority provides for the parents of children in need, and for their children. A child is not in care when they are being provided with accommodation. Nevertheless, the local authority has a number of duties towards children for whom it is providing accommodation, including the duty to discover the child's wishes regarding the provision of accommodation, and to give them proper consideration.

Accountability Being answerable for one's decisions and actions. Accountability cannot be delegated.

Added value A measure of productivity expressed in terms of the financial value of an item as a result of workforce. Often used loosely in the NHS.

Adolescents Young people in the process of moving from childhood to adulthood. Because of their age, adolescents may have special needs as patients.

Adoption Total transfer of parental responsibility from the child's natural parents to the adopters.

Advance directives A document which sets out the wishes of a patient if they are later unable to give or withhold consent for a particular treatment. This is particularly important when the patient's/user's wishes may conflict with clinical judgement.

Adversarial One of two kinds of court process: adversarial and inquisitorial. The adversarial system refers to a court process in which the parties bring competing claims so that the court decides the outcome on the merits of each case.

Advocate An individual acting on behalf of, and in the interests of, patients who may feel unable to represent themselves in their contacts with a healthcare or other facility.

Advisory boards Bodies established to ensure the National Programme for IT engages with stakeholders, such as patients, the public, and health and care professionals.

Affidavit Statement in writing and an oath sworn before a person who has the authority to administer it, e.g. a solicitor.

Amenity bed A bed in a single room or small NHS hospital ward for which a patient may be charged a small fixed amount for the hotel part of the cost, but not the cost of treatment, under section 12 of the 1977 NHS Act.

Analysis of expenditure by client group Analysis of expenditure over broad groups of service related to patient care groups, e.g. services for mentally ill people, services mainly for children, and general and acute hospital and maternity services.

 ▸ **Functional (objective):** The object for which the payment has been made – medical staff services, nursing staff services, transport services and so on.
 ▸ **Subjective:** According to the nature of the payment, e.g. salaries and wages, travel, drugs, etc.

Annual report A report, written annually, which details progress over the last year and plans for the following year. Includes financial and activity statements.

Apology A sincere expression of regret.

Appeal (Care of Child) Appeals in care proceedings are now to be heard by the High Court or, where applicable, the Court of Appeal. All parties to the proceedings will have equal rights of appeal. On hearing an appeal, the High Court can make such orders as may be necessary to give effect to its decision.

Application In computer technology this is a synonym for a program that carries out a specific type of task. Word processors or spreadsheets are common applications available on personal computers.

Arbitration The process of settling a disagreement between two or more parties by the introduction of an external body or person with authority to make and implement an agreement.

Arden syntax   A language created to encode actions within a clinical protocol into a set of situation-action rules for computer interpretation, and also to facilitate exchange between different institutions.

Area Child Protection Committee (ACPC)   Based on the boundaries of the local authority, it provides a forum for developing, monitoring and reviewing the local child protection policies, and promoting effective and harmonious co-operation between the various agencies involved. Although there is some variation from area to area, each committee is made up of representatives of the key agencies, who have authority to speak and act on their agency's behalf. ACPCs issue guidelines about procedures, tackle significant issues that arise, offer advice about the conduct of cases in general, make policy and review progress on prevention, and oversee interagency training.

Artificial intelligence (AI)   Any artefact, whether embodied solely in computer software or a physical structure like a robot, that exhibits behaviours associated with human intelligence. (*See also* Turing test.)

Artificial intelligence in medicine   The application of artificial intelligence methods to solve problems in medicine, e.g. developing expert systems to assist with diagnosis or therapy planning. (*See also* artificial intelligence and expert systems.)

Assessment   Process by which the capacities and incapacities of people who may require community care are established by social services departments, with appropriate services thereby identified.

Assessment (children)   Process of gathering together and evaluating information about a child, its family and circumstances. Its purpose is to determine children's needs, in order to plan for their immediate and long-term care and decide what services and resources must be provided. Childcare assessments are usually co-ordinated by social services, but depend on teamwork with other agencies (such as education and health).

Associates   Salaried doctors who support principals in hard-pressed areas, such as the London Implementation Zone Education Initiative area or remote parts of Scotland.

Asynchronous communication   Communication between two parties when the exchange does not require both to be an active participant in the conversation at the same time, e.g. sending a letter. (*See also* synchronous communication and email.)

Audit   Originally the process by which the probity of operations and activities of an organisation was examined (internal audit) and a report on the annual accounts produced (external audit). Now used more widely, e.g. clinical audit evaluates the effectiveness of clinical activities; and management audit evaluates the effectiveness and efficiency of organisational and management arrangements. It involves the process of setting or adopting standards and measuring performance against those standards, with the aim of identifying both good and bad practice and implementing changes to achieve unmet standards.

Audit Committee   A committee of an NHS trust or authority board, comprising non-executive members, which ensures probity in the corporate governance of the organisation. Following the Cadbury Report, NHS bodies should have such a body.

Audit trails   Anyone accessing a patient's record using the NHS Care Records Service is automatically recorded in an audit trail. This is like an electronic footprint that shows who they are, when they accessed the record and what they did.

Authorised person (children)   In relation to care and supervision proceedings, this is a person not from the local authority who is authorised by the Secretary of State to bring proceedings under section 31 of the Act. This covers the National Society for the Prevention of Cruelty to Children (NSPCC) and its officers. Elsewhere in the Act there is a reference to persons who are authorised to carry out specified functions, e.g. to enter and inspect independent schools.

Average daily available beds The average number of staffed beds in each department in which patients are being treated, or could be treated, each day without any changes being made in facilities or staff. Beds borrowed from other departments are included.

Average length of stay The average number of days a bed is occupied by each patient.

Bayes' theorem Theorem used to calculate the relative probability of an event given the probabilities of associated events. Used to calculate the probability of a disease given the frequencies of symptoms and signs within the disease and within the normal population.

Bed bureau An administrative unit that ensures that patients needing urgent admission are directed to a hospital which will admit them.

Bed days
> **Available bed days:** the sum of beds available for use each day during a specified period of time.
> **Occupied bed days:** the sum of the number of beds occupied by patients each day during a specified period of time. This total, divided by the number of discharges and deaths during the same period, gives the average length of stay.
> **Vacant bed days:** the number obtained when the total of occupied bed days is subtracted from the available bed days.

Bed norm A measure of the bed requirements for a given population, expressed as number of beds per 1000 people. Bed norms may be used in several different ways: age specific, as in the case of hospital accommodation for the elderly – 10 beds per 1000 aged 65 years and over; or by specialty, as in the case of orthopaedic beds – 0.35 per 1000.

Bed occupancy The number of beds occupied by patients at a particular time, usually midnight. It may be expressed as a percentage of available beds.

Bed state The number of beds, both occupied and vacant, at a particular time.

Bed turnover The average number of patients using each bed in a given period, such as a year.

Behavioural science The study of individuals and groups in a working environment. Issues may include communication, motivation, organisational structure and organisational change. The science is still being developed and relies on contributions from psychology and sociology.

Benchmarking Defined by the UK Benchmarking Centre (1993) as the continuous, systematic search for best practices, and the implementation that will lead to superior performance.

Benchmarks Benchmarks are sources of information (e.g. cost, quality outcomes, etc.) used as comparators to compare performance between similar organisations or systems.

Booked case An elective admission where the date has been arranged in advance with the patient. Waiting lists should include booked cases.

British Association of Medical Managers (BAMM) Aims to 'support the provision of quality healthcare by improving and supporting the contribution of doctors in management, together with all other activities which contribute to, further, or are ancillary to this principal aim'.

Broadband A type of data transmission in which a single (telephone) wire can carry several channels at once. Cable TV, for example, uses broadband transmission.

Budget A statement of the financial resources made available to a budget holder to provide an agreed level of service over a set period of time.

Business plan A plan setting out the goals of an organisation and identifying the resources and actions needed to achieve them. Usually prepared on an annual basis, the business plan seeks to balance planned activity with income so as to minimise financial risk.

Caldicott Guardian The member of staff in an NHS organisation who is responsible for ensuring that patient rights to confidentiality are protected.

Capital asset Land, property, plant or equipment valued at more than £5000.

Capital Asset Register A list of all the capital assets of an organisation. This contains information required to administer a capital asset replacement programme such as the purchase price, acquisition and replacement date of assets.

Capital Asset Replacement Programme A programme which uses depreciation accounting techniques to spread the cost of the replacement of capital assets.

Capital charges Since 1991, the use/ownership of capital in the NHS has incurred a cost, the capital charge. This was introduced so that NHS capital was no longer regarded as a free good or gift from the state. Capital charges consist of two elements: depreciation and interest on fixed assets. The interest rate currently applied is 6%. NHS trusts retain depreciation charges within the trust and are required to make a target rate of return equivalent to the interest rate.

Capital programme A plan over a period of time (normally five years) showing costs and starting and final dates of schemes of work to be charged to the capital allocation.

Career advice Providing information on career opportunities and training requirements.

Career counselling Discussing career options for which the individual may be most suited.

Care order (children) Order made by the court under s31 (1)(a) of the Children Act placing the child in the care of the designated local authority. A care order includes an interim care order except where express provision to the contrary is made.

Care pathway An approach to managing a specific disease or clinical condition that identifies what interventions are required, and sets out the various stages of care through which a patient passes and the expected outcome of treatment.

Care plan A written statement of community care services to be provided following assessment (q.v.). The document details the care and treatment that a patient receives and identifies who delivers the care and treatment. This term covers the term 'individual plan' (*See also* health record).

Care Programme Approach (CPA) The individual packages of care (care programmes), developed in conjunction with social services, for all patients accepted by the specialist psychiatric services. Care programmes may range from 'minimal' single-worker assessment and monitoring for individuals with less severe mental health and social needs, to complex and multi-professional assessments and treatment.

Care Record Development Board (CRDB) Established as an independent body to provide advice to NHS Connecting for Health on a variety of issues arising from the development of the NHS Care Records Service. The CRDB was replaced on 1 October 2007 by the National Information Governance Board for Health and Social Care, which will continue to publish and review the NHS Care Record Guarantee, formerly produced by the CRDB (*See also* National Information Governance Board for Health and Social Care).

Care Record Guarantee The commitment of the NHS in England to patients that it will use records about them in ways that respect their rights and promote their health and well-being. The Guarantee covers people's access to their own records, controls on others' access, how access will be monitored and policed, options to further limit access,

access in an emergency and what happens when someone cannot make decisions for him or herself.

Carer   A person who regularly provides help (without pay) to someone who requires domestic, physical, emotional or personal care as a result of illness or disability. This term also incorporates friends, relatives and partners. There are thought to be six million 'informal carers'.

Case-based reasoning   An approach to computer reasoning that uses knowledge from a library of similar cases, rather than by accessing a knowledge base containing more generalised knowledge, such as a set of rules. (*See also* artificial intelligence and expert system.)

Case conference (children)   Formal meeting attended by representatives from all the agencies concerned with the child's welfare. This increasingly includes the child's parents (and the Act promotes this practice).

Casemix   The mixture of clinical conditions and severity of condition encountered in a particular healthcare setting.

Cash limit   A limit imposed by the government on the amount of cash a public body may spend during a given financial year. Separate cash limits may be set for revenue and capital.

Causal reasoning   A form of reasoning based on following from cause to effect, in contrast to other methods in which the connection is weaker, such as probabilistic association.

Chairman (chairperson or chair is more politically correct)   A person who leads or conducts discussions. A chair's skill and technique may be used in a one-to-one meeting or by indirect communication methods, such as the telephone.

Change agent   A third party, who may be a trained behavioural scientist, and who acts as a catalyst in bringing about change by means of an organisation development programme.

Checklist   A means of recording observations relating to fixed criteria; used to check compliance with agreed procedures or standards.

Child   A person under the age of 18 years. There is an important exception to this in the case of an application for financial relief by a 'child' who has reached 18 years and is, or will be, receiving education or training.

Child assessment order   The order requires any person who can do so to produce the child for an assessment and to comply with the terms of the order.

Child Protection Register   Central record of all children in a given area for whom support is being provided via inter-agency planning. Generally, these are children considered to be at risk of abuse or neglect. The register is usually maintained and run by social service departments under the responsibility of a custodian (an experienced social worker able to provide advice to any professional making inquiries about the child). Registration for each child is reviewed every six months.

Child minder   Person who looks after one or more children under the age of eight for reward, for more than two hours in any one day.

Children in need   A child is in need if: (a) he or she is unlikely to achieve or maintain (or have the opportunity of achieving or maintaining) a reasonable standard of health or development without the provision for him or her of services by a local authority; or (b) his or her health or development is likely to be significantly impaired (or further impaired) without the provision for him or her of such services; or (c) he or she is disabled.

Children living away from home   Children who are not being looked after by the local authority but are nevertheless living away from home, e.g. children in independent schools. The local authority has a number of duties towards such children, e.g. to take reasonably practicable steps to ensure that their welfare is being adequately safeguarded and promoted.

Choice   Giving patients more choice about how, when and where they receive treatment is one cornerstone of the government's health policy. In the context of NHS reforms, this is the overarching policy term given to range of initiatives within the reform of the NHS designed to act as a driver for efficiency, quality and effectiveness.

Choose and Book   Allows a patient, in partnership with health and care professionals, to book first outpatient appointments at the most appropriate date, time and place for the patient.

Clinic session   A session held, and not merely scheduled, for, by or on behalf of one consultant, senior hospital medical officer or dental officer. Now extended to include sessions run by nurses and other clinical staff.

Clinical budgeting   The allocation of specific budgets to consultant clinical staff who are responsible for the budget management. A part of management budgeting.

Clinical directorate   A unit of management for specific clinical services. A clinical directorate is usually led by a clinical director, who is often a consultant working in that role for a number of sessions per week. They are supported by a nurse and/or business manager. The extent to which management responsibilities for budgets and staff are devolved to directorates varies.

Clinical guideline   An agreed set of steps to be taken in the management of a clinical condition.

Clinical pathway   *See* clinical guideline.

Clinical protocol   *See* clinical guideline.

Clinical responsibilities   Range of activities for which a clinician is accountable.

Clinical Risk and Safety Board   Local NHS boards responsible for establishing a framework for the safe implementation and continuing use of new IT systems in local NHS organisations. The board is made up of clinical representatives including doctors, nurses and other healthcare professionals.

Clinical Spine Application (CSA)   The web-based application that enables healthcare professionals who do not have access to local NHS Care Records Service systems and services to have controlled access to the Personal Demographics Service (PDS) and the Personal Spine Information Service (PSIS). It enables clinicians and other staff to access information held on the Spine.

Clinician's sealed envelope   *See* sealing.

Closed beds   Beds which have not been used (i.e. closed) for longer than one month for the purpose of redecoration or structural alterations, or because of a shortage of staff, but are scheduled to be reopened at a future date.

Code   In medical terminological systems, the unique numerical identifier associated with a medical concept, which may be associated with a variety of terms, all with the same meaning. (*See also* term.)

Cognitive map   A process of recording information in related groupings and intended to assist lateral thinking. (*See also* mind map.)

Cognitive science   A multidisciplinary field studying human cognitive processes, including their relationship to technologically embodied models of cognition. (*See also* artificial intelligence.)

Commissioner   An organisation or individual involved in purchasing healthcare. (*See also* purchaser.)

Commissioning   Relates to the purchasing and contracting of healthcare services. It is a broad term that can cover a range of activities but in principle a distinction can be drawn between two levels of commissioning. At one level, commissioning can involve service planning and design, through identifying population need; assessing the local priorities; understanding the market; and determining where and how services should be provided and by whom. On another level, commissioning can involve the daily purchasing of services, through managing contracts and spending budgets.

Commissioning a patient-led NHS   The letter and attachments (entitled *Commissioning a Patient-led NHS*) was sent to NHS Chief Executives and others at the end of July 2005. It builds on the *NHS Improvement Plan* and *Creating a Patient-Led NHS*. The details contained in the papers relate to the form and function of primary care trusts and strategic health authorities and was designed to begin to address the tension between providing services and commissioning services in PCTs. It was also intended to prompt cost savings of £250 million; deliver practice-based commissioning (PBC) by December 2006 at the latest; and SHAs will be reconfigured to move towards alignment with Government Office boundaries.

Communication   The two-way process of exchanging ideas, thoughts, feelings and facts.

Communication strategy   A written statement of objectives for effective communication and a plan for meeting those objectives. The strategy should be consistent with the business plan.

Community care   The assessment and commissioning of health and social care and treatment to patients/clients outside hospital, who have an identified physical or mental illness or disability. It is often more narrowly associated with patients being resettled from institutional care, e.g. from large psychiatric hospitals, or frail, elderly people who previously would have remained in hospital care.

Community Health Councils (CHCs)   'Patient watchdog' bodies established as part of the NHS reorganisation in 1974. Their role included assisting with complaints and visiting NHS premises. The government published the *NHS Plan for England* in 2000, which proposed the abolition of CHCs in England and their replacement by Patient and Public Involvement Forums and Patient Advocate and Liaison Services and established by each NHS trust, including primary care trusts in England. CHCs have been retained in Wales and Scotland.

Community health services   These divide into two main groups: patient care in the community – the treatment or care (outside hospital) of patients with identified physical or mental illness or disability; and services to the community – services of prevention or intervention that are provided to a population, such as immunisation, screening and health promotion.

Complainant   A person who expresses dissatisfaction. They may or may not be the patient concerned.

Complaint   An expression of dissatisfaction.

Complaints procedure (children)   The procedure that a local authority must set up in order to hear representations regarding the provision of services under Part III of the Children Act from a number of persons, including the child, the parents and 'such other person' as the authority considers has sufficient interest in the child's welfare to warrant his or her representations being considered by them.

Compliment   An expression of approval or satisfaction.

Computer-based patient record   *See* electronic medical record.

Computerised protocol Clinical guideline or protocol stored on a computer system so that it may be easily accessed or manipulated to support the delivery of care. (*See also* clinical guideline.)

Computer Sciences Corporation (CSC) The Local Service Provider (LSP) for the North West and West Midlands Cluster and North East and Eastern Clusters, delivering software developed by its main subcontractor iSoft.

Conciliation The process of a layperson assisting two parties in dispute to reach informal agreement through discussion and persuasion without any legally binding status.

Conciliatory The application of conciliation techniques particularly outside a formal conciliation process.

Concurrent jurisdiction (children) The High Court, a County Court and a Magistrates' Court (Family Proceedings Court) all have jurisdiction to hear proceedings under the Children's Act.

Connectionism The study of the theory and application of neural networks. (*See also* neural network.)

Consent to share Where a patient has explicitly consented to share information across organisations for the purpose of their healthcare, or has expressed no preference so consent is inferred. The sharing of information will be on a need-to-know basis. A Summary Care Record exists and is visible to an authorised user with a legitimate relationship to the patient. Consent may be given in two ways.

- **Implied consent:** When a patient has not expressed a preference so consent to share is inferred. For example, when a GP sends clinical information to a consultant following a patient referral to specialist care, the GP is assuming the patient's consent to send that information as part of the referral.
- **Express consent:** When a patient expresses permission for the sharing of their clinical information across NHS organisations.

Patients may also express dissent to the sharing of information.

- **Dissent to share:** Prevents confidential information maintained by one legal organisation being accessible by another legal organisation, unless the information is sent as part of a direct clinical communication like a referral or discharge note. A Summary Care Record will exist but will not be automatically visible to any authorised user, when combined with Consent to Store.

Constant prices A mechanism for comparing prices for goods and services over a number of years, which compensates for the distortion introduced by inflation.

Contact order (children) Order requiring the person with whom a child lives, or is to live, to allow the child to visit or stay with the person named in the order.

Continuing education Activities which provide education and training for staff. These may be used to prepare for specialisation or career development as well as facilitating personal development.

Continuing professional development (CPD) Defined as: 'A process of lifelong learning for all individuals and teams which enables professionals to expand and fulfil their potential and which also meets the needs of patients and delivers the health and healthcare priorities of the NHS'.

Contract/Agreement A document agreed between providers and purchasers of healthcare. Details activity, financial and quality levels to be achieved.

Contract currencies Agreed units of measurement for contracting, e.g. finished consultant episodes.

Contracts   The basis for agreement on the services that should be provided to patients, including specification of quality. Block contracts specify facilities to be provided, and may include workload agreements including patient activity targets within an agreed range. Cost and volume contracts specify the level of services required by the purchaser. Purchasers can link payment with agreed activity. Provider units will be able to match funding with workload and deploy resources more flexibly. Cost per case contracts cover the cost of treatment for specific patients.

Control measures   Ways in which risk can be controlled, including physical controls such as locking away drugs and valuable items, and system controls such as restricting access to hazardous areas to specific staff groups.

Convenor   A non-executive director of a trust, health authority or health board who decides whether or not to convene an independent panel to review a complaint against an NHS provider.

Corporate   Relating to the whole of an organisation, e.g. the management of an organisation.

Corporate seal   A seal used by organisations to certify documents used in legal transactions (such as the sale of land) so as to fulfil legal requirements.

Court welfare officer (children)   Officer appointed to provide a report for the court about the child and the child's family situation and background. The court welfare officer will usually be a probation officer.

Criterion   A measurable component of performance. A number of criteria need to be met to achieve the desired standard.

Cross-functional team   A team of people from different disciplines.

Cruse   A non-religious UK-based organisation specialising in bereavement. Email info@ crusebereavementcare.org.uk

Cybernetics   A name coined by Norbert Weiner in the 1950s to describe the study of feedback control systems and their application. Such systems were seen to exhibit properties associated with human intelligence and robotics, and so were an early contribution to the theory of artificial intelligence.

Cyberspace   Popular term (now associated with the Internet) which describes the notional information 'space' that is created across computer networks. (*See also* virtual reality.)

Cycle time   Time a patient is under treatment (in hospital). Thus, cycle time plus waiting time equals the lead time.

Database   A structured repository for data, usually stored on a computer system. The existence of a regular and formal indexing structure permits rapid retrieval of individual elements of the database.

Day care (children)   A person provides day care if they look after one or more children under the age of eight on non-domestic premises for more than two hours in any day.

Day cases   Patients who have an investigation, treatment or operation, but are admitted electively and discharged on the same day.

Decision support system   General term for any computer application that enhances a human's ability to make decisions.

Decision tree   A method of representing knowledge that makes structured decisions in a hierarchical tree-like fashion.

Deduction   A method of logical inference. Given a cause, deduction infers all logical effects that might arise as a consequence. (*See also* abduction, induction and inference.)

Designated person   A person within an NHS provider, or a department of an NHS provider, who is delegated responsibility to ensure that complaints are properly resolved locally.

Detailed records   At present patients have many detailed records. These include a GP record, usually held electronically but often supplemented by paper records. Where patients have visited a hospital or clinic, there will usually be an electronic patient administration record; a separate written clinical record in their local hospital; a separate paper record if they have been pregnant; a further separate paper record if they have received mental health treatment; another separate paper record if they have been treated in the sexual health clinic; and a separate record if they have attended Accident and Emergency. Each of these records will be repeated for each hospital or clinic the patient has attended. In addition, the patient may have a community record if receiving long-term care in the community (e.g. physiotherapy). The National Programme for IT has a clear objective to reduce this duplication of diverse records by providing a patient-centred electronic detailed record that spans these areas. As a minimum, this would be within a hospital but there are real benefits when providing a consistent record across a local health community and across the boundaries involved in care pathways for a patient. The overall objective is a single detailed record for an individual patient that is accessible by the GP and by community and local hospital care settings.

Dictionary of Medicines and Devices (dm+d)   The source of terminology and a common language for medicines and devices used in healthcare.

Direct credits   The income from the sale of meals to staff, renting accommodation to staff and so on.

Direct discrimination   Where someone is treated less favourably purely on grounds of marital status, sex, ethnic origin or similar criteria which do not affect the individual's ability to perform the job. (*See also* indirect discrimination)

Disabled (children)   A child is disabled if 'he or she is blind, deaf or dumb or suffers from a mental disorder of any kind or is substantially and permanently handicapped by illness, injury or congenital deformity or such other disability'.

Dissent to share   *See* consent to share.

Disclosure interview (children)   Term sometimes used to indicate an interview with a child, conducted as part of the assessment for suspected sexual abuse. It could be misleading (since it implies, in some people's view, undue pressure on the child to 'disclose') and therefore the latest preferred term is 'investigative interview'.

Discrimination   May be direct or indirect. For details see separate headings.

Distributed computing   Term for computer systems in which data and programs are distributed and shared across different computers on a network.

Dual registered homes   Homes for disabled or elderly people, registered as both a residential care home and a nursing home.

Duty to investigate (children)   A local authority is under a duty to investigate in a number of situations where they have a 'reasonable cause to suspect that a child who lives, or is found, in [its] area is suffering, or is likely to suffer, significant harm'.

Early Adopter Programme   A programme of work involving NHS Connecting for Health supporting the first primary care trusts to implement Summary Care Records for patients in their area. There were six Early Adopter PCTs that made up the Early Adopter Programme. The Early Adopter sites were independently evaluated so that lessons could be learned and business processes tested and refined before Summary Care Records started to roll out across England from 2008.

European Computer Driving Licence (ECDL)   A training course in essential IT skills available to all NHS staff to help them prepare for new ways of working and increase confidence in their use of IT. ECDL is an internationally recognised qualification that has been adopted as the NHS standard. Since replaced by Essential IT Skills.

Education supervision order (children)   Order which puts a child under the supervision of a designated local education authority.

Education welfare officer (EWO)   Social work support to children in the context of their schooling. While EWOs' main focus used to be the enforcement of school attendance, today they perform a wider range of services, including seeking to ensure that children receive adequate and appropriate education and that any special needs are met, and more general liaison between local authority education and social services departments.

Educational psychologist   A psychology graduate who has had teaching experience and additional vocational training. Educational psychologists perform a range of functions including assessing children's education, psychological and emotional needs, offering therapy and contributing psychological expertise to the process of assessment.

Electronic mail   *See* email.

Electronic medical record   A general term describing computer-based patient record systems. It is sometimes extended to include other functions, such as order entry for medications and tests, among other common functions.

electronic Government Interoperability Framework (eGIF)   Standards used to ensure the security of systems for registering system users and authenticating their identity. The eGIF defines the technical policies and specifications governing information flows across government and the public sector.

Electronic Patient Record (EPR)   EPR is a catch-all term covering the patient data held in digital form by computers. The National Programme for IT is delivering a number of EPRs. A Summary Care Record (SCR), Detailed Records, Diagnostic Test Order and Results, PACS images and all other clinical data held in computers are examples of EPRs.

Electronic transmission of prescriptions (ETP)   Enables GPs/prescribers to send prescriptions electronically to pharmacies.

Email/e-mail/electronic mail   A messaging system available on computer networks, providing users with personal mail boxes from which electronic messages can be sent and received.

Emergency admission   A patient admitted on the same day that admission is requested.

Emergency protection order (children)   That which a court can make if it is satisfied that a child is likely to suffer significant harm, or where inquiries are being made with respect to the child and they are being frustrated by the unreasonable refusal of access to the child.

Enterprise-wide arrangements   Arrangements with key suppliers in the IT industry. Given its size, the National Programme seeks to procure quality IT services from suppliers to the NHS on a greater scale and at a more competitive rate than any single NHS organisation.

Epidemiology   Study of the distribution and determinants of disease in human populations.

Epistemology   The philosophical study of knowledge.

Estates strategy   A written statement of objectives relating to estates management and a plan for meeting those objectives. The strategy should be consistent with the business plan.

European Directive   A requirement which binds an EU member state, e.g. the one designed to facilitate the free movement of doctors and the mutual recognition of their diplomas, certificates and other evidence of formal qualifications (Council Directive 93/16/EEC).

Evaluation   The study of the performance of a service (or element of treatment and care) with the aim of identifying successful and problem areas of activity.

Evidence-based medicine   A movement advocating the practice of medicine according to clinical guidelines, developed to reflect best practice as captured from a meta-analysis of the clinical literature. (*See also* clinical guideline, meta-analysis and protocol.)

Existing system provider   A supplier whose system is currently installed within the NHS and related care settings. NHS Connecting for Health's Existing Systems Programme works with these suppliers to make their systems compatible with National Programme systems and services that in turn ought to enable patients to benefit from the new services such as Choose and Book, the Electronic Prescription Service and GP2GP Record Transfer.

Expert system   A computer program that contains expert knowledge about a particular problem, often in the form of a set of if-then rules, that is able to solve problems at a level equivalent or greater than human experts. (*See also* artificial intelligence.)

Explicit consent   *See* consent to share.

External financing limit (EFL)   A cash limit set by the NHSE on net external financing for an NHS trust. A positive external financing limit is set where the agreed capital spending for an NHS trust exceeds income from internally generated resources. A zero external financing limit is set where the agreed capital spending programme for a trust equals internally generated resources. A negative external financing limit is set where the agreed capital spending programme for a trust is less than internally generated resources.

Extra-contractual referral (ECR)   The term used for referral of an individual for health services that were not covered in contracts that existed between the old system of purchaser and providers of services.

Family centre   Child and parents, or other person looking after a child, can attend for occupational and recreational activities, advice, guidance or counselling, and accommodation while receiving such advice, guidance or counselling.

Family Panel   Panel from which magistrates who sit in the new Family Proceedings Court are selected. These magistrates will have undergone specialist training on the Children's Act.

Family Proceedings Court   Court at the level of the magistrates' court to hear proceedings under the Children Act 1989. The magistrates will be selected from a new panel, known as the Family Panel, and will be specially trained.

Fieldworker (field social worker)   Conducts a range of social work functions in the community and in other settings (e.g. hospitals).

Financial strategy   A written statement of objectives relating to financial management and a plan for meeting those objectives. The strategy should be consistent with the business plan.

Financial target (for an NHS trust)   A real pre-interest return of 6% on the value of net assets, effectively a return on the average of the opening and closing assets shown in the accounts.

Finished consultant episode (FCE)   An episode where the patient has completed a period of care under a consultant and is either discharged or transferred to another consultant. The total number of episodes is a common measure of overall hospital activity.

Firewall   A security barrier erected between a public computer network like the Internet and a local private computer network.

Flexible training   Available for doctors who have 'well-founded individual reasons' for working less than full-time. The DoH runs two schemes to encourage flexible training for career registrars and senior registrars (PM(79)3). Flexible training for PRHOs and SHOs is available on a personal basis. In addition, a number of regions organise their own flexible training schemes.

Foster carer   Provides substitute family care for children. A child looked after by a local authority can be placed with local authority foster carers.

Foundation trusts (FTs)   First set up as a result of the Health and Social Care (Community Health and Standards) Act 2003. More hospitals have become foundation trusts since then and all Acute NHS Trusts will be required to attain FT status by the end of 2008. Although remaining part of the NHS, foundation trusts are subject to reduced control from central government. They differ from traditional NHS trusts in three main ways:
> they possess the freedom to decide locally how to meet their obligations (which can also involve borrowing money from private sources)
> they are accountable, through (mainly elected) governors, to their members, who are drawn from local residents, patients and staff
> they are authorised and monitored by Monitor, the Independent Regulator of NHS foundation trusts.

Frequently asked questions (FAQ)   Common term for information lists available on the Internet which have been compiled for newcomers on a particular subject, answering common questions that would otherwise often be asked by submitting email requests to a Newsgroup.

Front line staff   The employees of an NHS provider who have direct, face-to-face contact with patients and other NHS users.

Front Line Support Academy   Provides learning opportunities for staff involved in the implementation of IT in the NHS and social care. The Academy works with staff to change and improve patients' experience of their care.

Functional department   Examples would include X-ray, a ward, theatre, pharmacy, pathology, a clinic or outpatients.

Functional team   A team from within a single discipline.

General Practice Element   Usually referenced in relation to Summary Care Records, this is the information from the GP patient record that is included in a patient's Summary Care Record.

General Medical Services (GMS)   The rules used to manage payments to family doctors as part of the GP's contract.

General Medical Services Contract (GMS contract)   In 2003 GPs accepted a new contract, negotiated by the British Medical Association and the NHS Confederation. The terms of this contract meant that payments to GPs were more closely related to the quantity and quality of the services provided.

Go live   For the purposes of communications with the public, go live is when new systems and services start to be used to enable information to be linked so that it can be accessed by people in different organisations, e.g. a hospital can access information created by a GP.

GP fundholder   Term that was used for GP practice with a budget for the purchase of a range of hospital inpatient and outpatient (and certain nursing and paramedical) services. Ceased in April 1999.

GP2GP   A service that transfers electronic patient records from one GP practice to another when a patient changes GP practices. A secure way of transferring patient records from one GP practice to another.

Guardian *ad litem* (GAL)   Person appointed by a court to investigate a child's circumstances and to report to the court.

Guidance (children)   Authorities are required to act in accordance with the guidance issued by the Secretary of State. However, guidance does not have the full force of law but is intended as a series of statements of good practice and may be quoted or used in court proceedings.

Hawthorne effect   Term used to describe changes in productivity and employee morale as a direct result of management interest in their problems. Improvements may arise before any management action. Originates from a study of the Hawthorne Works, Western Electric Co, USA (1920s).

Hazard assessment procedures   The process by which the origins, frequencies, costs and effects of hazards are identified and strategies adopted to avoid or minimise their effects.

Hazards   The potential to cause harm, including ill health and injury, damage to property, plant, products or the environment, production losses or increased liabilities.

Health and safety policy   A plan of action for the health, safety and well-being of staff, patients, residents and visitors.

Healthcare Resource Groups (HRGs)   These are codes that signify clinically similar treatments that use common levels of healthcare resource. An information management tool, they have been developed to support Payment by Results.

Health economy or health community   These terms generally refer to all providers, purchasers and service users within a defined geographical area.

Health gain   The improvement of the health status of a community or population. It is sometimes described as 'adding years to life and life to years'.

Health level 7 (HL7)   A healthcare-specific communication standard for data exchange between computer applications.

Healthcare professional   A person qualified in a health discipline.

Health promotion   Enabling individuals and communities to increase control over the determinants of health and thereby improve their health.

Health record   Information about the physical or mental health of someone, which has been made by, or on behalf of, a health professional in connection with the care of that person. These must be kept for a statutory period of time after the patient is discharged from the service. Records will be held in addition to care plans.

Health Service Commissioner (HSC)   The Ombudsman, appointed by Parliament to protect the rights of users of the NHS. Responsible only to Parliament.

Health service price index   This index takes the NHS 'shopping basket' of goods and services (it excludes pay of employees) and weighs them according to use. The cost movement of these items is measured each month and the index updated to reflect these changes. It is used by the NHS to measure price movements and quite often to update allocations and budgets.

HealthSpace   A secure website which provides an online personal health organiser for patients. In time, and after completing the registration process for an advanced HealthSpace account, patients who have a Summary Care Record will be able to access it using HealthSpace.

Health status   A measure of the overall health experience of an individual or a defined population.

Hearing The process of perceiving sound or agreement to having heard a person's statement.

Herzberg's two-factor theory Herzberg maintained on the basis of research studies that in any work there are factors which satisfy and dissatisfy, but they are not necessarily opposites of each other. The latter are to do with conditions of work which he called hygiene or maintenance factors, and the former are achievement, recognition, responsibility and advancement, which he called motivators.

Heuristic A rule of thumb that describes how things are commonly understood, without resorting to deeper or more formal knowledge. (*See also* model-based reasoning.)

HMRL First of a series of hospital medical record forms. It is usually the front sheet of a patient's case notes and summarises personal, administrative and medical details. It is used for inpatients in all hospitals except those for mental illness and maternity.

Hospice NHS, voluntary or private residential premises for the provision of clinical and nursing care to residents who are terminally ill.

Hospital acquired infection An infection acquired by a patient during their stay in hospital, which is unconnected with their reason for admission.

Hospital information system (HIS) Typically used to describe hospital computer systems with functions such as patient admission and discharge, order entry for laboratory tests or medications, and billing functions. (*See also* electronic medical record.)

Hospital stay The number of days a patient stays on one hospital site during a hospital provider spell.

Hotel costs The costs of food, heating, maintenance and so on for keeping a patient in hospital, excluding all medical and treatment costs.

Human-computer interaction The study of the psychology and design principles associated with the way humans interact with computer systems.

Human-computer interface The 'view' presented by a program to its user. Often literally a visual window that allows a program to be operated, an interface could just as easily be based on the recognition and synthesis of speech or any other medium with which a human is able to sense or manipulate.

Human resource strategy A written statement of human resource objectives and a plan for meeting those objectives. The strategy should be consistent with the business plan.

Hygiene factor The element of work motivation concerned with the environment or context of job, i.e. salary, status and security, etc. To be distinguished from motivators, i.e. achievement recognition. Based on theory of Herzberg F. (*see* Herzberg 1959).

IG alert An alert to a Caldicott Guardian or Privacy Officer, which will be generated when a user has had to justify special access to confidential patient information, and access has been provided. The privacy officer will ensure that the reason given for access is genuine and justifiable.

Information Governance (IG) The structures, policies and practice used to ensure the confidentiality and security of health and social care services records, especially clinical records, and to enable the ethical use of them for the benefit of the individual to whom they relate and for the public good.

IG Statement of Compliance (IGSoC) An agreement between NHS Connecting for Health and any organisation wishing to use services provided through the National Programme for IT. The agreement stipulates the obligations that the organisation is expected to maintain to ensure patient data is safeguarded and only used appropriately.

Implied consent *See* consent to share.

In care (children)   Refers to a child in the care of the local authority by virtue of an order or under an interim order.

Incident   An event or occurrence, especially one that leads to problems. An example of this could be an attack on one person by another within a service.

Income and expenditure reports   An accountancy tool which describes and analyses the flow of funds into and out of an organisation in order to assess liquidity. Sometimes known as 'source and application of funds statements' or more commonly 'cash flow statements'.

Independent contractor   In primary care, this normally refers to a self-employed professional. The vast majority of GPs are self-employed – unlike hospital doctors who are normally directly employed by the hospital.

Independent review   The process of a panel of laypersons reviewing the case of a complaint where the complainant is not satisfied with the results of local resolution by an NHS provider.

Independent visitor (children)   A local authority in certain sets of circumstances appoints such a visitor for a child it is looking after. The visitor appointed has the duty of 'visiting, advising and befriending the child'.

Indirect discrimination   Where an unjustifiable requirement or condition is applied to the job which has a disproportionately adverse effect on one sex or group. For example, the career and life pattern of women is often different from that of men as a consequence of family responsibilities and child-bearing. Women may be less mobile than men. Another example of indirect discrimination is insisting on a conventional career path. (*See also* direct discrimination.)

Individual performance review (IPR)   A system of appraisal based on the setting of agreed objectives and targets between individual employees and their managers and the extent of the attainment of these targets. Normally, IPR is linked to development; within the NHS it is often associated with performance-related pay for senior managers.

Induction   A method of logical inference used to suggest relationships from observations. This is the process of generalisation we use to create models of the world. (*See also* abduction, deduction and inference.)

Induction programme   Learning activities designed to enable newly appointed staff to function effectively in a new position.

Industrial tribunals   Set up under the Industrial Training Act 1964, they consider cases of unfair dismissal, sex discrimination and disability.

Industry Liaison   Provides information and guidance to IT suppliers who would like to be involved in providing products and services to NPfIT. It also supplies information to the National Programme on product innovations and developments in IT.

Infant mortality rate   The deaths of infants under one year of age per 1000 live births.

Inference   A logical conclusion drawn using one of several methods of reasoning, knowledge and data. (*See also* abduction, deduction and induction.)

Information Governance Framework   The Information Governance Framework for Health and Social Care is formed by those elements of law and policy from which applicable information governance standards are derived, and the activities and roles which individually and collectively ensure that these standards are clearly defined and met. While a key focus of information governance is the use of information about service users, it applies to information and information processing in its broadest sense and underpins both clinical and corporate governance.

Information Standards Board (ISB)   Established in 2001 to provide an independent mechanism for the approval of information standards in the NHS.

Information superhighway   A popular term associated with the Internet and used to describe its role in the global mass transportation of information.

Information theory   Initially developed by Claude Shannon, this describes the amount of data that can be transmitted across a channel given specific encoding techniques and noise in the signal.

Informed consent   The legal principle by which a patient is informed about the nature, purpose and likely effects of any treatment proposed, before being asked to consent to accepting it.

Inherent jurisdiction (children)   Powers of High Court to make orders to protect a child.

Injunction   Order made by the court prohibiting an act or requiring its cessation.

Inpatient   A patient who has gone through the full admission procedure and is occupying a bed in a hospital inpatients' department.

Inquisitorial   One of two kinds of court process: adversarial and inquisitorial. The inquisitorial system is one where the role of the court is to inquire into the facts of a particular matter in order to reach a judgement. The Coroners Court is a good example.

Inspiration trap   The difficulty faced by a conciliator who can identify an obvious and sensible solution to a dispute but must ensure that the parties to the dispute reach the same conclusion without identifiable direction from the conciliator.

Integrated Services Digital Network (ISDN)   A digital telephone network that is designed to provide channels for voice and data services. Customer must be within about 3.4 miles of the telephone exchange otherwise expensive repeater devices are required.

Inter-agency plan (children)   Plan devised jointly by the agencies concerned in a child's welfare which co-ordinates the services they provide.

Interim Access Controls   All NHS organisations are working towards fulfilling all the commitments set out in the Care Record Guarantee. Until that time, interim measures will be put in place by organisations, in order to allow appropriate access to information while providing the necessary security and confidentiality.

Interim care order (children)   Made by court, placing the child in the care of the designated local authority.

International Classification of Disease (ICD-10)   Tenth edition published by the World Health Organization for the statistical classification of morbidity and mortality. It may be used in conjunction with another classification termed Read coding. Review of the WHO website suggests work is under way on ICD-11 and more information about the ICD can be found at www.who.int/research/en.

Investigative interview (children)   Preferred term for an interview conducted with a child as part of an assessment following concerns that the child may have been abused.

Investment appraisal   A means of assessing whether expenditure of capital (or revenue) on a project will show a satisfactory rate of return (e.g. lower costs or higher income), either absolutely or when compared with alternative projects.

Job description   Contains standard information for staff regarding conditions of service, location(s) of the post, duties of the post, accountability, education and training facilities, appraisal and the salary scale of the post. It should be available and made known to all potential applicants at the earliest possible stage and should be sent out with every application form. It contains details of accountability, responsibility, formal lines of communication, principal duties, entitlements and performance review. It is a guide for an individual in a specific position within an organisation. (*See also* person specification.)

Joint financing   A sum of money taken from the health allocation and then spent on projects which are agreed by a joint consultative committee. Such monies should normally be spent on personal social service projects to reduce demands on NHS services.

Judicial review An order from the divisional court quashing a disputed decision. The divisional court cannot substitute its own decision but can merely send the matter back to the offending authority for reconsideration.

Key worker The person responsible for co-ordinating the care plan for each individual patient, for monitoring its progress and for staying in regular contact with the patient and everyone involved. A key worker may be from a variety of different professional or non-professional backgrounds.

Kipling's serving men 'I keep six honest serving men (they taught me all I know). Their names are What and Why and When and How and Where and Who'.

Knowledge acquisition Subspecialty of artificial intelligence, usually associated with developing methods for capturing human knowledge and of converting it into a form that can be used by computer. (*See also* expert system, heuristic and machine learning.)

Knowledge-based system *See* expert system.

Korner data Korner relates to the review of NHS information requirements by the NHS/DHSS steering group on health services information which was chaired by Edith Korner. The group recommended a minimum set of data that should be collected in all districts for management purposes.

Lay person A person who is not, and preferably never has been, a professional in the field under dispute or any associated field.

Lead time Time between presentation to GP or perhaps A&E and discharge. Thus the lead time = cycle time + waiting time.

Lecture 50–55 minutes of largely uninterrupted discourse from a teacher with no discussion between students and no student activity other than listening and note taking.

Legacy systems suppliers These are the commercial companies that supply the current/existing IT systems and software in use in the NHS. Also known as existing systems suppliers.

Legitimate relationship (LR) Staff involved in a patient's care are considered to have a 'legitimate relationship' with that patient. Access to confidential information will be limited to those staff who have a 'legitimate relationship' with that patient.

Listen The process of actively hearing, accepting and understanding a verbal communication.

Local Improvement Finance Trust (LIFT) Local Improvement Finance Trusts are a method for funding primary care and community care estates modernisation, similar in some respects to PFI. The contracts involved in a LIFT scheme are for buildings and maintenance. It is an additional procurement route for developing primary care estates that currently includes the use of conventional public capital, premises built and operated under the national contract for general medical services (GMS), PFI and other public–private partnerships.

Local implementation An NPfIT management group and individual project teams who have responsibilities for implementation in each SHA. They co-ordinate and manage the progress of the programme by dealing with a variety of issues, including progress monitoring, problem solving, risk management, planning, good practice and allocating resources.

Local resolution The process of resolving a complaint against an NHS provider swiftly, at or very near to the point at which the issue complained about actually occurred.

Local Service Providers (LSPs) Responsible for working with the local NHS to deliver

National Programme for IT systems and services at a local level. They work to integrate local systems with national applications and to maintain common standards. LSPs also support local organisations to deliver and realise the benefits from their National Programme for IT systems and services.

Local voices initiative   Encourages gathering of the views and wishes of local people as a contribution to purchasing intelligence (q.v.).

Logical   To follow a sound set of rules and tests.

Looked after (children)   A child is looked after when in local authority care or is being provided with accommodation by the local authority.

Mailing list   A list of email addresses for individuals. Used to distribute information to small groups of individuals who may, for example, have shared interests. (*See also* email.)

Major incident (external)   A serious external incident which requires the organisation to implement contingency plans or change or suspend some normal functions. An example would be the aftermath of a rail crash.

Major incident (internal)   A serious incident occurring within the healthcare facility resulting in the changing or suspension of some normal functions or threatening of the organisation. This requires the drawing up of contingency plans. Examples of this would include the loss of electricity or telecommunications services or bomb threats.

Makaton symbols   A system of symbols used to communicate with some people who have severe learning disabilities.

Management by objectives   An approach to management which aims to integrate the organisation's objectives with the individual's objectives.

Management development   An approach for ensuring that the organisation meets its current and future needs for effective managers. Would include succession planning, performance appraisal and training.

Manpower planning   A method of ensuring that the organisation's human resources can be met now and in the future.

Market forces   May be characterised as any system of incentives which rely on market type mechanisms such as contracts, price or cost to create a desired behaviour from the various participants in that market. For example, competition, fixed or decreasing budget limits, bidding for contracts, and so on may all be seen as market forces.

Matrix management   A system of managing in a horizontal as well as a vertical organisation structure. Typically, a person reports to two superiors, a department or line manager and a functional or project manager.

Matrix team   People from different parts of the organisation and with no line authority.

Mediation   The process of resolving a dispute by the intervention of an expert person who closely guides the disputing parties towards agreement.

Mentoring and co-mentoring   An ancient process of learning facilitation by mutual professional support, traditionally given by a senior to a junior colleague. In co-mentoring the process of mentoring is non-hierarchical and involves co-mentees helping and supporting each other in learning.

Meta-analysis   Pooled statistical analysis of results from several individual statistical analyses of different experiments, searching for statistical significance which is not possible within the smaller sample sizes of individual studies.

Mind map   A process of recording information in related groupings which is intended to assist lateral thinking. (*See also* cognitive map.)

Minimum data sets   A group of statistics or other information that together comprise the minimum amount of information required to inform any management process, for example for contract monitoring.

Ministerial Taskforce An NHS Summary Care Record Taskforce was established in July 2006 to recommend how best to implement the Summary Care Record in the Early Adopter Programme. It reported to ministers in December 2006 and its recommendations are being implemented. The Taskforce considered a variety of perspectives including clinicians, hospital managers, patients and the ambulance service.

Mission statement Statement of the overall purpose of an organisation.

Model Any representation of a real object or phenomenon, or template for the creation of an object or phenomenon.

Model-based reasoning Approach to the development of expert systems that uses formally defined models of systems, in contrast to more superficial rules of thumbs. (*See also* artificial intelligence and heuristic.)

Modernisation Agency Created as part of the NHS Plan to help local clinicians and managers redesign local services around the needs and convenience of patients. It is discussed in more detail in Chapter 1, 'Understanding the NHS'.

Monitor An independent corporate body established under the Health and Social Care (Community Health and Standards) Act 2003. It is responsible for authorising, monitoring and regulating NHS foundation trusts.

Monitoring The systematic process of collecting information on clinical and non-clinical performance. Monitoring may be intermittent or continuous. It may also be undertaken in relation to specific incidents of concern or to check key performance areas. It is also used in respect of selection in recording data such as sex, ethnic origin and age, etc. on applicants, short-listed candidates and appointees for retrospective review to show whether an organisation's equal opportunities policies are being carried out successfully. Monitoring also includes analysing the information and data obtained to see if there are any discrepancies in treatment/success rates of different groups, identifying the reasons and taking remedial action where appropriate. Monitoring in respect of childcare is where plans for a child, and the child's safety and well-being, are systematically appraised on a routine basis. Its function is to oversee the child's continued welfare and enable any necessary action or change to be instigated speedily, and, at a managerial level, to ensure that proper professional standards are being maintained.

Morbidity The incidence of a particular disease or group of diseases in a given population during a specified period of time.

Mortality The number of deaths in a given population during a specified period of time.

Motivators Factors leading to job satisfaction and high employee morale. See Herzberg's theory of motivation, as described in some detail on p. 118 in Part 1. Also *see* Herzberg 1983.

Movement The stage in a conciliation or mediation process during which the parties modify their views and their opinions become closer to each other's.

Multi-professional A combination of several professions working towards a common aim.

National Application Service Providers (NASPs) Responsible for purchasing and integrating IT systems and services which are common to all users across the country including the Spine element of the NHS Care Records Service, Choose and Book, NHSmail and the National Network for the NHS (N3).

National clinical leads Appointed by NHS Connecting for Health to lead engagement about the National Programme for IT with their respective clinical professions at a national level. National clinical leads are in place for nurses, GPs and hospital doctors.

GLOSSARY OF NHS TERMINOLOGY **237**

They work closely with the clinical professional bodies and other organisations as well as the chief clinical officers at the DoH. They make sure that clinical involvement is central to all the work of NHS Connecting for Health.

National Programme for IT (NPfIT)   Responsible for procurement and delivery of the multi-billion-pound investment in new information and technology systems to improve the NHS.

National Information Governance Board for Health and Social Care   Provides leadership and promotes consistent standards for information governance across health and social care. It arbitrates on the interpretation and application of information governance policy and gives advice on matters at national level. The NIGB has taken over some of the responsibilities of the Care Record Development Board, which has now closed. It will continue to publish and review the NHS Care Record Guarantee.

National Network for the NHS (N3)   Provides fast, wide area networking services to the NHS, offering reliability and value for money. N3 replaced the private NHS communications network NHSnet. N3 is vital to the delivery of the National Programme for IT, providing the essential technical infrastructure to support the NHS Care Records Service, the Electronic Prescription Service, Choose and Book and Picture Archiving and Communications Systems.

National Service Frameworks (NSFs)   Set national standards and service models for a specific service or care group. They set up programmes of implementation and performance management against which progress in an agreed timescale can be measured. They may help decide which services are best provided in primary care, in hospitals and in specialist centres.

Natural team   For example, a boss with direct subordinates.

Neonatal death rate   The deaths of infants under four weeks of age per 1000 live births. The early neonatal death rate is the deaths of infants under one week of age per 1000 live births.

Neural computing   *See* connectionism.

Neural network   Computer program or system designed to mimic some aspects of neurone connections, including summation of action potentials, refractory periods and firing thresholds.

New outpatient   A patient attending for an outpatient appointment for the first time for a particular ailment. If transferred to another department, the patient is also a new outpatient on their first attendance there.

Newsgroup   A bulletin board service provided on a computer network like the Internet, where messages can be sent by email and be viewed by those who have an interest in the contents of a particular newsgroup. (*See also* email and Internet.)

NHS Care Records Service (NHS CRS)   A secure service that links patient information from different parts of the NHS electronically so authorised NHS staff and patients have the information they need to make care decisions. There are two elements to the NHS CRS: detailed records (held locally) and the Summary Care Record (held nationally). The NHS CRS enables each person's detailed records to be securely shared between different parts of the local NHS, such as the GP surgery and hospital. Patients will also be able to have a summary of their important health information, known as their Summary Care Record, available to authorised NHS staff treating them anywhere in the NHS in England. Patients will be able to access their Summary Care Record using the secure website HealthSpace.

NHS Code of Practice   Sets out the basic principles underlying public access to information about the NHS. It reflects the government's intention to ensure greater access by the public to information about public services and complements the Code of Access to Information which applies to the DoH.

NHS Connecting for Health (NHS CFH)   An agency of the DoH supporting the NHS to introduce the National Programme for IT. This will help the NHS to deliver better, safer care for patients. NHS CFH is also responsible for other existing business-critical IT systems in the NHS.

NHSmail   A secure national email and directory service. It was developed specifically to meet NHS and BMA requirements for clinical email between NHS organisations.

NHS Number   The NHS Number is fundamental to the National Programme for IT. It is the national unique patient identifier that makes it possible to share patient information across the whole of the NHS safely, efficiently and accurately.

NHS Plan   Recognises that the NHS has achieved much but needs to keep pace with change to meet patient needs. Increased investment and modernisation are the steps described in the document (it was published July 2000).

Non-principals   A generic term for doctors who wish to practise in general practice but who do not want the financial or time commitment of becoming a principal – includes retainers, returners, assistants and associates as well as the new salaried doctor opportunities available under Primary Care Act Pilots (PCAPs).

Non-recurrent expenditure   'One-off expenditure', e.g. provision of new buildings, major alterations and major pieces of equipment. Clearly, capital expenditure is non-recurrent expenditure but the purchase of minor pieces of equipment and the carrying out of maintenance work is non-recurrent, though chargeable to revenue.

Non-recurring measures   These are one-off measures which affect the year of account only, e.g. raising capital through the sale of land or via a one-off payment or loan from an external source such as the Strategic Health Authority NHS Bank.

Objective   A clearly identifiable and quantifiable target to be achieved in the future. A specific and measurable statement which also sets out how overall aims are to be achieved.

Office of Population, Census and Surveys (OPCS)   The central government office that collected information on the entire population. Now Office for National Statistics.

Official solicitor   Officer of the Supreme Court. When representing a child, the official solicitor acts as a solicitor as well as a guardian *ad litem*.

Ombudsman   Health Service Commissioner who investigates cases of maladministration in the health service.

Open-loop control   Partially automated control method in which a part of the control system is given over to humans.

Open system   Computer industry term for computer hardware and software that is built to common public standards, allowing purchasers to select components from a variety of vendors and to use them together.

Opinion   A belief which is held but may not be based on provable fact.

Organisation   A generic term used to describe an entire organisation, as opposed to the term service, which is used to describe one part of the organisation (*see also* service). Thus a hospital, a practice or a university or medical school may all be described as organisations.

Organisation and management development strategy   A written document which sets out the strategy for developing the organisational processes and management skills needed by an organisation.

Organisational chart A graphical representation of the structure of the organisation, including areas of responsibility, relationships and formal lines of communication and accountability.

Organisational development (OD) An educational strategy aimed at changing the beliefs, attitudes, values and structures within an organisation so that it can better adapt to changing requirements. The emphasis is on interventions, rather than the objective assessment of services. A systematic process of improving organisational effectiveness and adaptiveness on the basis of behavioural science knowledge.

Originating capital debt The amount owed by an NHS trust to the consolidated fund. This is equal to the value of the net assets transferred to an NHS trust when it is set up. Assets donated to the NHS since 1948 are not included.

Output-based specification (OBS) Each prospective supplier to the National Programme must meet rigorous technical requirements. These are set out in an output-based specification.

Outcome The effect on health status of a healthcare intervention or lack of intervention. The end result of care and treatment; that is, the change in health, functional ability, symptoms or situation of a person, which can be used to measure the effectiveness of care and treatment.

Outpatient A patient attending for treatment, consultation, advice and so on, but not staying in a hospital.

Output (or programme) budgets A system of analysing expenditure by reference to objectives to be met (e.g. increased level of day care; more operations) instead of under input headings such as staff and running expenses, etc.

Out-turn prices The prices prevailing when the expenditure occurs, as distinct from the estimated prices.

Paramedics Ambulance personnel with extended qualifications in providing pre-hospital care according to protocols.

Paramount principle The principle that the welfare of the child is the paramount consideration in proceedings concerning children.

Parental responsibility Defined as all the rights, duties, powers, responsibilities and authority which by law a parent of a child has in relation to the child and his property.

Part III accommodation Residential care homes provided by local authorities under Part III of the National Assistance Act 1948.

Parties Parties to legal proceedings under the Children's Act are entitled to attend the hearing, present their case and examine witnesses. The Act envisages that children will automatically be parties in care proceedings. Anyone with parental responsibility for the child will also be a party to such proceedings, as will the local authority. Others may be able to acquire party status.

Party A patient, carer, representative or NHS provider involved in a dispute.

Passcode An alphanumeric code unique to each member of NHS staff to use alongside their Smartcard to access patient information contained on the patient's care record.

Patient A person currently or previously under medical care.

Patient Advice and Liaison Service (PALS) Known as PALS, the Patient Advice and Liaison Service supports patients to ensure that the NHS listens to patients, their relatives, carers and friends; answers their questions and resolves their concerns as quickly as possible. PALS also helps the NHS to improve services by listening to what matters to patients and their carers and supporting the NHS to make changes, when appropriate.

Patient Administration System (PAS)   An administrative system typically used in hospitals and community service settings that contain essential non-clinical data, such as patient attendance lists, appointments and waiting times.

Patient and Public Involvement Forums (PPI Forums)   PPI Forums were set up following the NHS Reform and Health Care Professions Act 2002. There are 572 forums – one for each trust in England. They are the local voice of the community on health matters and have a wide range of responsibilities.

Patient costing   A system whereby costs are analysed in relation to specific patients or types of patient. This is the most complete analysis that can be undertaken and enables different combinations of costs to be made to fulfil any requirement. Particularly useful for evaluating proposed changes in service provision.

The Patient's Charter   A list of required national standards and rights set by central government for the NHS.

Patients' council/forum/group   This is a group led and determined by patients, meeting independently of staff with its own agenda and operations. There can be patient councils/forums/groups within inpatient services, day hospitals, residential or community-based services. They are different to users' groups that are separately funded and legal entities in their own right, e.g. charities such as the UK Advocacy Network.

Patient Safety Assessment Process   All new NHS CFH products and services are subject to this process, which operates to international standards. The patient safety assessment process is overseen by NHS CFH's national clinical safety officer working with the National Patient Safety Agency. The patient safety assessment process involves three key steps:

1 products are risk-assessed in the context in which they will be used
2 a safety case sets out how identified hazards would be mitigated
3 a safety closure report provides evidence that hazards have been addressed satisfactorily.

Patient's sealed envelope   *See* sealing.

Patterns of delivery   The way in which services are delivered, their structure and relationship to each other. This does not relate to the content of services.

Payment by Results (PbR)   A funding system for care provided to NHS patients, which pays healthcare providers on the basis of the work they do. It does this by paying a nationally set price or tariff for similar groups of treatments, known as healthcare resource groups (HRG), which itself is based on the historical national average cost of providing services to those HRGs. The fixed tariffs for specified HRGs are set by the DoH and are intended to avoid price differentials across providers that could otherwise distort patient choice. Payment is on a 'per spell' basis, where a spell is defined as a continuous period of time spent as a patient within a trust, and may include more than one episode. The aim of Payment by Results is to provide a transparent, rules-based system for paying NHS trusts. It hopes to reward efficiency, support patient choice and diversity, and encourage strategies for achieving sustainable reductions in waiting times.

Percentage occupancy   Occupied beds expressed as a percentage of the available beds during a given period.

Performance appraisal   A process for assessing performance to assess training needs, job improvement plans and salary reviews, etc.

Performance indicators   A standard of work that acts as a measurement of performance, e.g. response times to requests for work used to indicate the performance of the service. (*See also* quality indicator.)

Performance review   A systematic check on the achievement of the organisation and individuals compared with set objectives.

Perinatal mortality rate   Stillbirths and deaths of infants under one week of age per 1000 total births.

Period of study leave (PSL)   GPs can apply (in accordance with paragraph 50 of the Statement of Fees and Allowances) for financial assistance in connection with a period of study leave to undertake postgraduate education, which will result in benefit to the GP, primary care (in particular) and the NHS.

Permanency planning   Deciding on the long-term future of children who have been moved from their families.

Personal Demographics Service (PDS)   The national electronic database of NHS patient demographic details used within health and social care. Demographic information includes, for example, name, address, date of birth and NHS Number.

Personal Spine Information Service (PSIS)   The central database on the Spine containing clinical records for each NHS patient.

Personality   The distinctive and identifiable characteristics of an individual human being.

Person specification   Derived from the job description and outlines the qualifications, skills and experience required to perform the job. It lists what is essential and what is desirable and it should be used for shortlisting and interviewing. Person specifications should be available and made known to all those considering applying for a post so that they are aware of the criteria that will be used to judge them.

Picture Archiving and Communication Systems (PACS)   A system enabling images such as X-rays and scans to be stored and sent electronically so that doctors and other health professionals can access the information with the touch of a button.

Physician's workstation   A computer system designed to support the clinical tasks of doctors. (*See also* electronic medical record.)

Planning   The process by which the service determines how it will achieve its aims and objectives. This includes identifying the resources which will be needed to meet those aims and objectives.

Police protection   The Children Act allows police to detain a child or prevent his or her removal for up to 72 hours if they believe that the child would otherwise suffer significant harm.

Policy   An operation statement of intent in a given situation.

Portfolios   Personal professional development tools, aimed at encouraging reflection and self-direction in identifying training needs. They record and monitor opportunities for learning and provide tangible evidence of the outcomes. Content varies – for a job interview it will focus on practical skills, competencies and achievements, whereas for academic recognition it will reflect the ability to independently problem solve in the chosen field.

Positive action   Measures by which people from particular racial groups are either encouraged to apply for jobs in which they have been under-represented or are given training to help them develop their potential and so improve their chances when competing for particular work.

Postgraduate Education Allowance (PGEA)   GPs are eligible if they maintain a balanced programme of education and training geared towards providing the best possible care for their patients. Courses are approved (in advance) by the regional directors of postgraduate general practice education (or their staff) and can be classified in the following three areas: health promotion and prevention; disease management; and service management. GPs have to show that they have attended an average of five days' training a year. Any doctor who does not take part stands to lose financially as they will not be eligible for PGEA. The structure varies and approval may be given for, e.g.:

> lunchtime lecturettes (maybe a half or quarter session)
> in-house practice meetings on specific educational topics
> week-long courses at PG centres (including at overseas resorts)
> national meetings
> reading (free) weekly medical magazines and answering MCQs on the magazine content.

Postscript In computer technology the commercial language that describes a common format for electronic documents that can be understood by printing devices and converted to paper documents or images on a screen.

Practice-based commissioning (PBC) The term given to a form of practice-level commissioning which enables practices (usually this refers to primary care teams led by GPs, although there are some exceptions) to commission care and other services that are directly tailored to the needs of their patients. Practices can keep up to 100% of any savings made by agreement with the local PCT.

Practice parameter *See* clinical guideline.

Preliminary hearing (children) Hearing to clarify matters in dispute, to agree evidence, and to give directions as to the timetable of the case and the disclosure of evidence.

Prescription Pricing Authority (PPA) A national provider of managed services to the NHS. Its main functions are to calculate and make payments for amounts due to pharmacists and GPs for supplying drugs and appliances prescribed under the NHS. It also produces information for NHS organisations and stakeholders about prescribing volumes, trends and costs and manages a range of health benefits, e.g. the NHS Low Income Scheme.

Preventive maintenance and replacement programme A plan for the maintenance of machines to minimise the amount of time lost through breakdown by anticipating and preventing likely problems.

Primary Care Audit Group (i.e. multidisciplinary) Groups of professionals and managers in health authorities whose remit is to encourage and facilitate the undertaking and implementation of audit in primary care – the cyclical reappraisal of structure process and outcome.

Primary care centre (PCC) Centre for out-of-hours treatment, allowed under changes to the GP contract in 1994.

Primary Care Trust (PCT) Responsible for commissioning all healthcare in their community.

Principals Doctors who have been established in general practice by the traditional route, i.e. by means of appointment to the health authorities' GMS Principal List.

Private bed (pay bed) A bed occupied by a patient who pays the whole cost of accommodation and medical and other services.

Private Finance Initiative (PFI) Provides a way of funding major capital investments as an alternative to the public procurement route, which is funded directly by the Treasury. Private consortia, usually involving large construction firms, are contracted to design, build, and in some cases manage new projects. Contracts typically last for about 30 years, although some are longer, during which time the building is leased by a public authority. It remains a contentious issue with many critics who state that it does not offer value for money and effectively transfers ownership of NHS hospitals out of the

NHS. Others point to the relatively large number of new facilities built under the scheme that would not otherwise have been built.

Private patient   A patient who pays the full cost of all medical and other services.

Probation officer   Welfare professional employed as an officer of the court and financed jointly by the local authority and the Home Office.

Procedure   The steps taken to fulfil a policy. A particular and specified way of doing something.

Professional standards   Professionally agreed levels of performance.

Programmes for IT (PfIT)   Accountability for the delivery of the National Programme for IT (NPfIT) transferred to strategic health authorities on 1 April 2007, as part of the NPfIT Local Ownership Programme (NLOP). The SHAs operate as three Programmes for IT, each of which has a Local Service Provider. These are the London Programme for IT (LPfIT), the Southern Programme for IT (SPfIT) and the North, Midlands and East Programme for IT (NMEfIT).

Prohibited Steps Order (children)   Order that no step which could be taken by a parent in meeting his parental responsibility for a child, and which is of a kind specified in the order, shall be taken by any person without the consent of the court.

Project 2000   The system of nurse education which places increased emphasis on student-centred and research-based learning.

Protocol   The adoption by all staff of local or national guidelines to meet local requirements in a specified way. An alternative word for procedure. (*See also* clinical guideline.)

Provider   A healthcare organisation, such as an NHS trust, which provides healthcare and sells its services to purchasers.

Provider plurality   This term refers to the use of a range of different organisations from NHS and independent, private and 'not-for-profit' sectors in the delivery of services. In the context of NHS reforms, 'provider plurality' coupled with competition and patient choice is said to promote efficiency, effectiveness and value for money in the delivery of services.

PSL   *See* period of study leave.

Psychometric tests   Standardised question and answer papers designed to measure personality.

Public dividend capital (PDC)   A form of long-term government finance on which the NHS trust pays dividends to the government. PDC has no fixed remuneration or repayment obligations, but, in the long term, the overall return on PDC is expected to be no less than on an equivalent loan.

Public Information Programme   *See* Summary Care Record (SCR) Public Information Programme.

Public private partnership (PPP)   The umbrella name given to a range of initiatives which involve the private sector in the operation of public services.

Purchaser   A budget-holding body that buys health or social care services from a provider on behalf of its local population or service users.

Purchasing intelligence   The knowledge purchasers need in order to make informed decisions when purchasing healthcare on behalf of their resident population. Includes demographic data, information on healthcare services, and the views of local people (local voices).

Qualitative reasoning   A subspecialty of artificial intelligence concerned with inference and knowledge representation when knowledge is not precisely defined, e.g. 'back of the envelope' calculations.

Quality   A specified standard of performance.

Quality and Outcomes Framework (QOF)   As part of a new NHS contract, introduced in 2004, GP practices are rewarded for achieving clinical and management quality targets and for improving services for patients within a Quality and Outcomes Framework. It sets out a voluntary system of financial incentives for improving quality within the General Medical Services contract for GP payments.

Quality assurance (QA)   A generic term essentially meaning that one ensures not only that the right things get done, but also that none of the wrong things is done.

Quality improvement strategy   A written statement of objectives relating to quality improvement and a plan for meeting those objectives. The strategy should be consistent with the business plan.

Quality indicator   A standard of service which acts as a measurement of quality, for example incidence of infection used to indicate the quality of care. (*See also* performance indicator.)

Quality Management and Analysis Subsystem (QMAS)   To support the Quality and Outcomes Framework, NPfIT has commissioned British Telecom to develop and implement a new IT system called the Quality Management and Analysis Subsystem. It will provide reporting, forecasting and payment information for improving services within the Quality and Outcomes Framework.

Quango   A quasi-autonomous non-governmental organisation. A body with virtual statutory power.

RA01 Form   Used by a Registration Authority to register a user for access to patient information contained on the Spine. It is made up of two parts:

1   RA01 Part A Form contains the conditions a successful applicant has to agree to prior to becoming an authorised NHS Care Records Service (NHS CRS) user and being issued with a Smartcard

2   RA01 Part B Form is for the registering of users of NHS CRS applications.

Read coding   A hierarchically arranged thesaurus of clinical condition terms which provides a numeric coding system. The system was developed by Dr Read and is cross-referenced to other national and international classifications. Developed initially for primary care medicine in the UK, it was subsequently enlarged and developed to capture medical concepts in a wide variety of situations. (*See also* terminology.)

Reasoning   A method of thinking. (*See also* inference.)

Recovery order (children)   Order which a court can make when there is reason to believe that a child in care, who is the subject of an emergency protection order or in police protection, has been unlawfully taken or kept away from the responsible person, or has run away, is staying away from the responsible person, or is missing.

Recurrent expenditure   'Ongoing expenditure' such as salaries and wages, travelling expenses, drugs and dressings, and provisions.

Reflection   The process of returning verbal or body language communication to the original perpetrator to indicate agreement and acceptance.

Refuge (children)   Enables 'safe houses' to legally provide care for children who have run away from home or local authority care. A recovery order can be obtained in relation to a child who has run away to a refuge.

Registration Authority   Responsible for registering and verifying the identity of individuals who need to access the NHS Care Records Service. After proving their personal identity and being vouched for by a sponsor, the Registration Authority issues staff with a Smartcard and passcode with an approved level of access to patient information.

Regular day admission   A patient who attends electively and regularly for a course of treatment and care, but does not stay in hospital through the night.

Relate   A voluntary body, formerly known as the Marriage Guidance Council, which assists couples to resolve differences that threaten their relationship.

Representation   The method chosen to model a process or object. For example, a building may be represented as a physical scale model, drawing or photograph. (*See also* reasoning and syntax.)

Representations (childcare)   *See* complaints procedure.

Research and development (R&D)   Searching out knowledge and evidence about the relationship between different factors in the provision of services. Research does not require action in response to findings.

Residential care homes   Residential accommodation, other than group homes, providing board and lodging and personal care to the residents. Includes homes for elderly or physically disabled people.

Residential social worker (children)   Provides day-to-day care, support and therapy for children living in residential settings, such as children's homes.

Resource assumptions   Provisional estimates of cash resources (capital, revenue and joint finance) that may be made available over the next two to three years.

Resource management   The different definitions of resource management all emphasise the involvement of doctors, nurses and other clinical staff in the continuing improvement of the quality and quantity of patient care through better use of resources and information.

Respite care   Service giving family members or other carers short breaks from their caring responsibilities.

Responsibility   The obligation that an individual assumes when undertaking delegated functions.

Responsible person (children)   Any person who has parental responsibility for the child, and any other person with whom the child is living. With their consent, the responsible person can be required to comply with certain obligations.

Retainers   Doctors appointed to practices under the Doctors Retainer Scheme who are constrained from practising full-time or part-time usually by virtue of domestic commitments, but who wish to keep in touch with medicine.

Returners   Doctors wishing to return to clinical practice.

Revenue consequences of capital schemes (RCCS)   Annual running costs of capital schemes.

Review   The examination of a particular aspect of a service or care setting so that problem areas requiring corrective action can be identified.

Review (children)   Local authorities have a duty to conduct regular reviews in order to monitor the progress of children they are looking after.

Review meetings   The system whereby the NHSE regional offices monitor the performance of health authorities against planned objectives and set an action plan for further achievements.

Ringfencing   The identification of funds to be used for a particular purpose only – usually applied to funds earmarked by central government for a particular use within the NHS or local government, e.g. the mental illness specific grant.

Risk management   A systematic approach to the management of risk to reduce loss of life, financial loss, loss of staff availability, staff and patient safety, loss of availability of buildings or equipment or loss of reputation.

Risk management strategy   A written statement of objectives for the management of risk and a plan for meeting those objectives. The strategy should be consistent with the business plan.

Role-based access control (RBAC) Grants a view of a patient's record depending on the role the individual was assigned when they registered for their Smartcard. Authorised users using the NHS Care Records Service will only be able to access the information they need to carry out their role, e.g. a booking clerk will see less information than a doctor.

Safe discharge of patients A procedure for the discharge of patients who require care in the community which complies with DoH guidelines.

Satisfaction survey Seeking the views of patients through responses to pre-prepared questions and carried out through interview or self-completion questionnaires.

Sealing If a patient 'seals' information in their NHS Care Record, it can only be accessed with the patient's agreement, except in exceptional circumstances. Those outside the core team that created the information will see a 'flag' indicating that information is missing.

▸ **Seal and Lock** If a patient 'seals and locks' information in their NHS Care Record, no one will be able to look at the sealed information outside of the team that added it to the record. Other staff will not be informed that any 'sealed and locked' information exists. Information may be disclosed by the team that recorded it only where the law requires this to save others from serious harm, or where the information has been anonymised so that others will not know who it relates to.

▸ **Clinician Sealed Record** As now, clinicians can only withhold information from patients permanently in very exceptional circumstances. Those circumstances include where there is a clear danger that the information may cause serious harm to the patient or to someone else, or if it contains confidential information about other people. In those circumstances, it is intended that clinicians will be able to seal information from a patient's view. At the time of writing the process of achieving this is still being considered. Clinicians may also, with the patient's agreement, seal information until they can discuss it with the patient, e.g. an upsetting test result. This is particularly relevant as patients begin to be able to access their own Summary Care Record using HealthSpace. The Data Protection Act exempts clinicians from revealing the information that they have kept from patients for lawful reasons.

▸ **Patient Sealed Record** Allows a patient to place restrictions on access to parts of their records. (*See also* partial access.)

▸ **Partial access** As the NHS Care Records Service develops, but not right away, patients will be able to limit access to elements of their record by asking that certain information in the record is hidden from normal view. This will be known as a patient's 'sealed record'. Hidden information will only be accessible with the person's express permission, except in exceptional circumstances. In the future, patients will have two options for sealing information.

Secondary Uses Service (SUS) A single repository of person and care event level data relating to the NHS care of patients, which is used for management and clinical purposes other than direct patient care. These secondary uses include healthcare planning, commissioning, public health, clinical audit, benchmarking, performance improvement, research and clinical governance. The Information Centre for Health and Social Care is working in partnership with NHS Connecting for Health to develop and support the service so that it reflects user needs and requirements and protects patients' rights to confidentiality.

Section 8 orders (children)   The four new orders contained in the Children's Act, which, to varying degrees, regulate the exercise of parental responsibility.

Secure accommodation (children)   Provides for the circumstances in which a child who is being looked after by the local authority can be placed in secure accommodation. Such accommodation is provided for the purpose of restricting the liberty of the child.

Seeding   The process of 'planting' all or part of an idea or plan in the mind(s) of others such that those persons produce the plan as if it were their own original thought.

Semantics   The meaning associated with a set of symbols in a given language, which is determined by the syntactic structure of the symbols, as well as knowledge captured in an interpretative model. (*See also* syntax.)

Seminar   A session during which prepared papers are presented to the class by one or more students.

Sensitively flagged records   Indicates that a demographics record for certain people requires extra protection from unauthorised access, e.g. those in adoption cases and victims of domestic violence. Controls are in place to limit access to patient details that would allow such patients to be contacted. In these cases, the patient's address, telephone numbers and GP registration will not be visible on the Personal Demographics Service.

Service   The term used to describe part of an organisation, as opposed to the entire organisation. (*See also* organisation.)

Service contract   A legally binding contract between an organisation and an external supplier of goods or services. The contract sets out the agreed cost and quality for a given period.

Service level agreement   The term used to describe a document, agreed between organisations or services that will provide and receive a service, which sets out in detail how the service will be provided.

Significant harm (children)   'Whether harm suffered by the child is significant turns on the child's health or development; his [or her] health or development shall be compared with that which could reasonably be expected of a similar child'.

Skill mix   The balance of skill, qualifications and experience of nursing and other clinical staff employed in a particular area. The process of reassessing the skill mix required is known as reprofiling.

Slippage   The shortfall compared with planned spending caused by delays in the planning or execution of expenditure. Can be expressed in terms of money or time.

Smartcard   A plastic card containing an electronic chip (like a chip and PIN credit card) used to identify those who are authorised to use the NHS Care Records Service (NHS CRS). This is used together with an alphanumeric passcode. The chip on the Smartcard does not contain any personal information. It provides a secure link between the NHS CRS and the database holding the user's information and assigned access rights. The Smartcard is printed with the user's name, photo and unique identity number.

Smartcard passcode   *See* passcode.

Social worker   Generic term applying to a wide range of staff who undertake different kinds of social welfare responsibilities. (*See also* education welfare officer, fieldworker, probation officer and residential social worker.)

Specialty costing   The analysis of costs to clinical specialties, thus enabling comparisons to be made in the same institution over time or between different institutions.

Specific Issue Order (children)   Order giving directions for the purpose of determining a specific question which has arisen, or which may arise, in connection with any aspect of parental responsibility for a child.

Spine A national, central service that underpins the NHS Care Records Service. It manages the patient's national Summary Care Records. Clinical information is held in the Personal Spine Information Service (PSIS) and demographic information is held in the Personal Demographics Service (PDS). The Spine also supports other systems and services such Choose and Book and the Electronic Prescription Service (EPS).

Spine Directory Services (SDS) The main information source about NHS registered users and accredited systems and services. It ensures that transactions/messages are only processed from authorised users and systems. The Spine Directory Service also stores a record of each NHS organisation. It is a key component of the Spine.

Sponsor A member of staff appointed by an NHS organisation's Executive team to vouch for staff applying for a Smartcard and passcode to gain access to the NHS Care Records Service. Sponsors will usually be a member of staff's operational head, manager or administrator within a practice, clinic, ward or department. They may also be a member of the HR/personnel department.

Staffed allocated beds Staffed beds allocated to particular specialties including those which are available and those which are temporarily not available.

Staff Incident Reporting System A standardised system for reporting incidents and near misses. The NHSE recommends that no more than two types of forms are used for this.

Standardised mortality ratio (SMR) The number of deaths in a given year as a percentage of those expected. The expected number is a standard sex/age mortality of a reference period.

Standing financial instructions Specific instructions issued by the board of a hospital or trust to regulate conduct of the organisation, its directors, managers and agents in relation to all financial matters.

Standing orders A series of established instructions governing the manner in which business will be conducted.

Standards Standards are a means of describing the level of quality that healthcare organisations are expected to meet or to aspire to. The performance of organisations can be assessed against this level of quality.

Strategic Health Authority (SHA) SHAs are responsible for managing the NHS locally and acting as a conduit between NHS organisations and the DoH. They oversee the local implementation of national policy and are responsible for devising overarching local plans for the NHS to improve services and the health of their population. Accountability for the delivery of the National Programme for IT transferred to SHAs in April 2007, as part of the NPfIT Local Ownership Programme (NLOP).

Strategy A long-term plan.

Subject Access Request A written, signed request from an individual to see information held on them by an organisation, made under the Data Protection Act 1998.

Suggestion The process of putting a thought, plan or desire to another person.

Summary Care Record (SCR) A summary of a patient's health information. Patients will, over the next few years, have a Summary Care Record, which will be available to authorised healthcare professionals treating them anywhere in the NHS in England. At first, the information in the Summary Care Record will come from their GP record and will contain their current medications, adverse reactions and allergies. Later, it may be added to from other parts of the NHS. Initially, the Summary Care Record will contain only basic essential information such as current medications and allergies and bad reactions to medicines in the past. Patients will be able to request that sensitive information, for example relating to mental or sexual health, or other matters that they consider sensitive, is restricted.

Summary Care Record (SCR) Public Information Programme   A rolling programme to raise public awareness about linking electronic medical records and what it means for patients. The programme began in 2007 in early adopter areas for the Summary Care Record. Information and advice is being provided about how health records will be handled differently and patients' options for participating. It is important to ensure that NHS frontline staff and other patient-facing groups are trained to handle patient queries which may result from the Public Information Programme.

Supervision order (children)   Order including, except where express contrary provision is made, an interim supervision order.

Supervisor (children)   Person under whose supervision the child is placed by virtue of an order.

Supplier Attachment Scheme (SAS)   The Supplier Attachment Scheme is a new opportunity for NHS professionals to have a direct influence on the future of healthcare by working in one of a range of roles with a Local Service Provider.

Supplier Liaison   The function of Supplier Liaison is to assist IT suppliers to locate information on the National Programme and to provide contact details for those organisations that have been awarded contracts.

Supraregional Services   Specialist services for rarer conditions provided for a population significantly larger than that of an English region. They are specially funded.

Survey   The collection of views from a sample of people in order to obtain a representative picture of the views of the total population being studied.

Synchronous communication   A mode of communication when two parties exchange messages across a communication channel at the same time, e.g. telephones. (*See also* asynchronous communication.)

Synergy   The extent to which investment of additional resources produces a return which is proportionally greater than the sum of the resources invested. Sometimes known as the '2+2=5' effect.

Syntax   The rules of grammar that define the formal structure of a language. (*See also* semantics.)

Systematised Nomenclature of Human and Veterinary Medicine (SNOMED)   A commercially available general medical terminology, initially developed for the classification of pathological specimens. (*See also* terminology.)

Targets   Refer to a defined level of performance that is being aimed for, often with a numerical and time dimension. The purpose of a target is to incentivise improvement in the specific area covered by the target over a particular time frame.

Target Allocation   National share of the resources available calculated by reference to established criteria of need.

Team   Any group of people who must significantly relate with each other in order to accomplish shared objectives.

Teleconsultation   Clinical consultation carried out using a telemedical service. (*See also* telemedicine.)

Telemedicine   The delivery of healthcare services between geographically separated individuals, using telecommunication systems, e.g. video conferencing.

Temporarily closed beds   Staffed allocated beds closed for less than one month.

Term   In medical terminology an agreed name for a medical condition or treatment. (*See also* code and terminology.)

Terminal A screen and keyboard system that provides access to a shared computer system, e.g. a mainframe or mini-computer. In contrast to computers on a modern network, terminals are not computers in their own right.

Terminology A set of standard terms used to describe clinical activities. (*See also* term.)

T group Training group; refers to training in interpersonal awareness or sensitivity, where a group of people meet in an unstructured way to discuss the interplay of the relationships between them.

Theory X A theory about motivation expounded by Douglas McGregor, which suggests that people are lazy, selfish and unambitious, and need to be treated accordingly. It contrasts with Theory Y, the optimistic view of people.

Theory Z An expression coined by William G. Ouchi as a result of studying Japanese success in industry, to denote a process of organisational adaptation in which the management of the enterprise concentrates on co-ordinating people, not technology, in the pursuit of productivity.

Throughput The number of patients using each bed in a given period, such as a year. (*See also* bed turnover.)

Top slicing Usually used to refer to a proportional sum of money retained from budgets in a district or region to fund, e.g. region-wide initiatives, or supplement financial reserves.

Total Quality Management (TQM) Approach to management of organisations which aims to change organisational culture, so that continuous improvements in quality are achieved, by moving from a traditional command structure to one which encourages and empowers staff.

Training The process of modifying behaviour at work through instruction, example or practice.

Training and Development Strategy A written statement of objectives for the training and development of staff and a plan for meeting these objectives. The strategy should be consistent with the business plan.

Training Needs Analysis An approach to assessing the training or development needs of groups of employees aimed at clarifying the needs of the job and the needs of the individuals in terms of the training required.

Transfer of Undertakings – Protection of Employment (TUPE) A safeguard of employees' rights where businesses change hands between employers.

Transaction Messaging Service A message transfer service that forms part of the Spine. The service allows messages from NHS Care Records Service users to be securely routed to the service they are requesting and to manage the response to that request.

Treatment centre Centres are dedicated units that offer pre-booked day and short-stay surgery and diagnostic procedures in specialties such as ophthalmology, orthopaedics, hernia repair and gallbladder and cataract removal, among others. Treatment centres can be run by the NHS or the Independent Sector and exist mainly to provide additional capacity (including staff) to address waiting list targets.

Tribunal A court-like procedure for the resolution of disputes.

Turing Test Proposed by Alan Turing, the test suggests that an artefact can be considered intelligent if its behaviour cannot be distinguished by humans from other humans in controlled circumstances. (*See also* artificial intelligence.)

Turnover interval The average number of days that beds are vacant between successive occupants.

Tutorial A discussion session, usually dealing with specified content, or a recent lecture or practical. Chaired by the teacher, it may have any number of students from one to 20 or so.

Unbundling and bundling   Under the Payment by Results (PbR) system, trusts are reimbursed per spell, categorised by HRG (*see* PbR definition above). There are debates as to whether the HRG categories accurately reflect the cost of providing services, and whether they are flexible enough to incorporate varying treatment patterns. When people refer to 'unbundling' the tariff, they mean being able to clearly identify the individual elements which go to make up the cost of each component of the HRG. This would allow different organisations to carry out different parts of the treatment. For example, unbundling the tariff for an HRG that includes a hospital procedure and after care, means that the after care can be administered in the community, with both the hospital and community provider accurately reimbursed for the work that they do. Conversely, when people talk about 'bundling' the tariff, they mean budgeting for whole patient pathways or treatment programmes, which allows the individual components to be negotiated locally.

Unusual medications   Medications which are currently unlicensed or being used for an unlicensed indication. Patients must be informed before they receive such medications.

Underlying deficit   This is the total amount of one-off measures the health economy has had to find to achieve a break-even position at year end, i.e. the overall position after ignoring 'in-year' non-recurrent measures.

Valid consent   The legal principle by which a patient is informed about the nature, purpose and likely effects of any treatment proposed before being asked to consent to accepting it. (*See also* informed consent.)

Value analysis   Also known as value engineering. Term used to describe an analytical approach to the function and costs of every part of a product with a view to reducing costs while retaining the functional ability.

Virement   The transfer of resources from one budget heading to another. It is a means of using a planned and agreed saving in one area to finance expenditure in another area. Clear rules are needed about how virement operates so that, for instance, a budget for one-off purchases (e.g. purchase of equipment) is not spent on recurrent payments (e.g. employing staff).

Virtual reality   Computer-simulated environment within which humans are able to interact in some manner that approximates interactions in the physical world.

Vital services   In management terms those services that are essential to the normal operation of the organisation. Examples include electricity, water, medical gases and telecommunications.

Voice mail   Computer-based telephone messaging system, capable of recording and storing messages, for later review or other processing, e.g. forwarding to other users. (*See also* email.)

Waiting list   The number of people awaiting admission to hospital as inpatients.

Waiting time   The time that elapses between (1) the request by a general practitioner for an appointment and the attendance of the patient at the outpatients' department, or (2) the date a patient's name is put on an inpatients' list and the date they are admitted.

Ward of Court   A child who, as the subject of wardship proceedings, is under the protection of the High Court. No important decision can be taken regarding the child while they are a ward of court without the consent of the wardship court.

Wardship   Legal process whereby control is exercised over the child in order to protect the child and safeguard his or her welfare.

Weighted capitation Sum of money provided for each resident in a particular locality. The three main factors reflected in the formula are: age structure of the population; its morbidity; and relative cost of providing services.

Welfare Checklist (children) Refers to the innovatory checklist contained in the Children Act.

Welfare Report (children) The Children Act gives the court the power to request a report on any question in respect of a child under the Act.

Whole-time equivalents (WTEs) The total of whole-time staff, plus the whole time equivalent of part-time staff, which is obtained by dividing the hours worked in a year by part-timers, by the number of hours in the whole-time working year.

Wide area network (WAN) Computer network extending beyond a local area such as a campus or office. (*See also* local area network.)

Work in progress Waiting lists or queues waiting to be seen.

Work Measurement A work study technique designed to establish the time for a qualified person to carry out a specified job to a defined level.

Work Study Includes several techniques for examining work in all its contexts, in particular factors affecting economy and efficiency, with a view to making improvements.

Written agreement (children) Agreement arrived at between the local authority and the parents of children for whom it is providing services. These arrangements are part of the partnership model that is seen as good practice under the Children Act.

Related reading

Some useful sources of further information on these topics are to be found at the following websites.

Department of Health: www.dh.gov.uk

Healthcare Commission: www.healthcare-commission.org.uk

Herzberg F, Mausner B, Snyderman BB. *Herzberg on Motivation.* Cleveland, OH: Penton/IPC; 1983.

Herzberg F, Mausner B, Snyderman BB. *The Motivation to Work.* New York: Wiley; 1959.

King's Fund: www.kingsfund.org.uk

NHS Alliance: www.nhsalliance.org

Royal College of Nursing: www.rcn.org.uk

Useful health-related acronyms

The following list excludes virtually all the clinical acronyms. Fortunately, you don't need to know these acronyms but I felt a reference source might be useful. There has been a burgeoning of acronyms in recent years. I have removed some of the more obvious, such as degrees, diplomas and other medical qualifications and many very common clinical ones. Some have lapsed, although they are still to be found referred to in literature and thus have been included. Interestingly, some have appeared and disappeared in the interval between this and the previous edition! For interest's sake only, included are a handful of mildly amusing ones to be found, although you will need to look carefully for them. I hope that none cause offence, but the author is only reporting those in current use or as reported in current literature.

A
A&C administrative and clerical
A&E Accident and Emergency
AA Attendance Allowance
AAA Annual Accountability Agreement; abdominal aortic aneurysm
AAC Advisory Appointments Committee
AAGBI Association of Anaesthetists of Great Britain and Ireland
AAMS Association of Air Medical Services (US)
AAO American Academy of Ophthalmology
AAOS American Academy of Orthopaedic Surgeons
AAOX3 awake, alert and oriented to date, place and person
ABC activity-based costing
ABG arterial blood gases
ABHI Association of British Healthcare Industries
ABI area-based initiative
ABM activity-based management
ABN Association of British Neurologists
ABPI Association of the British Pharmaceutical Industry
ABS Adult Basic Skills
AC Audit Commission

ACA Area Cost Adjustment (part of the SSA)

ACAC Area Clinical Audit Committee

ACAD Ambulatory Care and Diagnostic Centre

ACAS Advisory, Conciliation and Arbitration Service (set up by the UK government to assist in the resolution of disputes between employers and employees)

ACBS Advisory Committee on Borderline Substances

ACC Adjusted Credit Ceiling (part of capital control framework)

ACCEA Advisory Committee on Clinical Excellence Awards

ACDA Advisory Committee on Distinction Awards (consultants)

ACDC Ambulatory Care and Diagnostic Centre

ACDM Association of Clinical Data Managers

ACDP Advisory Committee on Dangerous Pathogens

ACEVO Association of Chief Executives of Voluntary Organisations

ACF Association of Charitable Foundations

ACGT Advisory Committee on Genetic Testing

ACHCEW Association of Community Health Councils for England and Wales (now obsolete)

ACHMS Asian Community Mental Health Services

ACIE Association of Charity Independent Examiners

ACIG Academy of Medical Royal Colleges Information Group

ACLS Advanced Coronary Life Support

ACM Assessment and Care Management – Social Services community care purchaser division

ACME Advisory Committee on Medical Establishment (Scotland); Alliance for Continuing Medical Education

ACMT Advisory Committee on Medical Training (European); *American College of Medical Toxicology*

ACOST (Cabinet) Advisory Committee on Science and Technology

ACP American College of Physicians

ACPC Area Child Protection Committee

ACR American College of Radiology

ACRA (DoH) Advisory Committee on Resource Allocation

ACRA Advisory Committee on Resource Allocation (obsolete)

ACRPI Association of Clinical Research for the Pharmaceutical Industry

ACT Assertive Community Treatment

ACTAF Association of Community Trusts and Foundations Now Community Foundation Network

ACTR Additional Cost of Teaching and Research (in Scotland)

ACTS Agency for Community Team Support

ADA Americans with Disabilities Act

ADC automatic data capture

ADCU Anti-Drugs Co-ordination Unit

ADD Attention Deficit Disorder

ADH additional duty hours (junior doctors)

ADHD Attention Deficit Hyperactivity Disorder

ADI acceptable daily intake

ADL activities of daily living

ADMS Assistant Director of Medical Services

ADNS   Assistant Director of Nursing Services
ADP   automatic data processing
ADQ   average daily quantity (average amount of a medication prescribed for an adult in England)
ADR   adverse drug reaction; alternative dispute resolution
ADS   Attribution Data Set
ADSS   Association of Directors of Social Services
ADSU   Automatic Distress Signal Unit
AED   Automatic External Defibrillator
AEF   Aggregate External Finance
AELS   Advanced Endocrinological Life Support
AEN   Additional Educational Needs (part of SSA)
AES   Assigned Educational Supervisor
AFAIAA   as far as I am aware
A4A   Awards for All
AfC   Agenda for Change
AFOM   Association of the Faculty of Occupational Medicine
AFPP   Association for Perioperative Practice
AFR   annual financial return
AfS   Action for Sustainability
AFWG   Allocation Formula Working Group (part of Home Office)
AGH   Advisory Group on Hepatitis
AGM   annual general meeting
AGMETS   Advisory Group for Medical Education, Training and Staffing (an overarching body designed to co-ordinate all issues relating to staffing and educating doctors)
AGREE   Appraisal of Guidelines for Research and Evaluation in Europe
AGUM   Association for Genito-urinary Medicine
AHA   Associate of the Institute of Hospital Administrators (previously Area Health Authority)
AHCPA   Association of Health Centre and Practice Administrators
AHHRM   Association of Healthcare Human Resource Management
AHP   allied health professional
AHRQ   Agency for Healthcare Research and Quality
AHSC   Academic Health Science Centre
AI   artificial intelligence
AICD   Automatic Internal Cardiac Defibrillator
AIDS   Acquired Immune Deficiency Syndrome
AIF   area investment frameworks
AIM   activity information mapping; advanced informatics in medicine
AIMS   Association for Improvements in Maternity Services
AIOPI   Association of Information Officers in the Pharmaceutical Industry
AIP   approval in principle
ALA   Association of Local Authorities
ALAC   Artificial Limb and Appliance Centre (Now known as the DSC.)
ALARM   Association of Litigation and Risk Managers
ALBs   arm's length bodies
ALD   Adult with Learning Difficulties
ALF   activity-led funding

ALI   Adult Learning Inspectorate
ALM   Action Learning for Managers
ALMO   Arm's Length Management Organisation
ALOS   average length of stay
ALPBs   arm's length public bodies
ALPHA   Access to Learning for the Public Health
ALPHA   Access to Learning for the Public Health Agenda
ALS   Advanced Life Support
ALSOB   alcohol-like substance on breath
AM   Assembly Member (Wales)
AMA   against medical advice; American Medical Association; Association of Metropolitan
    Authorities
AME   annual managed expenditure
AMEE   Association for Medical Education in Europe
AMIA   American Medical Informatics Association
AMP   annual maintenance plan; asset management plan
AMPS   assessment of motor and process skills
AMQ   average monthly quantities (the assumed maintenance dose per month for an adult
    of a drug)
AMRA   Asset Management Revenue Account
AMRC   Academy of Medical Royal Colleges; Association of Medical Research Charities
AMS   Army Medical Services
AMSPAR   Association of Medical Secretaries, Practice Administrators and Receptionists
ANDPB   advisory non-departmental public bodies
ANH   artificial nutrition and hydration
ANP   advanced nurse practitioner
A/O   alert and orientated
AOB   alcohol on breath
AOC   Adult Opportunity Centre
AODP   Association of Operating Department Practitioners (formerly BAODA: British
    Association of Operating Department Assistants)
AOMRC   Academy of Medical Royal Colleges
AOP   Association of Optometrists
AOT   Assertive Outreach Team
APC   antigen-presenting cell; Area Prescribing Committee
APD   Advanced Professional Development
APH   aged persons home (aka EPH); Association of Public Health (now turned into
    UKPHA)
APHA   American Public Health Association
APHI   Association of Public Health Inspectors
APL   accredited prior learning
APLS   Advanced Paediatric Life Support
APMS   Alternative Primary Medical Services; Alternative Provider Medical Services
A/R   alert and responsive
APROP   Action for the Proper Regulation of Private Hospitals
APSE   Association for Public Service Excellence
AQ   Advancing Quality
AQH   Association for Quality in Healthcare

AQS   Air Quality Strategy
ARC   Arthritis and Rheumatism Council
ARCP   Annual Review of Competence Progression
ARF   Annual Retention Fee
ARG   Academic Review Group
ARM   Association of Radical Midwives
ARSH   Association of Royal Society of Health
ARVAC   Association for Research in the Voluntary and Community Sector
AS   associate specialist
ASA   Ambulance Service Association
ASAP   as soon as possible
ASB   anti-social behaviour
ASBAH   Association for Spina Bifida and Hydrocephalus
ASBO   Anti-Social Behaviour Order
ASC   Action for Sick Children
ASCT   Asylum Seeker Co-ordination Team
ASD   Autistic Spectrum Disorder
ASEC   Associate Specialist Education Committee
ASGBI   Association of Surgeons of Great Britain and Ireland
ASH   Action on Smoking and Health
ASIM   American Society of Internal Medicine
ASIT   Association of Surgeons in Training
ASME   Association for the Study of Medical Education
ASPFA   Asylum Seekers and People From Abroad (a Social Services team who pay out cash to people who cannot get Social Security Benefits)
ASPIRE   Action to Support Practices Implementing Research Evidence
ASSIST   Association for Information Management and Technology Staff in the NHS
ASTC   Associate Specialist Training Committee
ASTRO-PU   Age Sex Temporary Resident Originated Prescribing Unit
ASW   Approved Social Worker (A social worker approved to carry out Sections under the Mental Health Act.)
ASWCS   Avon Somerset and Wiltshire Cancer Services
ATLS   Advanced Trauma Life Support
ATMD   Association of Trust Medical Directors
ATU   Alcohol Treatment Unit
AUDGP   Association of University Departments of General Practice
AURE   Alliance of UK Health Regulators on Europe
AVG   Ambulatory Visit Group
AvMA   Action for Victims of Medical Accidents
AWMEG   All-Wales Management Efficiency Group

B

BAAF   British Agencies for Adoption and Fostering
BACCH   British Association for Community Child Health
BAC   blood alcohol content
BACS   British Association for Chemical Specialities
BACTS   British Association of Clinical Terminology
BACUP   British Association of Cancer United Patients

BAEM   British Association for Accident and Emergency Medicine
BAMM   British Association of Medical Managers (for clinicians in, or interested in, management)
BAMS   Benefits Agency Medical Service
BAN   British Approved Name
BAO   British Association of Otolaryngologists
BAOT   British Association of Occupational Therapists
BAP   British Association for Psychopharmacology
BAPS   British Association of Paediatric Surgeons; British Association of Plastic Surgeons
BAPT   British Association of Physical Training
BARQA   British Association of Research Quality
BASH   British Association for the Study of Headache
BASICS   British Association of Immediate Care
BASRaT   British Association of Sports Rehabilitators and Trainers
BASSAC   British Association of Settlements and Social Action Centres
BASW   British Association of Social Workers
BaTA   Blood and Transplant Authority
BAUS   British Association of Urological Surgeons
BBP   blood-borne pathogen
BBS   Bulletin Board System
BBV   blood-borne virus
BC   Block Contract[ing]; Borough Council
BCA   Basic Credit Approval (part of capital control framework)
BCCCF   Black Community Care Consultative Forum
BCD   black and culturally diverse
BCF   Boundary Change Factor (part of SSA)
BCHS   Better Care Higher Standards
BCODP   British Council of Disabled People
BCS   British Computer Society
BCSH   British Committee for Standards in Haematology
BDA   British Dental Association; British Diabetic Association (now called Diabetes UK); British Dietetic Association; British Dyslexia Association
BDD   body dysmorphic disorder
BDH   British Drug Houses (no longer trading)
BEAM   Biomedical Equipment Assessment and Management
BEHAF   British Ethnic Health Awareness Foundation
BGM   Board General Manager (an NHS in Scotland term)
BGS   British Geriatrics Society for Health in Old Age
BHAF   Black HIV and AIDS Forum
BHF   British Heart Foundation
BHS   British Hypertension Society
BIBRA   British Industrial Biological Association
BILD   British Institute of Learning Disabilities
BIM   British Institute of Management
BioRes   Biological and Biomedical Sciences Research (Internet resource)
BIR   British Institute of Radiology
BIVDA   British In Vitro Diagnostics Association
BLROA   British Laryngological, Rhinological and Otological Association

BLS   Basic Life Support
BMA   British Medical Association
BMCIS   building maintenance cost information system
BME   black and minority ethnic
BMI   Body Mass Index
BMIS   British Medical Informatics Society
BMJ   *British Medical Journal*
BMR   basal metabolic rate
BNF   *British National Formulary* (quarterly publication containing details of prescribed drugs)
BNI   British Nursing Index
BOA   British Orthopaedic Association
BOPCAS   British Official Publications Current Awareness Service
BOS   British Orthodontic Society
BP   *British Pharmacopoeia*
BPA   British Paediatric Association
BPAS   British Pregnancy Advisory Service
BPC   British Pharmaceutical Codex
BPD   borderline personality disorder
BPMF   British Postgraduate Medical Federation
BPPV   benign paroxysmal positional vertigo
BPR   business process re-engineering
BPS   British Pharmacological Society
BPSU   British Paediatric Surveillance Unit
BR   budget requirement
BrAC   breath alcohol content
BrAPP   British Association of Pharmaceutical Physicians
BRCS   British Red Cross Society
BSA   Basic Skills Agency
BSAD   British Sports Association for the Disabled
BSC   Business Service Centre (NHS Wales)
BSCC   British Society for Clinical Cytology
BSE   bovine spongiform encephalopathy; breast self-examination
BSEC   Basic Surgical Education Committee
BSH   British Society for Haematology
BSI   British Society for Immunology; British Standards Institution
BSL   British Sign Language
BSPED   British Society for Paediatric Endocrinology and Diabetes
BSR   British Society of Rheumatology
BSS   basic surgical skills
BST   basic surgical training; basic specialist training
BSTC   Basic Surgical Training Committee; Basic Surgical Training Course
BSVP   Better Services for Vulnerable People
BTEG   Black Training and Enterprise Group
BTS   Blood Transfusion Service; British Thoracic Society
BUPA   British United Provident Association
BVACoP   Best Value Accounting Code of Practice
BVPI   Best Value Performance Indicator

BVPP Best Value Performance Plan
BWS Beached Whale Syndrome

C

CAB Citizens Advice Bureau
CABA Compressed Air Breathing Apparatus
CABE Commission for Architecture and the Built Environment
CABG Coronary Artery Bypass Graft
CADO Chief administrative dental officer
CAEF Clinical Audit and Effectiveness Forum
CAF Charities Aid Foundation
CAFCASS Children And Family Court Advisory Support Service
CAIT Citizens Advocacy Information and Training
CAL Computer assisted learning
CALL Cancer Aid Listening Line
CAM Complementary and Alternative Medicine
CAMHS Child & Adolescent Mental Health Services – Joint Local and Health Authority
services to young people with mental health problems.
CAMO Chief administrative medical officer
CAMS Computer Aided Medical Systems
CAN Community Action Network
CANO Chief Area Nursing Officer
CAOX4 conscious, alert/awake and orientated to person, place, time and recent events
CAP College of American Pathologists
CAPD Continuous Ambulatory Peritoneal Dialysis for people with kidney failure
CAPM Capital Asset Pricing Model
CAPO Chief administrative pharmaceutical officer
CARE Clinical Audit and Research Evidence; Craniofacial Anomalies Register
CAS Controls assurance statement; Care Assessment Schedule; Chemical Abstracts;
Community Accountancy Service; Controls Assurance Statement
CASE Centre for Analysis of Social Exclusion
CASH Consensus Action on Salt and Health
CASP Critical Appraisal Skills Programme
CASPE Clinical Accountability Service Planning and Evaluation Specialist Healthcare
Training Group
CAT Computerised axial tomography; Critically Appraised Topic; Community Alcohol
Team
CATS Credit Accumulated Transfer Scheme (a national scheme)
CAWG Controls Assurance Working Group
CBA cost-benefit analysis; competence-based assessment
CbD case-based discussion
CBRN Chemical, Biological, Radioactive and Nuclear
CBS Common basic specification
CBT Cognitive Behavioural Therapy; Computer Based Training
CC Charity Commission; County Council; Chief Complaint; City Council
CCA Cost-Consequence Analysis; Current Cost Accounting
CCC NHS Centre for Coding and Classification.
CCCG Cochrane Colorectal Cancer Group

CCDC   Consultant in Communicable Disease Control
CCE   Completed consultant episode (*see* FCE)
CCEPP   Cochrane Collaboration on Effective Professional Practice – now called EPOC
CCETSW   Central Council for Education and Training in Social Work (abolished October 2001)
CCG   Community Care Grant
CCHR   Citizens Commission on Human Rights
CCIT   Consultant Contract Implementation Team
CCN   County Councils' Network; Change Control Notice
CCP   Community Care Plan; Change Control Procedure
CCR   Cross Cutting Review
CCrISP   Care of the Critically Ill Surgical Patient
CCRN   Comprehensive Clinical Research Network
CCSC   Central Consultants and Specialists Committee (a committee of BMA)
CCSI   Critical Care Skills Institute
CCSR   Cross Cutting Spending Review
CCST   Certificate of completion of specialist training for junior doctors
CCT   Certificate of Completion of Training; compulsory competitive tendering (a sort of Dutch auction of public services, now partly replaced by the Best Value process)
CCTR   Cochrane Controlled Trials Register
CCTV   Closed Circuit TeleVision
CCU   coronary care unit; critical care unit
CD   Clinical Director; Clinical Directorate; Controlled Drug; Civil Defence; Cluster of Differentiation
CDC   Center for Disease Control and Prevention (USA)
CDDS   Council of Deans of Dental Schools
CDER   Center for Drug Evaluation and Research (USA)
CDHN   Community Development and Health Network
CDM   Chronic disease management; Construction, Design and Management
CDO   Chief dental officer
CDS   Contract Data Set – A collection of information recorded by the NHS Trust that identifies a patient and their treatment which is sent to the Health Authority; Community Dental Service
CDSC   Communicable Disease Surveillance Centre
CDSM   Committee on Dental and Surgical Materials (abolished 1994)
CDSR   Cochrane Database of Systematic Reviews
CDU   Child Development Unit; Central Delivery Unit; Colourflow Duplex Ultrasound
CDX   Community Development Exchange
CE   chief executive
CEA   cost-effectiveness analysis
CEAC   Clinical and Excellence Awards Committee (Northern Ireland)
CEDP   Chief Executive Development Programme
CEEU   Clinical Effectiveness and Evaluation Unit of the RCP
CEF   Community Empowerment Fund
CEFET   Central England Forum for European Training
CEMACH   Confidential Enquiry into Maternal and Child Health, evolved into the Centre for Maternal and Child Enquiries (CMACE).
CEMD   Confidential Enquiry into Maternal Deaths

CEMVO   Council of Ethnic Minority Voluntary Sector Organisations
CEN   Comite Europeen de Normalisation (European Standards organisation)
CEN   Community Empowerment Network
CEO   chief executive officer
CEPOD   Confidential Enquiry into Peri-operative Deaths (*see* NCEPOD)
CERA   Capital Expenditure, Revenue Account
CERES   Consumers for Ethics in Research
CertHSM   Certificate in Health Services Management
CES   Charities Evaluation Services
CESDI   Confidential Enquiry into Stillbirths and Deaths in Infancy
CESH   National Confidential Inquiry into Suicide and Homicide By People With Mental Illness
CEX   Clinical Evaluation Exercise
CF   Cystic Fibrosis
CfH   Connecting for Health
CfI   Centre for Infections (part of HPA)
CFI   Community Finance Initiative
CFISSA   Centrally Funded Initiatives and Services and Special Allocations
CFN   Community Foundation Network
CFO   Chief Finance Officer; Conventionally Financed Option; Co-Financing Public Sector Intermediary Organisation
CfPS   Centre for Public Scrutiny
CFR   Capital Financing Reserve
CFRC   Children and Family Resource Centre
CFS   Chronic Fatigue Syndrome closely associated with ME
CFSMS   Counter Fraud and Security Management Service
CG   Clinical Governance
CGD   Chronic Granulomatous Disease
CGF   Child Growth Foundation
CGRDU   Clinical Governance Research and Development Unit
CGST   Clinical Governance Support Team
CHAI   Commission for Healthcare Audit and Improvement (obs now HC)
CHAIN   Contact Help Advice and Information Network
CHAOS   Chief Has Arrived on the Scene
CHART   Community Health Action Resource Team
CHC   Community Health Council (now only in Wales)
CHCP   community health and care partnership (Scotland)
CHD   coronary heart disease
CHDGP   Collection of Health Data from General Practice project
CHEST   Combined Higher Education Software Team
CHEX   Community Health Exchange
CHG   Community Hospitals Group (now taken over by BUPA)
CHI   Commission for Health Improvement; community health index
CHIA   Comprehensive Health Impact Assessment
CHIME   Centre for Health Informatics in Medical Education
CHiQ   Centre for Health Information Quality (patient information)
CHIR   Canadian Institutes of Health Research
CHIRP   Confidential Human Factors Incident Reporting Procedure

CHMS   Council for Heads of Medical Schools; central health and miscellaneous services
CHMU   Central Health Monitoring Unit (obsolete)
CHOU   Central Health Outcomes Unit
CHP   Community Health Partnership (Scotland); Combined Heat and Power
CHRC   Community Health and Resource Centres
CHRE   Council for Healthcare Regulatory Excellence
CHRE   The Council of Healthcare Regulatory Excellence
CHS   child health surveillance
CHS   Community Health Services; Child Health Surveillance
CHSA   Chest, Heart and Stroke Association
CI   Clinical Indicator
CIA   Chief Internal Auditor
CIC   Common Information Core; Charitable Incorporated Organisation
CIM   Capital Investment Manual
CIMP   Clinical Information Management Programme
CIMS   Coalition for Improving Maternity Services
CINAHL   Cumulative Index to Nursing and Allied Health
CIO   Confederation of Indian Organisations; Charitable Incorporated Organisation; Chief Information Officer
CIP   Cost Improvement Programme
CIP(S)   Capital Investment Programme(s)
CIPC   Centre for Innovation in Primary Care
CIPFA   Chartered institute of Public Finance and Accountancy
CIS   Clinical Information System
CISH   Confidential Inquiry into Suicide and Homicide by people with mental illness
CISP   Community Information Systems Project
CJC   Commissioning Joint Committee
CJD   Creutzfeld Jacob Disease
CKD   Chronic Kidney Disease
CLA   Commissioner for Local Administration (the ombudsman)
CLAPA   Cleft Lip and Palate Association
CLDT   Community Learning Disability Team
CLGMS   Cash Limited General Medical Services
CLib   Cochrane Library
CLIP   Central-Local Information Partnership; Clinical Improvements Database
CM   community midwife
CMA   Cost Minimisation Analysis
CMACE   Centre for Maternal and Child Enquiries
CMAJ   Canadian Medical Association Journal
CMB   Central Midwives Board
CMC   Central Manpower Committee (no longer exists)
CMD   Continuing Medical Development
CMDS   contract/core minimum data set
CME   continuing medical education
CMF   Capital Modernisation Fund
CMHN   community mental handicap nurse (obsolete)
CMHSD   Centre for Mental Health Services Development, Kings College London
CMHT   Community mental health team

CML   Chronic Myeloid Leukaemia
CMMS   Case mix management system
CMO   Chief Medical Officer; (DoH) Corporate Management Board
CMP   Civilian Medical Practitioner
CMPS   Centre for Management and Policy Studies
CMR   Computerised Medical Record
CMS   Community Midwifery Service; clinical management support; contract management system
CMT   Corporate Management Team
CN   charge nurse
CNM   clinical nurse manager
CNO   chief nursing officer
CNS   clinical nurse specialist; community nursing service; central nervous system
CNST   Clinical Negligence Scheme for Trusts
CO   Cabinet Office; Course Organiser; Complains Of; Chief Officer; Capital Out-turn
COAD   Chronic Obstructive Airways Disease – usually called COPD
COGIT   Chief Officers' Group of Information Technology
COGPED   Committee of General Practice Education Directors
COI   Central Office of Information
COIN   Circulars on the Internet (e.g. all the Health Service Publications available online as letters, regulations, circulars, CMO updates, advance letters etc.; Clinical Oncology Information Network)
COMA   Committee on Medical Aspects of Food Policy (abolished 2000)
COMARE   Committee on Medical Aspects of Radiation in the Environment
COMEAP   Committee On the Medical Effects of Air Pollutants
COPC   Community Oriented Primary Care
COPD   Chronic Obstructive Pulmonary Disease
COPDEND   Conference of Postgraduate Dental Deans and Directors of Education
COPE   Committee on Publication Ethics
COPMED   Conference of Postgraduate Medical Deans
COR   Capital Out-turn & Receipts return
CORE   Clinical Outcomes Research and Effectiveness
COREC   Central Office for Research Ethics Committees
COSHH   Control of Substances Hazardous to Health Legislation (1994 Regulations)
COSLA   Convention of Scottish Local Authorities
COT   Committee on Toxicity
CP   Community Plan; Cerebral palsy
CPA   Care Programme Approach (patients needs for care are assessed on a four point scale: Level 4 means that you are dangerously ill and need supervision; Level 1 means that you are not thought to need anything more than a bit of advice and counselling); Comprehensive Performance Assessment; Clinical Pathology Accreditation; critical path analysis
CPAG   Child Poverty Action Group; Capital Prioritisation Advisory Group
CPAP   Continuous Positive Airway Pressure
CPC   Cost Per Case
CPCCH   Consultant Paediatrician in Community Child Health
CPCME   Centre for Postgraduate and Continuing Medical Education
CPCU   Child Protection Co-ordination Unit

CPD   continuing professional development
CPEP   Clinical Practice Evaluation Programme
CPFA   Charted Public Finance Accountant
CPH   Certificate in Public Health
CPHL   Central Public Health Laboratory
CPHM   Certified Professional in Healthcare Materiel Management
CPHMCH   Committee Public Health Medicine and Community Health
CPHVA   Community Practitioners and Health Visitors Association – part of AMICUS
CPMP   Committee for Proprietary Medical Products (EU)
CPN   community psychiatric nurse
CPNA   Community Psychiatric Nurses Association – now the Mental Health Nursing Association
CPO   chief pharmaceutical officer
CPOD   Centre for Professional and Organisational Development
CPPIH   Commission for Patient and Public Involvement in Health (obsolete)
CPR   Child Protection Register; cardiopulmonary resuscitation; Capital Payments & Receipts return
CPS   Child Protection Services
CPSM   Council for Professions Supplementary to Medicine
CPU   Contracts & Purchasing Unit; central processing unit
CPWP   Capital Programmes Working Party
CQC   Care Quality Commission
CQI   Continuous quality improvement
CQSW   Certificate of Qualification of Social Work (abolished 1989)
CQUIN   Commissioning for Quality and Innovation
CQUIN AQ   Commissioning for Quality and Innovation Advancing Quality
CRAG   Clinical Research and Audit Group; Charging for Residential Accommodation Guide – guidance for local authorities on community care financial assessment; Clinical Resource and Audit Group – the lead body within the Scottish Executive Health Department promoting clinical effectiveness in Scotland
CRAGPE   Committee of Regional Advisers in General Practice Education
CRAGPIE   Committee of Regional Advisers in General Practice Education
CRANE   Craniofacial Anomalies Register
CRB   Criminal Records Bureau
CRC   Clinical Research Centre; Cancer Research Campaign
CRCF   Conference of Royal Colleges and their Faculties
CRD   Centre for Reviews and Dissemination
CRDB   Care Record Development Board
CRDC   Central Research and Development Committee
CRE   Commission for Racial Equality (monitors the effects of the Race Relations Act 1976)
CRED   Clinical Governance/Education and R&D subgroup
CRES   Cash Releasing Efficiency Savings
CRHP   Council for the Regulation of Healthcare Professionals (replaced by Council for Healthcare Regulatory Excellence [CHRE])
CRIO   Chief Registration & Inspection Officer – responsible for the Health and Social Service Registration and Inspection Units and Guidance-ad-Litem service
CRIR   Committee for Regulating Information Requirements

CRMD   Cochrane Review Methodology Database
CRT   Community Rehabilitation Team; Cathode Ray Tube
CS   Capital Strategy
CSA   Child Support Agency; Common Services Agency; Clinical Spine Application
CSAG   Clinical Standards Advisory Group
CSASHS   Common Services Agency for the Scottish Health Service
CSBS   Clinical Standards Board for Scotland
CSC   Community Sector Coalition; Computer Sciences Corporation
CSCI   Commission for Social Care Inspection
CSD   carbonated soda drinks
CSEC   Corporate Specialist Education Committee
CSF   Community Support Framework; Cerebro-spinal Fluid
CSM   Committee on Safety of Medicines; Christian Socialist Movement
CSMC   Civil Service Management Committee
CSO   Central Statistical Office; Civil Society Organisation (or NGO)
CSP   Chartered Society of Physiotherapy; Children's Services Plan
CSPG   Central Support Protection Grant
CSR   Comprehensive Spending Review
CSS   Children's Social Services; Certificate of Satisfactory Service; Cascading Style Sheets
CSSD   Central Sterile Services/Supplies Department; Central Support Service Department
CSTC   Corporate Specialist Training Committee
CSV   Community Service Volunteers
CT   computerised tomography
CTBSL   Council Tax Benefit Subsidy Limitation
CTD   close to death; circling the drain
CTG   cardiotocography electronic measurement of foetal heart and uterine contractions
CTN   Charity Trustees Network
CTO   Compulsory Treatment Order
CTPLD   Community Team for People with Learning Disabilities
CU   Casualties Union
CUA   Cost-Utility Analysis
CUE   Community Unit for the Elderly
CUV   current use value
CVCP   Committee of Vice Chancellors and Principals
CVE   Continuous Vocational Education
CVS   Council for Voluntary Service; Cardiovascular system
CYA   cover your arse
CYPF   Children and Young People's Fund
CYPS   Children and Young People's Services
CYPU   Children and Young People's Unit

D

D&T   drugs and therapeutics
D&TP   *Drugs and Therapeutic Bulletin*
DA   distributable amount; district audit
DAAT   Drug and Alcohol Team
DAN   Disabled People's Direct Action Network

DANS   duty assessment nurses
DAP   Deans Advisory Panel
DARE   Database of Abstracts of Reviews of Effectiveness
DART   Drug and Alcohol Resistance Training
DASG   Drugs and Alcohol Specific Grant
DASS   Director of Adult Social Services
DAT   digital audio tape; Disability Appeal Tribunal (obsolete); Drugs Action Team
DATA   Distress Awareness Training Agency
DB   database
D/C   discharge; discontinue
DCLG   Department for Communities and Local Government
DCT   Disabled Children's Team
DCFS   Directorate of Counter Fraud Services
DDA   Disability Discrimination Act 1995; Disabled Drivers' Association
DDD   defined daily dose
DDPHRCS   Diploma in Dental Public Health, Royal College of Surgeons of England
DDRB   Doctors' and Dentists' Review Body (also known as the Review Body on Doctors' and Dentists' Remuneration)
DEB   Dental Estimates Board
DEC   Development and Evaluation Committee (replaced by NICE in 2000)
DEFRA   Department for Environment, Food and Rural Affairs
DEL   Departmental Expenditure Limit
DENS   Doctor's Educational Needs
DFBO   design, finance, build and operate
DfEE   Department for Education and Employment (now renamed DfES)
DfES   Department for Education and Skills
DFT   Distance from Target (relating to HA's financial allocation)
DFFP   Diploma of Faculty of Family Planning
DFG   Disabled Facilities Grant
DG5   The Public Health part of the European Union
DGH   district general hospital
DGM   district general manager
DH   Department of Health (England) (*see* DoH)
DHA   district health authority (obsolete April 2002)
DHSC   Directorate of Health and Social Care (obsolete)
DHSS   Department of Health and Social Security (later split into DoH and DSS)
DHSSPS   Department of Health, Social Services and Public Safety
DHT   District Handicap Team
DI   Director of Information
DIA   Drug Information Association
DIAL   Disablement Information and Advice Lines
DIC   dead in car; disseminated intravascular coagulation
DID   dissociative identity disorder
DIG   Disablement Income Group
DIO   district immunisation officer
DIPEx   Database of Individual Patient Experiences
DIPG   Drug Information Pharmacists Group
DIPHSM   Diploma in Health Services Management

DipSW   Diploma in Social Work
DIS   Departmental Investment Strategy
DisCASS   Disabled Citizens Advice and Support Service
DISP   Developing Information System for Purchasers
DISS   Disability Information Service Surrey
DLA   Disability Living Allowance
DLCV   drugs of limited clinical value
DLF   Disabled Living Foundation
dm+d   Dictionary of Medicines and Devices
DMARD   disease modifying anti-rheumatic drug
DMC   district medical committee
DMD   Drug Misuse Database; Duchenne muscular dystrophy
DMF   Disabled Motorists Federation
DMFT   (number of) decayed, missing, filled teeth
DMHE   Department of Mental Health for the Elderly
DMO   district medical officer (obsolete)
DMT   Departmental Management Team
DMU   directly managed unit
DN   district nurse
DNA   did not arrive; did not attend
DNDRN   Dementias and Neurodegenerative Disease Research Network
DNGNet   Disability Network Group
DNI   do not intubate (similar to DNR)
DNR   do not resuscitate
DNS   director of nursing services
DNW   Drugs North West
DOA   date of accident (in A&E departments); date of admission; dead on arrival
DOB   date of birth
DoF   Director of Finance
DOGPE   Director of General Practice Education
DoH   Department of Health
DOPS   Direct Observation of Procedural Skills
DPB   Dental Practice Board (obsolete)
DPC   Data Protection Commissioner
DPGPE   Director of Postgraduate GP Education
DPH   Director of Public Health
DPI   Disabled Peoples' International
DPR   Data Protection Registrar; directorate performance review
DPTC   Disabled Person's Tax Credit (now abolished)
DRC   depreciated replacement cost; Disability Rights Commission
DRF   direct revenue funding
DRG   diagnosis/diagnostic related group
DRS   Dental Reference Service
DSC   Directory of Social Change; Disablement Service Centre
DSCA   Defence Secondary Care Agency
DSCN   Data Set Change Notice
DSD   Decontamination Services Department
Dsh   deliberate self harm

DSL   Doctors' Support Line
DSO   Direct Service Organisation
DSON   Detailed Statement of Need
DSPD   dangerous and severe personality disorder
DSS   decision support systems; Department of Social Security (now the DWP)
DSU   day surgery unit
DTA   Development Trusts Association
DTB   Drug and Therapeutic Bulletin
DTC   Day Treatment Centre; Diagnostic and Treatment Centre; Drug and Therapeutics Committee
DTD   document type definition
DTF   Diversity Task Force
DTI   Department of Trade and Industry
DTNI   daytime net inflow
DTTO   Drug Testing and Treatment Order
DTP   Diphtheria Tetanus Pertussis (a vaccine)
DUI   driving under the influence
DV   deo volente (God willing); dependent variable; domestic violence; domiciliary visit (by consultant)
DVTA   Dental Vocational Training Authority (obsolete)
DWA   Disability Working Allowance (a benefit for people working at least 16 hours a week who have a disability affecting their working ability, now replaced by DPTC)
DWM   dead white male
DWP   Department for Work and Pensions

E
EAC   estimated annual cost
EAG   Expert Advisory Group
EAGA   Expert Advisory Group on AIDS
EAN   European article number
EAPN   European Anti Poverty Network
EASR   European age standardised rate (a measure of the incidence of disease)
EBD   emotional and behavioural difficulties
EBH   evidence-based healthcare
EBL   evidence-based learning
EBM   evidence-based medicine
EBMH   evidence-based mental health
eBNF   The BNF on CD-ROM
EBOC   evidence based on call
EBP   evidence-based practice
EBS   Emergency Bed Service (London)
EBV   Epstein-Barr virus
EC   European Community; Experience Corps
ECCA   English Community Care Association
ECDL   European Computer Driving Licence
ECN   Emergency Care Network
ECP   Emergency Care Practitioner
ECR   Extra-contractual Referral (now replaced by OATS)

ECTS   European credit transfer scheme

ED   economic development; enumeration district (the smallest unit for census data – about 200 homes)

EDA   Erectile Dysfunction Association

EDI   electronic data interchange (exchanging information electronically, not including faxing)

EDIFACT   Electronic Data Interchange for Administration, Commerce and Transport (Electronic Data Interchange is a particular structure which complies with ISO 9735; this is the standard for EDI adopted by the NHS)

EDIT   Elderly Dementia Intervention Team

EDP   Education Development Plan; emotionally disturbed person

EDS   Ehlers-Danlos syndrome

EDT   Emergency Duty Team (Social Services Departments)

EEA   European Economic Area

EEC   European Economic Community

EFGCP   European Forum for Good Clinical Practice

EFL   external financing limit

EFM   electronic foetal monitoring

EFMI   European Federation for Medical Informatics

EFQM   European Foundation for Quality Management

EGFR   epidermal growth factor receptor; estimated glomerular filtration rate

eGIF   Electronic Government Interoperability Framework

EHMA   European Healthcare Management Association

EHO   environmental health officer

EHP   Education and Health Partnership

EHR   electronic health record

EHS   extremely hazardous substance

EIA   European Information Association

EL   Executive Letter (has year and number with it)

eLIB   Electronic Libraries Programme

ELP   Essential Lifestyles Planning (person-centred planning tool emphasising rhythms and routines of daily life used in Learning Disability Services)

EM   electronic mail (email)

EMA   Education Maintenance Allowance; emergency medical admission

EMAG   Ethnic Minority Achievement Grant

EMAS   Employment Medical Advisory Service

EMEA   European Medicines Evaluation Agency

EMG   electromyogram

EMI   elderly mentally ill; elderly mentally infirm

EMIS   Egton Medical Information System

EMLC   European Midwives Liaison Committee

EMO   Examining Medical Officer

EMR   electronic medical record

EMS   emergency medical services

EMW   early morning wakening

EMWA   European Medical Writers Association

ENB   English National Board for Nursing, Midwifery and Health Visiting (obsolete)

ENDPB   executive non-departmental public bodies

ENHPA European Network of Health Promotion Agencies
ENIL European Network on Independent Living
ENP emergency nurse practitioner
EO Employers' Organisation
EOC Equal Opportunities Commission (set up under the Sex Discrimination Act 1975 to monitor sex discrimination)
EP emergency planning; English Partnerships
EPACT Electronic Prescribing Analysis and Costs
EPCS Environmental, Protective and Cultural Services
EPH elderly persons' home
EPHR electronic patient health record
EPICS Elderly Persons Integrated Care Scheme
EPO emergency planning officer
EPP Expert Patient Programme
EPR electronic patient record
EQUIP Education and Quality in Primary Care; Effectiveness and Quality in Practice Group (within DoH, chaired by CMO and CNO)
ERA-ETDA European Renal Association-European Dialysis and Transplant Association
ERDIP Electronic Record Development Implementation Programme
ERG electroretinogram
ERI Edinburgh Research and Innovation Limited
ERIC Estates Returns Information Collection
EROS Electronic Records in Office Systems
ERS External Reference Group (relating to NSFs)
ES educational supervisor; Employment Service
ESAT Emergency Services Action Team (obsolete)
ESF Education Standards Fund; European Social Fund
ESMI elderly severely mentally infirm or ill
ESOL English for speakers of other languages
ESP Economic and Social Partnership
ESRA European Society of Regulatory Affairs (now TOPRA)
ESRC Economic and Social Science Research Council
ESRI Economic and Social Research Institute (Ireland)
ESV Employer Supported Volunteering
ET environmental technologies; executive team
ETA estimated time of arrival
ETF Environment Task Force
ETP electronic transmission of prescription; Employer Training Pilot
ETT endotracheal tube
EU European Union
EWC expected week of confinement
EWO educational welfare officer
EWTD European Working Time Directive
EYDCP Early Years Development and Childcare Plan
EYDP Early Years Development Partnership
EYPD Early Years and Play Department
EYST Early Years Surgical Training
EZ Employment Zone

F

FA   Friedreich's ataxia
FAB   Family Action Benchill
FACS   Fair Access to Care Services
FAM   Fraud Awareness Month (an annual event)
FAQs   frequently asked questions
FARR   Fixed Asset Restatement Reserve
FAWN   Funding Advice Workers Network
FBC   full business case
FC   factor cost; family credit (now replaced by tax credits); fixed cost
FCAS   Federation of Charity Advice Services
FCDL   Federation for Community Development Learning
FCE   finished consultant episode (*see* CCE)
FCS   financial control system
FDA   US Food and Drug Administration
FDIU   foetal death in utero
FDL   finance directorate letter
FDTL   Fund for the Development of Teaching and Learning
FE   further education
FEC   Further Education College
FEFC   Further Education Funding Council (disbanded 2001, replaced by the Learning and Skills Council)
FENTO   Further Education National Training Organisation
FES   Family Expenditure Survey
FESC   Framework for Procuring External Support for Commissioning
FFCE   first finished consultant episode
FFP   fresh frozen plasma
FHom   Faculty of Homeopathy
FHR   foetal heart rate
FHS   Family Health Services (the primary healthcare providers, including GPs, dentists, pharmacists and opticians)
FHSA   Family Health Service Authority (role now taken over by the Health Authority)
FHSAA   Family Health Services Appeal Authority
FHSCU   Family Health Services Computer Unit
FHT   foetal heart tones
FIAC   Federation of Independent Advice Centres
FIBD   found in bed dead
FIG   Food Initiatives Group
FIP   financial information project
FIPO   Federation of Independent Practitioner Organisations
FIS   Family Income Supplement (became WFTC); Financial Information Service (run by IPF); financial information system
FIT   Focused Individualised Training
FITTA   fixed-term training appointment
FIU   Fraud Investigation Unit
FM   facilities management
FMD   foot and mouth disease
FMIP   financial management information project

FMIS financial management information systems

FMP financial management programme

FMR functions and manpower review

FOM Faculty of Occupational Medicine of Royal College of Physicians

FORD found on road dead

FP10 a prescription form

FPA Family Planning Association

FPC Family Planning Clinic; Family Practitioner Committee (which was replaced by the FHSA)

FPharmM Faculty of Pharmaceutical Medicine

FPHM Faculty of Public Health Medicine

FPS Family Planning Services; Family Practitioner Services

FR financial regulation

FRED Financial Reporting Exposure Draft (draft FRS)

FRS Fellow of the Royal Society; Financial Reporting Standard

FRSH Fellow of the Royal Society of Health

FSA Financial Services Authority; Food Standards Agency

FSID Foundation for the Study of Infant Deaths

FSM free school meals

FSO Forum Support Organisations

FSS Forensic Science Service

FSSA Federation of Surgical Speciality Associations

FSU Family Support Unit (now known as Family Unit – FU).

FT NHS foundation trust; full-time

FTC Federal Trade Commission

FTE full-time equivalent

FTP fitness to practice

FTR Foundation Training Report

FTSTA Fixed Term Specialty Training Appointment

FTTA Fixed Term Training Appointments

FU Family Unit (a mixture of residential and outreach service for children and young people and their families); follow-up

FWATAG Flexible Working and Training Advisory Group

FWN further work needed

FY full year

FY1 Foundation Year 1

FY2 Foundation Year 2

FYC full-year cost

FYE full-year effect; full-year equivalent

G

GAAP Generally Accepted Accounting Practice

GAD Government Actuary's Department

GAG getting ahead of the game

GAL guardian *ad litem* (usually an independent social worker)

GALRO Guardian Ad Litem Reporting Officer (these are appointed to represent the best interests of the child)

GAPS Genetic Information and Patient Services

GATB   Global Alliance for TB Drug Development
GATS   General Agreement on Trade in Services
GBP   pounds sterling (for people who don't have a £ sign on their computer, etc.)
GBS   Guillain-Barré syndrome
G-CAT   Government IT Catalogue
GCC   General Chiropractic Council
GCS   Glasgow Coma Score
GCSE   General Certificate of Secondary Education
GDA   guideline daily amount
GDC   General Dental Council
GDP   general dental practitioner; gross domestic product
GDS   general dental services
GENECIS   General Clinical Information System
GHG   General Healthcare Group
GHQ   General Health Questionnaire
GHS   General Household Survey
GIDA   Government Intervention in Deprived Areas
GIGO   garbage in, garbage out
GIS   Geographical Information System (computers designed to create, manipulate, ana-
   lyse and display geographical data)
GLACHC   Greater London Association of Community Health Councils
GLAD   Greater London Association of Disabled People
GLADD   Gay and Lesbian Association of Doctors and Dentists
GM   Geiger-Muller; general manager
GMC   General Medical Council
GMCDP   Greater Manchester Coalition of Disabled People
GMO   genetically modified organisms
GMP   general medical practitioner; good medical practice
GMS   general medical services
GMSC   General Medical Services Committee
GNP   gross national product
GNVQ   General National Vocational Qualifications
GO   Government Office for the Regions
GOC   General Optical Council; Gynaecological Oncology Centre
GOK   God only knows
GOMER   get out of my emergency room (US slang for an unwelcome patient)
GOP   General Optical Council
GOS   General Ophthalmic Service
GOSC   General Osteopathic Council
GOSH   Great Ormond Street Hospital for Children
GP   general practitioner; Green Paper
GP2GP   the transfer of electronic patient records from one GP to another when a patient
   changes practices
GPAS   General Practice Assessment Survey (produced by the NPCRDC)
GPASS   General Practice Administration System Scotland
GPC   General Practitioners Committee
GPCC   GP Commissioning Consultant
GPCG   GP Commissioning Group (*see* HSC 1998/030)

GPEC   GP Emergency Centre
GPFC   General Practice Finance Corporation
GPFH   General Practitioner Fundholder (obsolete)
GPIAG   General Practice Airways Group
GPMSS   General Practice Minimum System Specification
GPPS   General Professional Practice of Surgery (manual that replaces MBST)
GPR   General Practice Registrar
GPWA   GP Writers Association
GPWSI   GPs with a special interest
GRE   grant related expenditure (replaced by NRE)
GREA   Grant Related Expenditure Assessment (replaced by SSA)
GRIPP   Getting Research Into Purchasing and Practice
GSCC   General Social Care Council
GSI   Government Secure Intranet
GSL   General Sales List (a medicine which can be sold anywhere)
GSM   Global System of Mobility
GSOH   good sense of humour (as important in the health service as on the lonely hearts pages)
GSW   gunshot wound
GTAC   Gene Therapy Advisory Committee
GTLRC   Gypsy and Traveller Law Reform Coalition
GTN   Government Telephone Network
GUCH   Grown Up Congenital Heart Patients Association
GUI   graphical user interface
GUM   genito-urinary medicine (where STDs are treated)
GWC   General Whitley Council

H

H&S   health and safety
HA   health authority; housing association
HaCCRU   Health and Community Care Research Unit (based at Liverpool University)
HAG   Housing Association Grant
HAI   hospital-acquired infection
HARP   Hulme Action Research Project (works with people with mental health problems)
HAS   Health Advisory Service; human activity system
HASHD   hypertensive arteriosclerotic heart disease
HASSASSA   Health and Social Services and Social Security Adjudication Act
HAT   Housing Action Trust
HAWNHS   Health at Work in the NHS
HAZ   Health Action Zones (obsolete)
HB   Health Board (in Scotland); Housing Benefit
HBAI   households below average income
HBG   Health Benefit Group
HC   health circular; Healthcare Commission; Health Council; Huntingdon's chorea
HCA   historic cost accounting; Home Care Assistant (social care worker who provides domiciliary care; formerly known as home helps); Hospital Caterers Association
HCAG   Hospital Consultants Advisory Group (a steering body for projects on work patterns for consultants)

HCAI healthcare associated infection

HCFA Health Care Financing Administration (the federal agency that administers the Medicare, Medicaid and Child Health Insurance Programs in the US)

HCG human chorionic gonadotrophin

HCHS hospital and community health services (hospital services, ambulances and certain community health services such as district nursing; these services are provided mostly by NHS Trusts)

HCIA Health Care Information (an American company which analyses health data; now part of Solucient)

HCS Holiday Care Service

HCSP Health Care Service for Prisoners

HCW Health Care Worker (provides nursing support in clinical areas; NVQ qualified)

HDA Health Development Agency (obsolete; now the National Institute for Health and Clinical Excellence [NICE]); Huntington's Disease Association

HDL high-density lipoprotein

HDM house dust mite

HDU High Dependency Unit (one step down from the ITU)

HE health education; higher education

HEA Health Education Authority (now replaced by the HAD); Health Equity Audit

HEASIG High Ethnicity Authorities' Special Issues Group

HEBS Health Education Board for Scotland

HEED Health Economic Evaluations Database

HEFC Higher Education Funding Council

HEFCE Higher Education Funding Council for England

HEFMA Health Estates and Facilities Management Association

HEI higher education institution

HEIF Higher Education Innovation Fund

HELMIS Health Management Information Service (Nuffield Institute, Leeds)

HEO health education officer

HEP Health Education Partnership

HEPA high efficiency particulate air

HERO Higher Education and Research Opportunities in the UK

HEROINE Health Electronic Resources Online in Northern England

HES Hospital Episode Statistics; Hospital Eye Service

HEVU Health Education Video Unit

HFEA Human Fertilisation and Embryology Authority

HfHT Help for Health Trust (obsolete)

HFMA Healthcare Financial Management Association

HGAC Human Genetics Advisory Commission

HGC Human Genetics Commission

HHT hand-held terminal

HIA health impact assessment; Housing Improvement Agency

HIBCC Health Index Bar Code Council; Health Index Business Communications Council

HImP Health Improvement Programme

HIP Health Investment Programme

HIPE Hospital In-Patient Enquiry Scheme

HIS health service indicators

HIS hospital information system

HISN High Individual Support Needs
HISS hospital information and support system
HIU Health Inequalities Unit
HIV human immunodeficiency virus
HIYE Health in Your Environment
HJSC Hospital Junior Staff Committee (of BMA)
HL7 Health Level 7 (a healthcare-specific communication standard for data exchange between computer applications)
HLC Healthy Living Centre
HLF Heritage Lottery Fund
HLI Healthy Living Initiative
HLPI high level performance indicator
HM HNA Health Needs Assessment
HMIC Health Management Information Consortium
HMO health maintenance organisation (US); house in multiple occupation
HMR hospital medical record
HMSO Her Majesty's Stationery Office (now TSO)
HNI Housing Needs Index
HO Home Office; House Officer
HoN Health of the Nation White Paper on Prevention
HoNOS Health of the Nation Outcomes Scale
HOWIS Health of Wales Information Service (the official website for NHS in Wales)
HP health promotion
HPA Health Protection Agency
HPC Health Professions Council
HPC Health Professions Council
HPE Health Promotion England (obsolete); higher professional education
HPERU Health Policy and Economic Research Unit
HPH health-promoting hospital
HPMA Healthcare People Management Association
HPR health process re-design
HPSS Health Promotion Specialist Service; Health and Personal Social Services
HPU Health Protection Unit
HR human resources (personnel)
HRD human resource development
HRD-MET Human Resources Directorate-Medical Education and Development
HRG Healthcare Resource Group
HRQOL health-related quality of life
HSAC Health Service Advisory Committee (of HSE)
HSC Health Select Committee; Health and Safety Commission; Health Service Circular (management letters from the DoH replacing ELs, HSGs, FDLs and FHSLs); Health Service Commissioner
HSCA Health and Social Care Authority (Northern Ireland)
HSCI Health Service Cost Index
HSCIC Health and Social Care Information Centre
HSCT Health and Social Care Trust (Northern Ireland)
HSDU hospital sterile and disinfection unit
HSE Health and Safety Executive

HSG   health service guidance; Health Strategy Group; Housing Support Grant
HSJ   *Health Services Journal*
HSMC   Health Services Management Centre (University of Birmingham)
HSP   Healthy Schools Programme; heart sink patient
HSPI   Health Service Prices Index
HSPSCB   High Security Psychiatric Services Commissioning Board (obsolete)
HSSB   Health and Social Services Board (Northern Ireland)
HSSC   Health and Social Services Council (Northern Ireland)
HST   higher surgical trainee (a senior registrar in old speak); higher surgical training
HSTAT   Health Services/Technology Assessment Text
HSV   herpes simplex virus
HSW   health and safety at work
HSWA   Health and Safety at Work Act 1974
HTA   Health Technology Assessment; Human Tissue Authority
HTAI   Health Technology Assessment International
HTCS   Hospital Travel Cost Scheme
HTH   hope this helps
HTM   high technology medicine
HV   health visitor; home visit
HVA   Health Visitors Association
HVHSC   Human and Veterinary Healthcare Sectoral Consultation (bringing together interested bodies in the public and private sectors to draw up key principles concerning biotechnology and genetically modified organisms)
HWI   Healthy Workplace Initiative
HWRC   Household Waste Recycling Centre

I

I&D   incision and drainage
IADL   instrumental activities of daily living
IAG   information age government
IAGI   intended average gross income (of GPs) (the total money paid on average to GPs, i.e. inclusive of indirectly reimbursed expenses)
IAMRA   International Association of Medical Regulatory Authorities
IANI   intended average net income (of GPs) (the total money paid on average to GPs, exclusive of indirectly reimbursed expenses)
IANR   intended average net remuneration
IAPO   International Alliance of Patients' Organisations
IAVI   International Aids Vaccine Initiative
IBD   interest-bearing debt
IBMS   Institute of Biomedical Science
IBNR   incurred but not reported (clinical negligence liability)
IC   Information Commissioner
ICA   Invalid Care Allowance (now replaced by Carers Allowance)
ICAS   Independent Complaints Advocacy Service
ICC   Integrated Child Credit
ICD   The WHO's International Statistical Classification of Diseases and Related Health Problems (now in its 10th revision)
ICE   Intercollegiate Examination

ICES Institute for Clinical Evaluative Sciences
ICFM Institute of Charity Fundraising Managers Trust
ICHS International Centre for Health and Society
ICIDH International Classification of Impairment, Activities and Participation
ICN infection control nurse; integrated care network
ICP integrated care pathway; Integrated Care Pilots; intra-cranial pressure
ICRC International Committee of the Red Cross
ICRS Integrated Care Records Service
ICT infection control team; information communication technology
ICU intensive care unit
ICW Indigenous Community Worker; integrated clinical workstation
ICWS integrated clinical workstation
ID2000 Indices of Deprivation 2000
IDA Improvement Development Agency
IDDM insulin-dependent diabetes mellitus
IdeA Improvement and Development Agency
IDF International Diabetes Federation
IELTS International English Language Testing Service
IEMC Inter-Balkan European Medical Centre
I4H Information for Health
IFM Information for the Management of Healthcare
IFPMA International Federation of Pharmaceutical Manufacturers Associations
IFRS International Financial Reporting Standards
IG information governance
IGSoC Information Governance Statement of Compliance
IHA Independent Healthcare Association of 600 independent hospitals and homes
IHCD Institute of Health and Care Development
IHE Institute of Hospital Engineering; International Health Exchange
IHEEM Institute of Healthcare Engineering and Estate Management
IHF International Hospital Federation
IHM Institute of Healthcare Management
IHRIM Institute of Health Record Information and Management
IHSM Institute of Health Service Managers (now part of the IHM)
IIP Investors in People (initiative)
ILA Individual Learning Account
ILAF Independent Local Advisory Forum
ILCOR International Liaison Committee on Resuscitation
ILD Index of Local Deprivation (replaced by IMD)
ILF Independent Living Fund
ILP Independent Living Project
ILSI International Life Sciences Institute
IM&T information management and technology
IMA Irish Medical Association
IMC Information Management Centre
IMCA independent mental capacity advocate
IMD Index of Multiple Deprivations
IMG international medical graduates
IMGE Information Management Group of NHS Executive

IMHO in my humble opinion; in my honest opinion
IMLS Institute of Medical Laboratory Sciences
IMR infant mortality rate
INASP International Network for the Availability of Scientific Publications
INES International Network of Engineers and Scientists for Global Responsibility
INSET in-service training
IOP Institute of Psychiatry
IoS Item of Service (something that GPs get paid for on a itemised basis under the terms of the Red Book)
IP inpatient
IPF Institute of Public Finance
IPH Improvement Partnership for Hospitals
IPM Institute of Personnel Management
IPPC Integrated Pollution Prevention Control
IPPF International Planned Parenthood Federation
IPPR Institute for Public Policy Research
IPR independent professional review; individual performance review; intellectual property rights
IPS Indicative Prescribing Scheme; Integrated Personnel System
IPU Information Policy Unit (DoH)
IQI Indicators for Quality Improvement
IRIS interactive resource information system
IRL Initial Resource Limit
IRO industrial relations officer
IRP Independent Reconfiguration Panel
IRR internal rate of return
IS Income Support (formerly Supplementary Benefit, before that National Assistance, before that the Poor Law)
ISB Information Standards Board (NHS); Intercollegiate Speciality Examinations Board; Invest to Save Budget
ISBN International Standard Book Number
ISCAP Integrating Surgical Curriculum and Practice
ISCP Intercollegiate Surgical Curriculum Project
ISD Information and Statistics Division (Scotland)
ISDD Institute for the Study of Drug Dependence
ISDN Integrated Services Digital Network
ISE individualised sensory environment
ISG Information Services Group
ISIP Integrated Service Improvement Programme
ISO Infrastructure Support Organisation; International Organization for Standardization
ISPOR International Society for Pharmacoeconomics and Outcomes Research
ISQua International Society for Quality in Health Care
ISS International Sponsorship Scheme (formerly ODTS)
ISSM Institute of Sterile Services Management
IST Intensive Support Team
ISTAHC International Society of Technology Assessment in Health Care
ISTC independent sector treatment centres
IT information technology

ITC   independent treatment centre
ITN   invitation to negotiate
ITS   Independent Tribunal Service (now replaced by the Appeals Service)
ITT   invitation to tender
ITU   intensive therapy/treatment unit
IUHPE   International Union for Health Promotion and Education
IV   independent variable; intravenous
IWL   Improving Working Lives
IYF   inter-year flexibility

J

J   judge (in law reports)
JAMA   *Journal of the American Medical Association*
JANET   Joint Academic Network
JCB   Joint Commissioning Board
JCC   Joint Consultative Committee; Joint Consultants Committee
JCCO   Joint Council for Clinical Oncology
JCE   Joint Commissioning Executive
JCHMT   Joint Committee for Higher Medical Training
JCHST   Joint Committee for Higher Surgical Training
JCPTGP   Joint Committee on Postgraduate Training in General Practice
JCVI   Joint Committee on Vaccination and Immunisation
JDC   Junior Doctors Committee
JE   job evaluation
JEMS   *Journal of Emergency Medicine*
JEWP   Job Evaluation Working Party
JFC   Joint Formulary Committee
JFSSG   Joint Food Safety and Standards Group
JHU   Joint Health Unit
JIF   Joint Investment Fund (Scotland)
JIGSAW   project designed to reduce the need for hospital beds; co-ordinated by GMAS
JIP   Joint Investment Plan (what you have to write in your BSVP group)
JISC   Joint Information Systems Committee
JIT   just in time (supplies delivery)
JLDS   Joint Learning Disability Service (runs CLDTs)
JNC(J)   Joint Negotiating Committee (on junior doctors terms and conditions of service)
JPAC   Joint Planning Advisory Committee (replaced by SWAG)
JRCT   Joseph Rowntree Charitable Trust
JRF   Joseph Rowntree Foundation
JRG   Joint Review Group
JSA   Job Seeker's Allowance
JSE   Joint Strategy Executive
JSG   Joint Strategy Group
JSOG   Joint Senior Officers Group

K

KED   Kendrick extrication device
KF   King's Fund

KFOA King's Fund Organisational Audit
KI key indicator (social services)
KIGS key indicators, geographical system
KISS keep it simple stupid
KSF Knowledge and Skills Framework (part of Agenda for Change)
KTD Kendrick traction device
KTP Knowledge Transfer Partnership
KVO keep veins open

L

LA local authority
LAA Local Area Agreement; Local Authority Association
LAC Local Authority Circular; Local Authority Company; looked after children
LACOTS Local Authorities Co-ordinating Body on Food and Trading Standards
LAD Local Authority District
LAF Local Advisory Forum
LAFS Local Authority Financial Settlement
LAG local advisory group
LAL local authority letter
LAN local area network
LAP local area partnership; local action plan
LAPIS Locality and Practice Information System
LARIA Local Authorities Research and Intelligence Association
LAS Locum Appointment Service; London Ambulance Service
LASA London Advice Services Alliance
LASFE Local Authorities' Self-Financed Expenditure
LASS Local Authority Social Services
LASSL Local Authority Social Services Letter
LAT locum appointment for training
LATF Local Asthma Taskforce
LATS London Academic Training Scheme (part of LIZEI)
LAWDC Local Authority Waste Disposal Company
LCFS Local Counter Fraud Specialist
LCMG local communications user group
LD learning difficulties; Liberal Democrat; local democracy
LD/MH learning difficulties/mental handicap
LDA Local Development Agency; London Development Agency
LDAF Learning Disabilities Award Framework
LDC Local Dental Committee (the statutory body of GDPs that represents dental practices in the local area)
LDP Local Delivery Plan
LDSAG Local Diabetes Service Advisory Group
LEA Local Education Authority
LEC Local Enterprise Company
LEI Local Employment Initiative
LEL lower explosive limit
LEO Leading Empowered Organisations
LETS Local Exchange Trading Scheme

LFS   Labour Force Survey
LGA   Local Government Association
LGBT   lesbian, gay, bisexual and transgender
LGC   Local Government Chronicle
LGFR   Local Government Finance Report
LGFS   Local Government Financial Settlement; Local Government Financial Statistics
LGHA   Local Government & Housing Act 1989
LGIB   Local Government International Bureau
LGIU   Local Government Information Unit
LGMB   Local Government Management Board
LGPS   Local Government Pension Scheme
LHB   local health boards (Wales)
LHC   Local Health Council
LHCC   Local Health Care Co-operative (Scottish variety of PCG)
LHG   Local Health Group (a sort of Welsh PCG)
LHP   Local Health Plan
LHSCG   Local Health and Social Carte Group (Northern Ireland)
LIF   Local Initiatives Fund
LIFT   Local Improvement Finance Trust
LIG   local implementation group
LIMS   laboratory information management systems
LINC   Library and Information Commission (obsolete)
LINks   Local Involvement Networks
LIO   Local Implementation Officer; Local Infrastructure Organisation
LIP   Local Implementation Plans
LIS   library information system; Local Implementation Strategy
LISI   Low Income Scheme Index (measure of deprivation based on claims for exemption from prescription charges on grounds of low income)
LIT   Local Implementation Team
LIZ   London Initiative Zone
LIZEI   London Implementation Zone Education Initiative
LLL   lifelong learning
LLSC   Local Learning and Skills Council
LLTI   limiting long-term illness
LMC   Local Medical Committee (statutory local committee for all GPs in the area covered by the health authority)
LMCA   Long-term Medical Conditions Alliance
LMWAG   Local Medical Workforce Advisory Groups (formed in 1996 to co-ordinate postgraduate medical education between groups of trusts; there are five or six in each NHS Region)
LNC   Local Negotiating Committee
LNRS   Local Neighbourhood Renewal Strategy
LOBNH   lights on but nobody home
LOS   length of stay (a measure of activity in hospital wards)
LPC   Local Pharmaceutical Committee (a committee of pharmacists)
LPfIT   London Programme for IT
LPI   labour productivity index
LPM   litres per minute

LPS   Local Pharmaceutical Services
LPSA   Local Public Service Agreement
LR   legitimate relationship
LRD   Labour Research Department
LREC   Local Research Ethics Committee
LRR   Local Reference Rent
LRS   Local and Regional Services
LSC   Learning & Skills Council; Legal Services Commission
LSCG   Local Specialised Commissioning Group
LSCS   lower segment Caesarean section
LSHTM   London School of Hygiene and Tropical Medicine
LSP   local service provider(s); local strategic partnership
LSVT   Large Scale Voluntary Transfer
LTA   long-term agreement
LTC   long-term condition
LTM   Learning to Manage Health Information
LTP   Local Transport Plan
LTPS   Liability to Third Parties Scheme
LTSA   long-term service agreement
LTVS   long-term ventilatory support
LURG   local user representative group
LWPG   Local Winter Planning Group
LYS   life years saved

M

MA   Maternity Allowance
MAA   Medical Artists Association of Great Britain
MAAG   Medical Audit Advisory Group; Multi-disciplinary Audit Advisory Group
MAAQ   Multidisciplinary Audit and Quality Group (replaced by the ACTS)
MAB   Metropolitan Asylums Board (obsolete)
MAC   Medical Advisory Committee
MACA   Mental After Care Association
MADEL   Medical and Dental Education Levy
MADEN   Medical and Dental Education Network
MAF   Management Accountancy Framework
MAGGOT   medically able, go get other transportation
MALDA   Multi-agency Learning Disability Assessment
MANCAS   Manchester Care Assessment Schedule
MAP   management action plan
MaPSaF   Manchester Patient Safety Framework
MAR2C   Matching Resources to Care (a mental health information system for caseload monitoring devised to study cases of serious mental illness; IT can compare data from Social Services, Health Services and the voluntary sector)
MARMAP   Multi-agency Risk Management Assessment Process
MARP   Multi-agency Risk Assessment Panel (decides whether mentally ill people are dangerous)
MAS   minimal access surgery
MASC   Medical Academic Staff Committee; Medical Advisors Support Centre

MAST   Multi-agency Support Team
MASTA   Medical Advisory Services for Travellers Abroad
MAT   Medical Appeal Tribunal
MAVIS   Mobility Advice and Vehicle Information Service
MBA   Master of Business Administration
MBTI   Myers-Briggs Type Indicator (Myers-Briggs Personality Type Inventory)
MC   Medicines Commission
MCA   Medicines Control Agency; motorcycle accident
MCCD   Medical Certificate of Cause of Death
MCI   mass casualty incident
MCN   managed clinical network
MCO   managed care organisation
MCP   male chauvinist pig (obsolete?); medical care practitioner
MCRG   Medical Career Research Group
MCSP   Member of the Chartered Society of Physiotherapy
MDA   Medical Devices Agency
MDAP   Multi-Deanery Appointment Process
MDD   Medical Devices Directorate
MDDUS   Medical and Dental Defence Union of Scotland
MDG   Management Development Group (Scotland); Muscular Dystrophy Group
MDI   metered dose inhaler
MDM   medical decision making
MDO   mentally disordered offender
MDR   multiple drug resistant
MDS   minimum data set
MDT   mobile data terminal; multi-disciplinary team
MDU   Medical Defence Union
ME   Management Executive
MEC   Management Education for Clinicians; Management Executive Committee
MEDITEL   GP information system
MEDLARS   Medical Literature Analysis and Retrieval System
MEDS   Medical Deputising Service
MEE   Medical Education for England
MEL   Management Executive Letter (Scotland)
MENCAP   Royal Society for Mentally Handicapped Children and Adults
MEQ   modified examination question
MeReC   bulletin published by the National Prescribing Centre on evidence based
   therapeutics
MERV   Medical Emergency Response Vehicle
MESB   Medical Education Standards Board
MeSH   Medical Subject Headings
MESOL   Management Education Scheme by Open Learning
MFF   market forces factor
MFS   market forces supplement
MGA   Myasthenia Gravis Association
MGRG   Management Guidance Review Group
MHA   Mental Health Act 1983
MHAC   Mental Health Act Commission

MHC   major histocompatability complex
MHE   Mental Health Enquiry
MHG   Mental Health Grant
MHIG   Mental Health Information Group
MHIS   Mental Health Information Strategy
MHMDS   Mental Health Minimum Data Set
MHPAF   Mental Health Performance Assessment Framework
MHPSS   Manchester Health Promotion Specialist Service
MHRA   Medicines and Healthcare Products Regulatory Agency
MHRT   Mental Health Review Tribunal (convened to hear appeals against detention under the MHA)
MHT   Mental Health Task Force
MIA   Medical Insurance Agency
MIDIRS   Midwife Information and Resource Service
MIE   Medical Informatics Europe
MIG   Medical Information Group
MIMMS   Major Incident Medical Management and Support
MIMS   Monthly Index of Medical Specialties
MINAP   Myocardial Infarction National Audit Project
MIND   organisation of mental health users
MINI   Mental Illness Needs Index
Mini-CEX   Mini Clinical Evaluation Exercise
Mini-PAT   Peer Assessment Tool (360-degree)
Mini-PBA   Procedure-based Assessment (single procedure)
MIQUEST   A method of extracting information from GP computer systems
MIS   management information systems
MISG   Mental Illness Specific Grant (government subsidy to supplement spending by local authorities on social care for mentally ill people living in the community)
MIT   Massachusetts Institute of Technology; minimally invasive therapy
MITAG   Medical Information and Technology Advisory Group
MIU   minor injuries unit
MLA   medical laboratory assistant; Museums, Libraries and Archives Council
MLA   Member of the Legislative Assembly (Northern Ireland)
MLCF   Medical Leadership Competency Framework
MLD   mild learning disability
MLSO   Medical Laboratory Scientific Officer
MMC   Modernising Medical Careers
MMR   measles, mumps, rubella
MMS   Medical Management Services
MMSAC   Medical Manpower Standing Advisory Committee (representatives from BMA, Royal Colleges, Regional Manpower committees, Medical Research Council and Council of Deans)
MNC   Modernising Nursing Careers
MO   Medical Officer
MOD   Ministry of Defence
MOH   Medical Officer of Health (a predecessor of the DPH)
MOI   mechanism of injury
MOP   Mobile Optical Practice

MOR   Millennium Operating Regime
MoU   memorandum of understanding
MPA   Masters in Public Administration; Medical Prescribing Adviser
MPC   Medical Practices Committee (abolished 2002)
MPDS   Medical Priority Dispatch System
MPET   Multi-professional Education and Training levy
MPIG   minimum practice income guarantee
MPS   Medical Protection Society; Modernising Public Services Group
MPT   maximum part time
MPU   Medical Practitioners Union
MRC   Medical Research Council
MREC   Multi-centre Research Ethics Committee
MRFIT   Multiple Risk Factor Intervention Trial
MRI   magnetic resonance imaging
MRO   Medical Records Officer
MRP   Minimum Revenue Provision (part of capital control framework)
MRSA   methicillin-resistant *Staphylococcus aureus*
MSAC   Maternity Services Advisory Committee
MSD   Merck Sharp & Dohme Ltd
MSDS   Material Safety Data Sheet
MSEB   Medical Standards Education Board (replacing JCPTGP and STA)
MSF   union for skilled and professional workers, including many NHS employees (formerly ASTMS, now joined into AMICUS; Medicine Sans Frontières; multi-source feedback)
MSGP-4   National Study of Morbidity in General Practice
MSI   Marie Stopes International
MSLC   Maternity Services Liaison Committee (brings together professions involved in maternity services with laypeople to agree procedures and monitor their effectiveness as they appear to individual women)
MSP   Member of the Scottish Parliament
MSPCG   Most Sparsely Populated Councils Group
MSU   medium secure unit; short for MSSU
MTA   Management Team Assistant
MTAS   Medical Training Application Service
MTFP   Medium Term Financial Plan
MTO   Medical Technical Officer
MUSCLE   Multi-Station Clinical Examination
MV   Millennium Volunteer
MWC   Mental Welfare Commission
MWCS   Mental Welfare Commission for Scotland
MWEP   Medical Workforce Expansion Programme
MWF   Women's Medical Federation
MWSAC   Medical Workforce Standing Advisory Committee (working for the education committee of the GMC on appraising doctors and dentists in training for SCOPME and on general clinical training during the pre-registration year)
MWSAG   Medical Workforce Standing Advisory Group

N

N3   New National Network (Broadband)
N&MC   Nursing and Midwifery Council
NA   Nursing Auxiliary
NAAS   National Association of Air Ambulance Services
NAB   National Assistance Board (1948–66)
NAC   National Abortion Campaign
NACAB   National Association of Citizens Advice Bureaux
NACC   National Association for Colitis and Crohn's Disease
NACEPD   National Advisory Council on Employment of People with Disabilities
NACGP   National Association of Commissioning GPs
NACPME   National Advice Centre for Postgraduate Medical Education
NACRO   National Association for the Care and Resettlement of Offenders
NACT   National Association of Clinical Tutors
NACVS   National Association of Councils for Voluntary Service
NAFHP   National Association of Fundholding Practices (obsolete)
NAGPT   National Association of GP Tutors
NAGS   NICE Appraisal Groups
NAGST   National Advisory Group for Scientists and Technicians
NAHAT   National Association of Health Authorities and Trusts (obsolete)
NAHCSM   National Association of Health Care Supplies Managers
NAHSSO   National Association of Health Service Security Officers
NAHWT   National Association of Health Workers and Travellers
NALHF   National Association of Leagues of Hospital Friends
NANOS   North American Neuro-Opthalmology Society
NANP   National Association of Non-Principals (now NASGP)
NANT   National Appraisal of New Technologies
NAO   National Audit Office
NAPC   National Association of Primary Care (formed from the embers of Fundholding
    National Association to represent interests of PCGs)
NAPMECA   National Association of Postgraduate Medical Education Centre Administration
NAPP   National Association for Patient Participation
NAPS   National Anti-Poverty Strategy (Ireland)
NAS   National Autistic Society
NASEN   National Association for Special Educational Needs
NASGP   National Association of Sessional GPs (representing Locums, Freelance GPs and
    Salaried GPs, i.e. Non Principals)
NASP   National Application Service Provider
NASS   National Asylum Support Service
NATN   National Association of Theatre Nurses; National Association of Training Nurses
NatPaCT   National Primary and Care Trust (development programme)
NAVB   National Association of Volunteer Bureaux
NAVHO   National Association of Voluntary Help Organisations
NAW   National Assembly for Wales
NAWO   National Alliance of Women's Organisations
NBA   National Blood Authority (England)
NBAP   National Booked Admissions Programme
NBG   lacking evidence of effectiveness

NBI   National Beds Inquiry
NBS   National Board for Nursing, Midwifery and Health Visiting for Scotland (obsolete)
NBTS   National Blood Transfusion Service (obsolete)
NBV   net book value
NCAA   National Clinical Assessment Authority
NCAS   National Clinical Assessment Service (formerly NCAA National Clinical Assessment Authority)
NCASP   National Clinical Audit Support Programme
NCBV   National Coalition for Black Volunteering
NCC   National Consumer Council
NCCA   National Centre for Clinical Audit (now absorbed into NICE); National Community Care Alliance
NCCG   Non-Consultant Career Grade
NCCHTA   National Co-ordinating Centre for Health Technology Assessment
NCCSDO   National Co-ordinating Centre for NHS Service Delivery and Organisation Research and Development (at the London School of Hygiene and Tropical Medicine)
NCE   National Confidential Enquiry; net current expenditure
NCEPOD   National Confidential Enquiry into Patient Outcome and Death (formerly CEPOD)
NCG   National Commissioning Group
NCH   National Children's Home, now known as Action For Children
NCI   National Captioning Institute
NCI   National Confidential Inquiry; NHS Centre for Involvement
NCIL   National Centre for Independent Living
NCIS   National Criminal Intelligence Service
NCISH   National Confidential Inquiry into Suicide and Homicide by people with Mental Illness
NCL   National Civic League
NCMO   National Casemix Office
NCSC   National Care Standards Commission (abolished 2004)
NCSSD   National Counselling Service for Sick Doctors
NCT   National Childbirth Trust
NCV   National Centre for Volunteering (obsolete)
NCVCCO   National Council of Voluntary Child Care Organisations
NCVO   National Council for Voluntary Organisations
NCVQ   National Council for Vocational Qualifications
NCVYS   National Council for Voluntary Youth Services
ND   New Deal
NDC   National Disability Council; New Deal for Communities
NDPB   non-departmental public body
NDPHS   National Disabled Persons Housing Service
NDT   National Development Team for People with Learning Disabilities
NDTMS   National Drug Treatment Monitoring System
NDU   Nurse Development Unit
NDYP   New Deal for Young People
NEAT   new and emerging applications of technology
NED   non-executive director
NEET   not in education, employment or training

NEJM *New England Journal of Medicine*
NeLH National Electronic Library for Health
NERC Natural Environment Research Council
NES NHS Education for Scotland
NESTA National Endowment for Science Technology and the Arts
NET new and emerging technologies
NF Nuffield Foundation
NFA no fixed address
NFAP National Framework for Assessing Performance
NFI National Fraud Initiative
NFP not-for-profit
NFR not for resuscitation
NFW no further work
NGfL National Grid for Learning
nGMS New General Medical Services (contract)
NGO non-governmental organisation
NHAIS National Health Authority Information Systems
NHD notional half day (consultants)
NHF National Heart Forum
NHFA Nursing Homes Fees Agency
NHIS National Health Intelligence Service
NHLI National Heart and Lung Institute, Imperial College
NHS CFH NHS Connecting for Health
NHS CRS NHS Care Records Service
NHS EED NHS Economic Evaluation Database
NHS EHU NHS Ethnical Health Unit
NHS FAM NHS Fraud Awareness Month
NHS IMC NHS Information Centre
NHS KSF NHS Knowledge and Skills Framework
NHS LIFT NHS Local Improvement Finance Trust
NHS PSA NHS Purchasing and Supply Agency
NHS QIS NHS Quality Improvement Scotland
NHS National Health Service
NHS(S) National Health Service in Scotland
NHS/N3 replaced the private NHS communications network NHSnet
NHSAC National Health Service Appointments Commission
NHSAR National Health Service Administrative Register
NHSBSA NHS Business Services Authority
NHSBSP NHS Breast Screening Programme
NHSCA NHS Consultants Association
NHSCCA NHS and Community Care Act (1990)
NHSCCC NHS Centre for Coding and Classification
NHSCR NHS Central Register
NHSCSF NHS Counter Fraud Service
NHSCSFMS NHS Counter Fraud and Security Management Service
NHSCTA NHS Clinical Trials Adviser
NHSE NHS Estates; NHS Executive (abolished 2002)
NHSFT NHS Foundation Trust

NHSI NHS Institute for Innovation and Improvement
NHSIA NHS Information Authority (abolished 2005)
NHSIII NHS Institute for Innovation and Improvement
NHSL NHS Logistics
NHSLA NHS Litigation Authority
NHSmail NHS email and directory service
NHSME National Health Service Management Executive (Scotland)
NHSME NHS Management Executive (in England; now called the NHSE)
NHSMEE NHS Medical Education England
NHSnet Intranet for the NHS
NHSOE NHS Overseas Enterprises
NHSP NHS Partners
NHSPA NHS Pensions Agency (now merged as part of the NHS Business Services Authority, NHSBSA)
NHSPA NHS Pensions Authority
NHSS NHS Scotland; NHS Supplies; National Healthy Schools Standard
NHSSMS NHS Security Management Service
NHST NHS Trust
NHSTD NHS Training Directorate; NHS Training Division
NHSTF NHS Trust Federation
NHSTU NHS Training Unit
NHSU National Health Service University (obsolete)
NI National Insurance
NIA Northern Ireland Assembly
NIACE National Institute of Adult and Continuing Education
NIAS Northern Ireland Ambulance Service
NIC National Insurance Contribution; net ingredient cost (the basic price of a drug)
NICARE Northern Ireland Centre for Health Care Co-operation and Development
NICE National Institute for Clinical Excellence; National Institute for Health and Clinical Excellence; Northern Institute for Continuing Education
NICEC National Institute for Carers and Educational Counselling
NICON NHS Confederation in Northern Ireland
NICS Northern Ireland Civil Service
NICU Neonatal Intensive Care Unit
NICVA Northern Ireland Council for Voluntary Action
NIH National Institute of Health; Nuffield Institute for Health (Leeds)
NIHR National Institute for Health Research
NIHSS Nosocomial Infection National Surveillance Scheme
NILO National Investment and Loans Office
NIMHE National Institute for Mental Health in England
NINo National Insurance Number
NISW National Institute of Social Work (obsolete)
NJC National Joint Council
NLC (DoH) National Leadership Council
NLDB National Leadership Development Bodies
NLH National Library for Health
NLIAH National Leadership and Innovation Agency for Healthcare (Wales)
NLM National Library of Medicine

NLN The National Leadership Network for Health and Social Care
NLOP NPfIT Local Ownership Programme
NMAC National Medical Advisory Committee
NMAP Nursing Midwifery and Allied Health Professionals (Internet resource)
NMC Nursing and Midwifery Council
NMDS nursing minimum data set
NMEfIT North, Midlands and East Programme for IT
NMET Non-medical Education and Training
NMIS Nurse Management Information System
NMS National Minimum Standards
NNH number needed to harm
NNT number needed to treat
NOF National Opportunities Fund
NOMDS National Organ Matching and Distribution Service (*see* UHTSSA)
NOMIS National Online Manpower Information Service
NOP National Opinion Polls
NOS National Occupation Standards
NP Non-Principal
NPA National Pharmaceutical Association
NPAT National Patients' Access Team
NPC National Prescribing Centre (based in Liverpool; formerly known as MASC; publishes *MeReC Bulletin* which is distributed to all GPs on request); net present cost
NPCRDC National Primary Care Research and Development Centre (based in the University of Manchester)
NPfIT National Programme for IT (in the NHS)
NPG Modernising Health and Social Services: National Priorities Guidance
NPHS National Public Health Service (Wales)
NPHT Nuffield Provincial Hospitals Trust
NPIS National Poisons Information Service
NPL National Physical Laboratory
NPN National PALS Network
NPRB Nurses Pay Review Body
NPSA National Patient Safety Agency
NPT near patient testing
NPV net present value
NR nearest relative
NRAC NHS Scotland Resource Allocation Committee
NRC National Regionalisation Consortium
NRCI national reference cost index
NRE non-recurring expenditure
NRES National Research Ethics Service
NRLS National Reporting and Learning Service
NRPB National Radiological Protection Board
NRR National Research Register
NRS Neighbourhood Renewal Strategy
NRT nicotine replacement therapy
NSC National Screening Committee (UK)

NSCAG   National Specialist Commissioning Advisory Group (succeeded by The National Commissioning Group, NCG)

NSCG   The National Specialised Commissioning Group

NSEC   National Smoking Education Campaign

NSF   National Schizophrenia Fellowship (now called Rethink); National Service Framework; National Stakeholder Forum

NSFMH   National Service Framework – Mental Health

NSMI   National Sports Medicine Institute (UK)

NSPCC   National Society for the Prevention of Cruelty to Children

NSRC   National Schedule of Reference Costs

NSS   National Services Scotland

NSTS   NHS Strategic Tracing Service

NSU   non-specific urethritis (common STD)

NSV   National Supplies Vocabulary

NTA   National Treatment Agency

NTN   National Training Number

NTO   National Training Organisation

NTT   nuchal translucency thickness (screening method for Down's syndrome)

NTTRL   National Tissue Typing Reference Laboratory

NVP   newly vulnerable person

NVQ   National Vocational Qualification

NWCS   Nation Wide Clearing Service (all trusts must submit data about admitted patient care which is then forwarded to HAs)

NWIPP   National Workforce Information and Planning Programme

NWN   NHS-wide networking

NWSI   Nurse with a Special Interest

NYCDOHMH   New York City Department of Health and Mental Hygiene

O

O&M   organisation and methods

OAPS   Objective Assessment of Professional Skills

OAT   Out of Area Treatment (the replacement for ECR)

OBC   outline business case

OBD   occupied bed day

OBS   output based specification

OCD   obsessive compulsive disorder

OCMO   Office of the Chief Medical Officer (Wales)

OCN   Open College Network

OCPA   Office of the Commissioner for Public Appointments

OCR   optical character reader; optical character recognition

OCS   order communication system; Organisational Codes Service

OD   once daily; organisational development; outside diameter; overdose

ODA   Operating Department assistant; Overseas Development Agency; Overseas Doctors Agency

ODO   Operating Department orderly

ODP   Operating Department practitioner

ODPM   Office of the Deputy Prime Minister

ODTS   Overseas Doctors Training Scheme (of appropriate Royal College)

OECD   Organisation for Economic Co-operation and Development
OEL   occupational exposure limit
Ofsted   Office for Standards in Education
OGC   Office for Government Commerce
OH   occupational health
OHAG   Oral Health Advisory Group
OHE   Office of Health Economics (London)
OHN   *Our Healthier Nation* (Cm3852, www.ohn.gov.uk)
OHS   Occupational Health Service
OIC   Officer in Charge
OIE   Office International des Epizooties
OIHCP   Office for Information on Health Care Performance
OISC   Office of the Immigration Services Commissioner
OJEC   *Official Journal of the European Community*
OME   Office of Manpower Economics
OMNI   Organising Medical Networked Information
OMP   Ophthalmic Medical Practitioner
OMV   open market value
OMVEU   open market value in existing use
ONS   Office for National Statistics (the result of a merger in April 1996 of the Central Statistical Office and the Office of Population Censuses and Surveys)
OO   optometrist
OOH   out of hours
OOP   Out of Programme
OOPC   Out of Programme for career break
OOPE   Out of Programme for experience
OOPR   Out of Programme for research
OOPT   Out of Programme for clinical training
OP   outpatient
OPAC   Online Public Access Catalogue
OPCS   Office of Population, Census and Surveys (system for classifying disease and treatment; now Office for National Statistics, ONS)
OPD   Outpatient Department
OPHIS   Office for Public Health in Scotland
OPM   Office of Public Management
OR   operation research (a scientific method which uses models of a system to evaluate alternative courses of action with a view to improving decision making)
OSB   Other Services Block (now replaced by EPCS)
OSC   Overview and Scrutiny Committee (local authority)
OSCE   Observed Structured Clinical Examination
OSCHR   Office for the Strategic Coordination of Health Research
OSDLS   Open Source Digital Library System
OST   Office of Science and Technology
OT   occupational therapist; occupational therapy
OTC   over the counter (medicines not requiring a prescription)
OU   Open University
OVE   occlusive vascular event
OWAM   Organisation with a Memory

OWW   One World Week
OXERA   Oxford Economic Research Associates

P

P&T   professional and technical
PA   Patients Association (patient's mechanism to communicate with medical services); personal assistant; physician assistant (US); Police Authority
PABX   Public Area Branch Exchange
PAC   Public Accounts Committee
PACE   Police & Criminal Evidence Act 1984; Promoting Action on Clinical Effectiveness; Property Advisers to the Civil Estate
PACS   Picture Archiving and Communication System
PACT   Placing, Assessment and Counselling Team; Prescribing Analysis and Costs (GPs get regular PACT reports from the PPA giving details of their recent prescribing, comparing them with local and national averages)
PAD   peripheral arterial disease
PAF   Performance Assessment Framework; Public Audit Forum
PAGB   Proprietary Association of Great Britain
PALS   Patient Advice and Liaison Service
PAMIS   Parliamentary Monitoring and Intelligence Service
PAMP   pathogen associated molecular pattern
PAMs   professions allied to medicine (physiotherapists, occupational therapists, etc.)
PAR   programme analysis and review
PARN   Professional Associations Research Network
PAS   Patient Administration System (a main hospital database); physician-assisted suicide
PASA   Purchasing and Supply Agency
PASG   pneumatic anti-shock garment
PAT   Personnel Accountability Tag; Policy Action Team
PAYE   pay as you earn
PBA   Procedure Based Assessment (may be in parts; *see* Mini-PBA)
PBC   practice-based commissioning; Public Benefit Corporation
PBL   problem-based learning
PBMA   programme budgeting and marginal analysis
PbR   payment by results
PBR   Pre-Budget Report
PBRS   Public Benefit Recording System
PBx   Private Branch Exchange (type of internal telephone network)
PC   Patients' Council; Parish Council; personal computer; politically correct; primary care; public convenience
PCA   patient controlled analgesia (usually a morphine pump)
PCAG   Primary Care Audit Group (i.e. multi-disciplinary)
PCAPs   Primary Care Act Pilots (the NHS (Primary Care) Act 1997 allowed NHS Trusts, NHS employees, qualified bodies and suitably experienced medical practitioners to submit proposals to provide general medical services under a contract with the health authority)
PCC   primary care centre
PCG   Primary Care Group (obsolete, *see* HSC 1998/230)
PCHR   Personal Child Health Record

PCIP   Primary Care Investment Plan

PCL   Provision for Credit Liabilities

PCMCN   Peninsula Cardiac Managed Clinical Network

PCO   primary care organisation (generic term for PCT in England, Health and Social Services Board in Northern Ireland, Local Health Board in Wales and Primary Care Division within Area Health Board in Scotland)

PCP   person-centred planning; personal communication profile

PCRC   Primary Care Resource Centre

PCRTA   Primary Care Research Team Assessment

PCS   Public and Commercial Services Union

PCS/E   Patient Classification System/Europe

PCT   primary care trust

PDC   public dividend capital (a form of long-term government finance on which the NHS trust pays dividends to the government. PDC has no fixed remuneration or repayment obligations, but in the long term the overall return on PDC is expected to be no less than on an equivalent loan)

PDD   pervasive development disorder; prescribed daily dose (the average daily dose which is actually prescribed)

PDF   Partnership Development Fund

PDO   property damage only

PDP   personal development plan; practice development plan

PDR   Personal Development Review

PDS   Parkinson's Disease Society; Personal Demographics Service; Personal Dental Services

PDSA   plan, do, study, act

PE   physical examination; pulmonary embolism

PEA   pulseless electrical activity

PEAT   Patient Environment Action Team

PEC   Professional Executive Committee

PECS   Picture Exchange Communication System

PEDC   Potential Elderly Domiciliary Clients (part of SSA)

PEDW   Patient Episode Database Wales

PEG   percutaneous endoscopic gastrostomy

PEM   prescription event monitoring

PES   Public Expenditure Survey

PESC   Public Expenditure Survey Committee (obsolete)

PESR   Potential Elderly Supported Residents (part of SSA)

PET   positron emission tomography

PETA   People for the Ethical Treatment of Animals

PETS   Paediatric Emergency Transfer Service

PEWP   Public Expenditure White Paper

PF   Patients' Forum

PFC   patient-focused care; Professional Fees Committee

PFI   Private Finance Initiative (now replaced by PPP)

PfIT   Programmes for IT

PFMA   Practice Fund Management Allowance (Allowance given to GP fundholders to manage their allocation. The allowance is primarily spent upon staff and equipment.)

PFU   Private Finance Unit

PGCME   Postgraduate and Continuing Medical Education
PGD   Patient Group Directions; Postgraduate Dean
PGEA   Postgraduate Education Allowance
PGMDE   Postgraduate Medical and Dental Education
PGY3   Postgraduate Year 3 (= ST1)
PHA   Public Health Alliance (now part of UKPHA)
PHAB   physically disabled and able-bodied
PHANYC   Public Health Association of New York City
PHC   primary healthcare
PHCDS   public health common data set
PHCSG   Primary Health Care Specialist Group
PHCT   Primary Health Care Team
PHeL   Public Health Electronic Library
PHIS   Public Health Institute of Scotland
PHL   Public Health Laboratory
PHLS   Public Health Laboratory Service
PHO   Public Health Observatory
PHOENIX   Primary Healthcare Organisations Exchanging New Ideas for Excellence
PHP   public health practitioner
PHPU   Public Health Policy Unit
PHRRC   Public Health Research and Resource Centre (at the University of Salford)
PHSS   Personal Health Summary System
PI   parallel imports; performance indicator
PIA   Partnership in Action; patient impact assessment; personal injury accident
PICKUP   Professional, Industrial and Commercial Updating
PICS   Platform for Internet Content Selection
PICU   Paediatric ICU; Psychiatric ICU
PIDA   Public Interest Disclosure Act
PIF   Patient Information Forum
PIG   Policy Implementation Groups; professional interest group; Promoting Independence Grant
PIL   patient information leaflet
PIMS   product information management system
PIN   personal identification number; prior identification notice
PIU   Performance and Innovation Unit
PLAB   Professional and Linguistic Assessment Board
PLICS   patient-led information and costing systems
PLP   personal learning plan
PLPI   Product Licence Parallel Import
PLT   Protected Learning Time
PM   project management
PMA   Personal Medical Attendant (what insurance companies etc. call a doctor who writes a report for them)
PMCPA   Prescription Medicines Code of Practice Authority
PMD   Performance Management Directorate
PMD   Prescribing Monitoring Document
PMETB   Postgraduate Medical Education and Training Board
PMF   Performance Management Framework

PMI private medical insurance
PMLD Profound and Multiple Learning Disabilities
PMR physical medicine and rehabilitation; progressive muscle relaxation
PMS personal medical service; post marketing surveillance; Primary Medical Services Contract
PND post-natal depression
PNL Prior Notification List (of patients for screening)
POC point of care
POCT point of care testing
PODS patient's own drugs
POINT Publications on the Internet (Department of Health)
POISE Procurement of Information Systems Effectively (The standard procedure followed for procurement of information systems.)
POLIS Parliamentary Online Indexing Service
POLST Physicians Orders for Life Sustaining Treatment
POM prescription-only medicine
POMR problem-oriented medical records
POPPs Partnerships for Older People Projects
POPUMET Protection of Persons Undergoing Medical Examination (regulations)
POSIX Portable Operating System Interface
POU Pulmonary Oncology Unit (chest cancers)
POVA Protection of Vulnerable Adults from Abuse
PPA Prescription Pricing Authority (costed all prescriptions dispensed in England in order to pay chemists for the costs of the drugs etc. they dispense; now done by NHSBSA)
PPBS Planning, Programming & Budgeting System
PPC promoting patient choice
PPDP Practice Professional Development Plans
PPDR Practice Profession Development and Revalidation
PPE personal protective equipment
PPF Priorities and Planning Framework
PPG Planning Policy Guidance; Principal Police Grant
PPI Patient and public involvement; proton pump inhibitor
PPIF Patient and public involvement forum (replaced by LINks)
PPM planned preventative maintenance
PPO preferred provider organisation
PPP Private Patients Plan; public private partnership
PPPFC Private Practice and Professionals Fees Committee
PPPP Public-Private Partnership Programme (aka 4Ps)
PPRD programme for provisionally registered doctors
PPRS Pharmaceutical Price Regulation Scheme
PPU Private Patients Unit
PQ parliamentary question; post qualification
PQASSO Practical Quality Assurance System for Small Organisations
PR per rectum; public relations (no known connection?)
PRA preventing and responding to aggression
PRB Pay Review Body
PREPP Post Registration Education and Preparation for Practice (nurses)

PRHO Pre-Registration House Officer
PRIAE Policy Research Institute on Ageing and Ethnicity
PRIMIS Primary Care Information Services
PRINCE Projects in Controlled Environments (a standard project management methodology used in all NHS Information systems projects)
PRO Public Record Office
PRODIGY Prescribing RatiOnally with Decision-support In General-practice studY
PRP performance-related pay
PRT personal risk training
PRU Police Resources Unit (part of Home Office)
PSA prostate-specific antigen; public service agreement
PSBR Public Sector Borrowing Requirement
PSC Public Sector Comparator
PSFD Public Sector Financing Deficit
PSG Prescribing Strategy Group
PSHE Personal Social and Health Education
PSI Policy Studies Institute (London)
PSIS Personal Spine Information Service
PSL period of study leave (GPs can apply in accordance with paragraph 50 of the Statement of Fees and Allowances for financial assistance in connection with a period of study leave to undertake postgraduate education, which will result in benefit to the GP, primary care in particular and the NHS)
PSM Professions Supplementary to Medicine
PSNC Pharmaceutical Services Negotiating Committee (represents chemists in negotiations with the DoH)
PSNCR Public Sector Net Cash Requirement
PSND Public Sector Net Deficit
PSNI Pharmaceutical Society of Northern Ireland
PSRCS Police Standard Radio Communication System
PSS Personal Social Services
PSSRU Personal Social Services Research Unit
PSU Prescribing Support Unit
PSX Public Service Expenditure
PT part-time
PTCA percutaneous transluminal coronary angioplasty
PTL Patient Targeting List
PTS Patient Transport Services
PTSD post-traumatic stress disorder
PU prescribing unit (developed to take account of elderly patients' greater need for medication; patients over 65 count as 3 PUs and those under 65 as one)
PUNS patient's unmet needs
PVC prime vendor contract
PVS persistent vegetative state
PWLB Public Works Loans Board
PYE part-year effect

Q
QA quality assurance

QAA   Quality Assurance Authority
QABME   Quality Assurance of Basic Medical Education
QALY   quality adjusted life year
QC   quality control; quick connect
QCA   Qualifications and Curriculum Authority
QMAS   Quality Management and Analysis System
QOF   Quality and Outcomes Framework
QOL   quality of life
QR   quick release
QSW   Qualified Social Worker
QUANGO   quasi-autonomous non-governmental organisation

R

R&D   research and development
R&S   recruitment and selection
RA   regional advisor; Regional Assembly; research associate; revenue account; rheumatoid arthritis
RA(SG)   Revenue Account (Specific Grants)
RAB   Resource Accounting and Budgeting
RADAR   Royal Association for Disability and Rehabilitation
RAE   Research Assessment Exercise
RAFT   Regulatory Authority for Fertility and Tissue
RAG   Research Allocation Group (NHS Executive)
RAGE   Radiotherapy Action Group Exposure
RAM   Risk Allocation Matrix
RAO   Referral and Advice Officer (first point of contact for inquiries about Social Services)
RAP   Referrals, Assessments and Packages of Care in Adult Personal Social Services
RAPt   Rehabilitation for Addicted Prisoners Trust
RARM   Remote and Rural Medicine
RARP   Resource Allocation Resource Paper
RASP   Resource Allocation and Service Planning
RATE   Regulatory Authority for Tissue and Embryos
RAWP   Resource Allocation Working Party (the working party devised a method of distributing resources to health authorities equitably in relation to need, which was used from 1977 to 1989; the system has been superseded by weighted capitation payments)
RB   Representative Body (BMA)
RBAC   role-based access control
RBE   relative biological effectiveness
RBMS   Referral Booking and Management System
RCA   root cause analysis; Royal College of Anaesthetists
RCC   Rural Community Council
RCCO   revenue contributions to capital outlay
RCCS   Reid Clinical Classification System; revenue consequences of capital schemes
RCGP   Royal College of General Practitioners
RCH   Residential Care Home
RCM   Royal College of Midwives
RCN   Royal College of Nursing
RCO   Refugee Community Organisations

RCOG   Royal College of Obstetricians and Gynaecologists
RCOphth   Royal College of Ophthalmologists
RCP   Royal College of Physicians
RCPath   Royal College of Pathologists
RCPCH   Royal College of Paediatrics and Child Health
RCPE   Royal College of Physicians of Edinburgh
RCPHIU   Royal College of Physicians Health Informatics Unit
RCPiLab   Royal College of Physicians Information Laboratory
RCPSG   Royal College of Physicians and Surgeons of Glasgow
RCPsych   Royal College of Psychiatrists
RCR   Royal College of Radiologists
RCS   Royal College of Surgeons
RCSE   Royal College of Surgeons of Edinburgh
RCSLT   Royal College of Speech and Language Therapists
RCT   randomised control trial
RCU   Regional Co-ordination Unit
RDA   Regional Development Agency; Rural Development Area
RDBMS   Relational Database Management System
RDC   Rural District Council (obsolete except in former UK colonies); Rural Development
   Commission
RDF   Resource Description Framework
RDN   Resource Discovery Network
RDPGPE   Regional Director of Postgraduate General Practice Education
RDRD   Regional Director of Research and Development
RDS   respiratory distress syndrome
RDSU   Research and Development Support Unit
RDU   Regional Dialysis Unit
REA   Regional Education Adviser
REACH   Research and Education for Children in Asthma; Retired Executives Action
   Clearing House
REAL   Research, Education, Audit, Libraries
REC   Racial Equality Council; Research Ethics Committee
REDG   Regional Education and Development Group
RES   Regional Economic Strategy
RFA   Requirements for Accreditation (GP computers)
RFC   request for comment
RFDS   Royal Flying Doctor Service
RG   Registrar-General
RGD   Revenue Grants Distribution
RGD(RG)   Revenue Grants Distribution (Review Group)
RGN   Registered General Nurse
RGPEC   Regional General Practice Education Committee
RHA   Regional Health Authority (obsolete)
RHB   Regional Hospital Board (obsolete)
RHI   Regional Head of Information
RHV   Registered Health Visitor
RIDDOR   Reporting of Injuries, Diseases and Dangerous Occurrences Regulations
RINN   recommended international non-proprietary name

RIPA   Royal Institute of Public Administration
RIPHH   Royal Institute of Public Health and Hygiene
RIS   Radiology Information System
RITA E   Extended RITA
RITA   Record of Individual (In-training) Training Assessment
RIU   Regulatory Impact Unit
RJDC   Regional Junior Doctors Committee
RLG   NHS Regional Librarians Group
RLQ   right lower quadrant
RLS   restless legs syndrome
RM   resource management
RMA   refuse[s] medical assistance
RMC   Regional Manpower Committee (obsolete)
RMI   resource management initiative
RMN   Registered Mental Nurse
RMO   Resident Medical Officer; responsible medical officer
RN   Registered Nurse
RNCC   Registered Nursing Care Contribution
RNHA   Registered Nursing Home Association
RNIB   Royal National Institute for the Blind
RNID   Royal National Institute for Deaf People
RNMH   Registered Nurse for the Mentally Handicapped
RO   NHS Regional Office; revenue out-turn
ROC   Retained Organs Commission (obsolete); return on capital
ROCE   return on capital employed
ROCR   Review of Central Returns
ROE   Regional Office for Europe (WHO)
ROS   return on sale
ROSPA   Royal Society for the Prevention of Accidents
RoW   Rights of Women
RP   Reporting Party
RPC   Regional Planning Conference (often now part of Regional Assembly)
RPGD   Regional Postgraduate Dean
RPHTF   Regional Prison Health Task Force
RPPG   Regional Policy Planning Guidance
RPSGB   Royal Pharmaceutical Society of Great Britain
RR   relative risk
RRMS   relaxing and remitting multiple sclerosis
RS   Rescue Squad
RSC   Royal Society of Chemistry
RSCG   Regional Specialised Commissioning Group
RSCN   Registered Sick Children's Nurse
RSH   Royal Society of Health
RSI   rapid sequence induction; repetitive strain injury; Rough Sleepers Initiative
RSIN   Rural Stress Information Network
RSM   Royal Society of Medicine
RSS   Royal Statistical Society
RSU   Regional Secure Unit; Rough Sleepers Unit

RSVP Retired and Senior Volunteers Programme
RSW Residential Social Work
RTA road traffic accident
RTF Regional Task Force
RTIA Receipts Taken Into Account (part of capital control framework)
RVSN Regional Voluntary Sector Network
RxList Internet Drug Index

S

SABA supplied air breathing apparatus
SAC Specialist Advisory Committee (of the Royal Colleges) (oversee higher medical training)
SACDA Scottish Advisory Committee on Distinction Awards
SACN Scientific Advisory Committee on Nutrition
SAD seasonal affective disorder
SAED semi-automatic external defibrillator
SaFF *Service and Finance Framework* (document setting out commissioning intentions for the following year)
SAGNIS Strategic Advisory Group for Nursing Information Systems
SAHC Scottish Association of Health Councils
SALT speech and language therapist
SAMH Scottish Association of Mental Health
SAMM Safety Assessment of Marketed Medicines (guidelines)
SAP Single Assessment Process
SAPHE Self-assessment in Professional and Higher Education (1996–99)
SAR search and rescue; subjective analysis return
SARS severe acute respiratory syndrome
SAS Scottish Ambulance Service; Staff and Associate Specialists; standard accounting system; Supplier Attachment Scheme
SASM Scottish Audit of Surgical Mortality
SAT Service Action Team
SAZ Sport Action Zone
SBS Small Business Service
SBU Swedish Council on Technology Assessment in Health Care
SCA Supplementary Credit Approval (part of capital control framework)
SCBA self-contained breathing apparatus
SCBU Special Care Baby Unit
SCCD Standing Conference on Community Development
SCD sickle cell disease
SCF Safer Communities Fund; Save the Children Fund; Scottish Council Foundation
SCG Specialised Commissioning Group
ScHARR School of Health and Related Research (University of Sheffield)
SCHIN Sowerby Centre for Health Informatics at Newcastle
SCI Self Certificate for first week of an Illness
SCID severe combined immune deficiency
SCIE Social Care Institute for Excellence
SCIEH Scottish Centre for Infection and Environmental Health
SCM Specialist in Community Medicine

SCMH Sainsbury Centre for Mental Health
SCMO Senior Clinical Medical Officer
SCODA Standing Conference on Drug Abuse
SCOPE Society for People with Cerebral Palsy
SCOPME Standing Committee on Postgraduate Medical and Dental Education
SCORPME Standing Committee on Regional Postgraduate Medical Education
SCOTH Scientific Committee on Tobacco and Health
SCP Shared Care Protocol; Short Course Programme; single capital pot; Society of Chiropodists and Podiatrists; Spinal Column Point (position on pay-scale); Surgical Care Practitioner
SCPMDE Scottish Council for Postgraduate Medical and Dental Education
SCR Social Care Region; Summary Care Record
SCS Senior Civil Service
SCT supervised community treatment; Society of County Treasurers
SCVO Scottish Council for Voluntary Organisations
SCVS Scottish Council for Voluntary Service
SDA Service Delivery Agreement; Severe Disability Allowance (obsolete); Sex Discrimination Act
SDO Service Delivery Organisation
SDP Service Delivery Practice (NHS web database); Sub-Divisional Partnership; Severe Disability Premium
SDS Spine Directory Services
SDU service delivery unit
SEA significant event audit
SEAC Spongiform Encephalopathy Committee (advises HMG on BSE)
SEACAG South East Ambulance Clinical Audit Group
SEC Specialist Education Committee; Standards and Ethics Committee
SEG socio-economic group
SEHD Scottish Executive Health Department
SEMI severe and enduring mental illness
SEN special educational needs; State Enrolled Nurse
SEO Society of Education Officers
SEPHO South East Public Health Observatory
SERNIP Safety and Efficiency Register of New Interventional Procedures run by the Medical Royal Colleges
SERPS State Earnings Related Pension Scheme
SEU Sentence Enforcement Unit; Social Exclusion Unit
SFA Statement of Fees and Allowances (the GP's Red Book)
SFDF Scottish Food and Drink Federation
SFF *Service and Finance Framework* (document setting out commissioning intentions for the following year)
SFI Social Fund Inspector; Standing Financial Instructions (financial procedures and framework for the Health Authority)
SG staff grade
SG1 (2; 3) Sector Group 1 etc. (part of CLP covering best value)
SGHT Standing Group on Health Technology
SGML Standard General Mark-up Language
SGPC Scottish General Practitioners Committee (part of the BMA)

SGR Scientists for Global Responsibility
SGUMDER Standing Group on Undergraduate Medical and Dental Education and Research
SHA Socialist Health Association; special health authority; strategic health authority
SHACE Strategic Health Authority Chief Executive
SHACIO Strategic Health Authority Chief Information Officer
SHAPE Strategic Health Asset Planning and Evaluation
SHARE Scottish Health Authorities Revenue Equalisation
SHAS Scottish Health Advisory Service
SHEPS Society of Health Education and Health Promotion Specialists
SHIFT Substitution of Hospital and other Institutional-focused Technology
SHMO Senior Hospital Medical Officer
SHO Senior House Officer (obsolete)
SHOT serious hazards of transfusion
SHOW Scottish Health on the Web
SHRINE Strategic Human Resources Information Network
SHTAC Scottish Health Technology Assessment Centre
SI Statutory Instrument
SIA Spinal Injuries Association
SIDS sudden infant death syndrome
SIFT Service Increment for Teaching (cash to hospitals for training medical students)
SIFTR Service Increment for Teaching and Research (the costs of undergraduate medical and dental education and research in teaching hospitals is met through SIFTR; it is intended to prevent some NHS trusts being at a disadvantage in cost terms by having to include these elements in contract prices)
SIG special interest group
SIGN Scottish Intercollegiate Guidelines Network
SIMS Standardised Incident Management System
SING Sexuality Issues Network Group
SIS Statistical Information Service (run by IPF); Supplies Information Service
SISTC Selection into Surgical Training Centres
SITF Social Investment Task Force
SLA Service Level Agreement
SLI specific learning incident
SLIPS Safety and Leadership for Interventional Procedures and Surgery
SLS Selected List Scheme (for drugs which are restricted to particular conditions)
SMA spinal muscular atrophy
SMAC Standing Medical Advisory Committee
SMART specific, measurable, attainable, relevant, timed (of objectives)
SMAS Substance Misuse Advisory Service
SMC Scottish Medicines Consortium (a sort of Scottish NICE)
SMI severe mental impairment (people with SMI do not have to pay Council Tax)
SMO Senior Medical Officer
SMP Statutory Maternity Pay
SMR standardised morbidity ratio; standardised mortality ratio
SN staff nurse
SNAFU situation normal, all fouled up
SNMAC Standing Nursing and Midwifery Advisory Committee

SNOMED Systematised Nomenclature of Human and Veterinary Medicine
SNP Scottish Nationalist Party; single nucleotide polymorphism (a marker of genetic difference)
SNTN Scottish National Training Number
SO Standing Orders
SOAP Shipley Ophthalmic Assessment Service
SOCITM Society of Information Technology Managers
SODoH Scottish Department of Health (obsolete)
SofS Secretary of State
SOHHD Scottish Home Office and Health Department (obsolete)
SON Statement of Need
SOP Standard Operational Procedure
SoS Secretary of State
SOSIG Social Science Information Gateway
SP strategic plan
SPA Scottish Prescribing Analysis; Small Practices Association; structured professional activities
SPAIN Social Policy Ageing Information Network
SPC Summary of Product Characteristics
SPfIT Southern Programme for IT
SPG (NHS) Security Policy Group
SPIN Sandwell Public Information Network
SPP Statutory Paternity Pay
SpR Specialist Registrar
SPRAT Sheffield Peer Review Assessment Tool
SPS Standard Payroll System
SpT Specialist Trainee
SPV special purpose vehicle; Statement of Personal Values
SQC Service Quality Committee
SQP suitably qualified person
SR Senior Registrar (obsolete); Sister; Society of Radiographers; Spending Review
SRB Single Regeneration Budget
SRD State Registered Dietician
SRE Sex and Relationship Education
SRG Stakeholder Review Group
SRSAG Supra Regional Services Advisory group
SS spreadsheet
SSA Standard Spending Assessment
SSAP Statement of Standard Accounting Practice (now being replaced by FRS)
SSARG Standard Spending Assessment Reduction Grant
SSAT Social Security Appeal Tribunal
SSC Sector Skills Council; Shared Services Centre
SSCF Safer and Stronger Communities Fund
SSD Social Services Department
SSDP Strategic Service Development Plan
SSHA Society of Sexual Health Advisers
SSI Social Services Inspectorate Transferred to Commission for Social Care Inspection 2004; Standard Spending Indicator (part of SSA)

SSIP   Strategic Service Implementation Plan,
SSIS   Social Services Information System
SSM   Special Study Module; System Status Management
SSP   Statutory Sick Pay; Sub-regional Strategic Partnership
SSR   Service Strategy and Regulation
SSRADU   Social Services Research and Development Unit
SSRG   Social Services Research Group
SSSI   Site of Special Scientific Interest
STA   Specialist Training Authority of Royal Colleges
STAR   Short Term Assessment and Rehabilitation Team (social services teams which provide up to four weeks of care for people leaving hospital and residential homes and returning home)
STAR-PU   Specific Therapeutic Group Age-Sex Related Prescribing Unit
StBOP   Shifting the Balance of Power
STC   Specialty Training Committee (of local postgraduate dean)
STEIS   Strategic Executive Information System
STEP   Surgeons in Training Education Programme
STG   Special Transitional Grant (DoH money given to Social Services to change to Community Care; now defunct)
StN   Student Nurse
STP   short-term programme
StR   Specialty Registrar
STR   Structured Training Report
STrAP   Speciality Training Assessment Process (sometimes STRAP)
STSS   Short Term Support Services (planned residential respite care for people with learning disabilities)
SU   Strategy Unit (Cabinet Office); Students Union
SUI   serious untoward incident
SURE   Service User Research Enterprise
SUS   Secondary Uses Service
SWAG   Specialist Workforce Advisory Group (a group focused on the number of doctors required to provide the service)
SWG   Service Working Group; Settlement Working Group; Specialty Working Group
SWOT   An analysis of strengths, weakness, opportunities and threats (usually relates to organisations but could apply equally to an individual)

T

T&CS   terms and conditions of service (*see also* TCS)
T&O   Trauma and Orthopaedics
TAB   Team Assessment of Behaviour
TAG   Technical Advisory Group
TALOIA   there's a lot of it about
TAP   Trainee Assistant Practitioner
TATT   tired all the time
TBA   to be announced; to be arranged
TC   total communication; Town Council
TCBL   Temporary Capital Borrowing Limit (part of capital control framework)
TCI   to come in

TCP Total Commissioning Project
TCS terms and conditions of service (*see also* T&CS)
TDHC The Doctors Healthcare Company
TEACCH Treatment and Education of Autistic and Related Communication Handicapped Children
TEC Training and Enterprise Council (obsolete)
TEETH tried everything else, try homoeopathy
TEL Trust Executive Letter
TICK teamwork, integrity, courage, knowledge
TIE Theatre In Education
TIP Trust Implementation Plan (Scotland)
TIS Technical Information Services
TLA three-letter abbreviation (acronym like this one)
TMB too many birthdays
TME total managed expenditure
TME Trust Management Executive
TNA training needs analysis
TOD took own discharge
TOIL time off in lieu
TOPRA The Organisation for Professionals in Regulatory Affairs
TOPS Termination of Pregnancy Service
TOPSS Training Organisation for Personal Social Services
TPC Teenage Pregnancy Co-ordinator
tPCTs Teaching PCTs
TPD Training Programme Director
TPP Total Purchasing Project
TPQ Threshold Planning Quantity
TPU Teenage Pregnancy Unit
TQM total quality management
TR Technical Release (term used by Audit Commission)
TRBL Temporary Revenue Borrowing Limit (part of capital control framework)
TRiP Turning Research into Practice
TRIPS Trade Related Intellectual Property Rights
TRO time ran out
TSC Technical Sub-Committee
TSE Transmissible Spongiform Encephalopathies
TSG Transport Supplementary Grant
TSO The Stationery Office (formerly HMSO)
TSP Training Support Programme
TSS Total Standard Spending
TSSU Theatre Sterile Supplies Unit
TtT Train The Trainers (sometimes as TTT)
TUBE totally unnecessary breast examination
TUPE Transfer of Undertakings (Protection of Employment) Regulations 1981
TV transfer value
TWG Technical Working Group

U

UA   Unitary Authority (a council which carries out all the functions in its area)
UASC   unaccompanied asylum-seeking children
UASSG   Unlinked Anonymous Surveys Steering Group
UB   Unemployment Benefit (now JSA)
UCAS   Universities College Admission Service
UEL   upper explosive limit
UEMS   European Union of Medical Specialists
UGM   Unit General Manager
UKADCU   UK Anti-Drugs Co-ordination Unit (formerly Drugs Co-ordination Unit)
UKAN   United Kingdom Advocacy Network
UKCC   United Kingdom Central Council for Nursing, Midwifery and Health Visiting (abolished 2002); UK Cochrane Centre
UKCHHO   UK Clearing House on Health Outcomes (Leeds)
UKCRC   UK Clinical Research Collaboration
UKCRN   UK Clinical Research Network
UKDIPG   UK Drug Information Pharmacists Group
UKHFAN   UK Health for All Network
UKOLN   The UK Office for Library and Information Networking
UKPFO   The UK Foundation Programme Office
UKPHA   UK Public Health Alliance
UKTSSA   UK Transplant Support Service Authority
UKXIRA   UK Xenotransplantation Interim Regulatory Authority
ULC   unit labour cost (staff cost required to provide a given unit of activity)
ULTRA   Unrelated Live Transplant Regulatory Authority
UMLS   Unified Medical Language System
UNICEF   United Nations Children's Fund
UNISON   Trades Union for public sector workers, incorporating COHSE, NALGO and NUPE
UPA   Underprivileged Area (a measure of deprivation; 0 is the mean for England)
URL   Universal (or Uniform) Resource Locator (on Internet)
UTD   Unit Training Director
UTG   Unified Training Grade (now SpR)
UTH   University Teaching Hospital

V

VA   voluntary action; voluntary-aided; Vote Account
VAMP   a GP information system supplier user group
VB   Volunteer Bureau
VC   variable cost; voluntary-controlled
VCO(s)   Voluntary and Community Organisation(s)
VCS   Voluntary and Community Sector
VCT   Voluntary Competitive Tendering
VDRFAMP   Vascular Disease Risk Factor Assessment and Management Process
VFM   value for money
VFMU   Value for Money Unit
VHI   Voluntary Health Insurance (Ireland)
VOCOSE   Voluntary, Community and Social Economy

VPE   Virtual Private Exchange (type of internal telephone network)
VSA   volatile substance abuse
VSC   Voluntary Service Co-ordinator
VSNTO   Voluntary Sector National Training Organisation
VSO   Voluntary Sector Option (New Deal); Voluntary Service Overseas
VSPG   Voluntary Sector Policy and Grants
VSpR   Visiting Specialist Registrar
VTE   venous thromboembolism
VTN   Visiting Training Number
VTR   Vocational Training Record
VTS   Vocational Training Scheme (the mandatory scheme of structured experience and training in hospitals and the community for doctors planning a career in general practice)

W

WAA   Working Age Agency
WADEM   World Association for Disaster and Emergency Medicine
WAHAT   Welsh Association of Health Authorities and Trusts
WAIS   wide area information server
WAN   wide area network
WAT   Workforce Action Team
WBA   workplace-based assessment
WCH   Wales Centre for Health
WCVA   Wales Council for Voluntary Action
WDC   Workforce Development Confederation
WeBNF   web-accessible BNF
WEST   Winter and Emergency Services Team
WF   Work Foundation (formerly Industrial Society)
WFP   Working for Patients
WFTC   Working Families Tax Credit (now replaced by Tax Credits)
WGSMT   Working Group on Specialist Medical Training
WHCSA   Welsh Health Common Services Agency (obsolete; now part of Welsh Health Estates)
WHDI   Welsh Health Development International
WHE   Welsh Health Estates
WHO   World Health Organization
WiC   Walk in Centre
WIGS   women in grey suits
WIH   work in hand
WIMS   Works Information Management System
WIsH   Welsh Innovations in Healthcare
WIST   Women in Surgical Training Scheme
WM   workload measure (e.g. OBD, LOS, FCE)
WMA   World Medical Association
WMQI   West Midlands Quality Observatory
WNAB   Workforce Numbers Advisory Board
WNC   Women's National Commission
WO   Welsh Office

WONCA World Organisation of National Colleges Academies and Academic Associations of General Practitioners/Family Physicians

WP White Paper; word processor

WP10 Working Paper 10 (now NMET)

WPA Western Provident Association

WPBA workplace-based assessments

WRC Women's Resource Centre

WRT Workforce Review Team

WRVS Women's Royal Voluntary Service

WTC Working Tax Credit

WTD Working Time Directive

WTEP whole time equivalent posts

WTEs whole-time equivalents (the total of whole-time staff, plus the whole time equivalent of part-time staff, which is obtained by dividing the hours worked in a year by part-timers by the number of hours in the whole-time working year)

WTI Waiting Time Initiative

WU Women's Unit

Y

YCS young chronic sick

YDU Young Disabled Unit

YHYCYS *Your Health, Your Care, Your Say*

YOT Youth Offender Team

Z

ZBB Zero-Base Budgeting

Index

Please seek additional information in the Glossary and List of Acronyms. Entries in **bold** denote figures.